NEUROLOGY - LABORATORY AND CLINICAL RESEARCH DEVELOPMENTS

DEMENTIA

PREVALENCE, RISK FACTORS AND MANAGEMENT STRATEGIES

NEUROLOGY - LABORATORY AND CLINICAL RESEARCH DEVELOPMENTS

Additional books in this series can be found on Nova's website
under the Series tab.

Additional e-books in this series can be found on Nova's website
under the e-book tab.

NEUROLOGY - LABORATORY AND CLINICAL RESEARCH DEVELOPMENTS

DEMENTIA

PREVALENCE, RISK FACTORS AND MANAGEMENT STRATEGIES

PAMELA TANNER
EDITOR

NOVA BIOMEDICAL

New York

For permission to use material from this book please contact us:
Telephone 631-231-7269; Fax 631-231-8175
Web Site: http://www.novapublishers.com

Library of Congress Cataloging-in-Publication Data

ISBN: 978-1-63321-928-1
Library of Congress Control Number: 2014948899

Published by Nova Science Publishers, Inc. † New York

Contents

Preface

Dementia is a distressing, progressively disabling, financially burdening and, most of all, self-erasing illness. The nature of the disease presents patients, families and care providers from multiple domains with numerous, multi-faceted challenges. As a rule, these challenges morph into new and distinctive challenges as patients move through various stages of the disease. Caring for persons with dementia represents one of the most challenging medical issues of the 21st century. A sense of urgency related to the problem of dementia has recently intensified, as the number of patients receiving a new dementia diagnosis is rapidly on the rise. This book explores the prevalence, risk factors and the management strategies available for dementia patients.

Chapter 1 – Over the past five years, studies exploiting high-throughput genome technologies have significantly advanced the knowledge on the genomic underpinnings of Alzheimer's disease (AD) by identifying more than 20 disease-associated loci. The cumulative population attributable fraction (PAR) associated with these genetic variants amounts to ~80%. High throughput sequencing studies have started to map specific causative variants in these genes and have provided instrumental evidence for an involvement of rare variants in AD overturning the common-disease-common variant hypothesis. The ongoing translational studies and next generation whole genome or whole exome sequencing efforts hold the promise to map the specific causative variants in these genes, to identify several additional risk variants and to identify novel targets for genetic testing, prevention and treatment.

Chapter 2 – Dementia is a distressing, progressively disabling, financially burdening, and, most of all, self-erasing illness. The nature of the disease presents patients, families, and care providers from multiple domains with numerous, multi-faceted challenges. As a rule, these challenges morph into new and distinctive challenges as patients move through various stages of the disease. In general., the service needs of the patient with dementia tend to intensify as severity of the disease increases. Due to the fact that most patients with dementia receive care and support from multiple providers, the risk of fragmentation in care provision is very real. Providers are called to search for better ways to ensure a continuum of care as the patient with dementia moves from living in the home to a long-term care facility. Also, end-of-life (EOL) care presents its own unique set of challenges and should be considered a key phase in planning for care continuum. Additionally, providing adequate and appropriate care and support to caregivers should be considered a central element of treatment planning.

Similar to the patients themselves, caregivers require different forms of support, in varying degrees, as time and the disease progress. As the number of veterans being diagnosed with this complex medical issue increases, the Veterans Health Administration (VHA) looks to its Office of Geriatrics and Extended Care, a central body that provides policy direction for the development, coordination, and integration of geriatrics and long-term care clinical programs, and for the advancement of geriatrics and long-term care through research, education and evaluation of clinical models. A myriad of important programs and services exist within the Office of Geriatrics and Extended Care, including 20 "GRECCS" (Geriatric Research, Education and Clinical Centers), institutional care programs, non-institutional care programs, inpatient dementia units, and outpatient dementia clinics. This chapter will first present the many facets of dementia care, highlighting the complex nature of the illness as it occurs across disease stages. The chapter will subsequently reveal past and current efforts of the largest medical system in the United States as it works to provide comprehensive, coordinated care for veterans with dementia.

Chapter 3 – *Introduction:* Florida has the second highest percentage of persons with advanced dementia in the United States. While sleep disturbances are common in older persons in general., sleep disturbances can be more pronounced for persons with dementia (PWD) and can be stressful for caregivers of PWDs. Sleep disturbances among PWD, including unsupervised wandering and pacing, can be dangerous for PWDs, and may increase the risk of physical and psychological morbidity for both the PWD and caregiver. This chapter covers a brief epidemiology of sleep in Alzheimer's disease and related disorders, describes the burden of sleep disturbances for PWDs and caregivers, and reviews non-pharmacologic interventions that have been developed to improve sleep for non-institutionalized PWDs. One such program is NITE-AD (Nighttime Insomnia, Treatment, and Education for Alzheimer's disease), a home based caregiver training program that includes light exposure, exercise, and sleep hygiene education to improve sleep among PWD. The authors describe a six-week community–informed group delivery modification of NITE-AD conducted with caregivers of PWD attending adult-day care programs. The results will be outlined and discussed.

Chapter 4 – Apathy is common across a variety of neurological disorders. However, apathy is one of the earliest and probably most persistent neuropsychiatric symptoms in patients with Alzheimer's disease and other dementing disorders. It affects approximately 70% of patients in the mild to moderate stages of Alzheimer's disease. It is defined as the absence or lack of feeling, emotion, interest, concern, and motivation and manifested by diminution of goal directed cognition and behavior relative to the individual's previous level of functioning. Apathy is linked with a faster progression of cognitive, functional., and emotional impairment. It is also associated with decreased insight. As a result, patients with apathy rely on caregivers to provide more care and it subsequently causes increased stress for caregivers. Neuropathological changes in Alzheimer's disease may result in apathy by affecting the orbitofrontal and anterior cingulate circuits. Although apathy is increasingly recognized in patients with neuropsychiatric symptoms, no official diagnostic classification systems offer a definition of apathy. In this chapter, treatment strategies of apathy in dementia patients are discussed along with a brief review of pathophysiological correlates, neuroimaging, and diagnosis.

Chapter 5 – With an ageing population worldwide, the incidence of dementia and associated care costs are rising. As there is currently no cure, identifying effective preventative lifestyle interventions has been the focus of much recent research to reduce risk and delay onset. Risk factors for dementia overlap with those for cardiovascular disease and the cardiovascular benefits of physical activity are well documented. Thus, the scope for physical activity to improve cognitive abilities and reduce the risk of dementia has been increasingly investigated. Physical activity is also a targetable behaviour for older adults as the majority do not meet the minimum level recommended for health benefits. Reviewing the literature is challenging due to the wide variety of ways that this relationship has been investigated, such as study design, specific components of exercise, cognitive outcome measures and participant characteristics. Previous reviews have identified components of exercise which appear to afford the largest cognitive improvements and also moderators of the effect. However, there are inconsistent findings across reviews and meta-analyses as to which aspects of cognitive performance demonstrate the largest effect with exercise. A biopsychosocial approach to dementia in this context is argued to be more appropriate than a traditional medical or disease model due to the evidence of the impact of the social environment on cognitive improvement or decline. Physical activity does not occur independently of the environment. However, psychosocial factors in the relationship between physical activity and cognitive ability in older adults have largely been neglected despite evidence for their effect in non-physical activity contexts. It is suggested that future work should investigate the role of psychosocial factors to further understand their impact on cognitive outcomes in a physical activity context. A better understanding of this would assist with exercise intervention design to maximise cognitive benefits.

Chapter 6 – Frontotemporal lobar degeneration (FTLD) is an umbrella term covering a heterogeneous set of neurodegenerative disorders whose clinical presentation may be cognitive, behavioural., motor, or mixed. These syndromes frequently combine during the course of the disease. FTLD syndromes show considerable phenotypic overlap and variable histopathological and genetic correlations. Current neuropathological classification is based on specific types of protein deposits and their related genes. Although infrequent in the general population, FTLD is nearly as common as Alzheimer's disease in patients below 65 years of age. Its scope extends from sporadic (60%) to familial forms (40%), some of the latter having an autosomal dominant inheritance pattern. Numerous mutations of several implicated genes have been described. FTLD represents a diagnostic challenge owing to its mixed features. Implementation of various methods is required and consists of a clinical assessment, neuropsychological testing, structural or functional neuroimaging and, sometimes, genetic analysis looking for mutations. Additional CSF and blood biomarkers, some of them still under study, may provide information about FTLD genetic risk factors or exclude other diseases. To date, only an autopsy allows a definite diagnosis.

No therapies are currently available to cure or alter the evolution of FTLD disorders. Management strategies include pharmacological treatment of the signs and symptoms and non-pharmacological interventions for the patients, for instance skill-based compensation methods, environmental modifications or activity groups. Caregivers should be integrated in the process and offered support when needed (educational programmes, psychological follow-up, respite facilities, etc.). Genetic counselling may prove useful.

Research aims at a better understanding of the biochemical pathways of the proteinopathies which will potentially lead to more efficient diagnosis tools and innovative drug strategies.

Chapter 7 – A large number of possible risk factors have been associated with Alzheimer's disease (AD). This chapter discusses the validity of the major risk factors that have been identified including age, genetics, exposure to aluminum, head injury, malnutrition and diet, mitochondrial dysfunction, vascular disease, immune system dysfunction, and infection and proposes a hypothesis to explain how these various risk factors may cause AD pathology. Rare forms of early-onset familial AD (FAD) are strongly linked to the presence of specific gene mutations, viz. mutations in *amyloid precursor protein (APP)* and *presenilin (PSEN1/2)* genes. By contrast, late-onset sporadic AD (SAD) is a multifactorial disorder in which age-related changes, genetic risk factors, such as allelic variation in *apolipoprotein E (Apo E)* gene, vascular disease, head injury and risk factors associated with diet, immune system, mitochondrial function, and infection may all be involved. These risk factors interact to increase the rate of normal aging ('allostatic load') which over a lifetime results in degeneration of neurons and blood vessels and as a consequence, the formation of abnormally aggregated 'reactive' proteins such as β-amyloid (Aβ) and tau leading to the development of senile plaques (SP) and neurofibrillary tangles (NFT) respectively. Life-style changes that may reduce the allostatic load and therefore, the risk of dementia are discussed.

Chapter 8 – Dementia is a progressive global cognitive dysfunction resulting in cognitive and functional impairment. An accurate prognosis is helpful for the patient, family, healthcare professionals and also for planning of future health and social care resources. The incidence and prevalence of dementia is rising. Alzheimer's disease (AD) accounts for 60-80% of dementia cases, with vascular dementia (VaD) the next most common. There is also an increased mortality in patients with dementia with Lewy bodies and frontotemporal dementia.

Median survival from time of onset of dementia is 3.3-11.7 years and from diagnosis is 3.2-6.6 years. There is an increased risk of death with dementia (hazard ratio (HR) 2-4) which can result from the disease itself, and comorbidities which may be associated with the disease process. Typical risk factors predicting outcomes in dementia, such as age of onset, gender and education, are often not supported by studies with varying outcomes. Increased mortality is associated with older age, but more life years will be lost in younger sufferers. Male gender is associated with a higher mortality (HR 1.2-1.9). Ethnicity and education do not have strong associations with mortality. People who carry the APOE ε4 allele have an increased risk of developing AD (RR 3.2) and mortality doubles when AD is present. Reviewing the often heterogeneous study data on dementia makes comparisons difficult. Excess mortality in AD patients may be associated with the disease itself (adjusted HR 1.55 in AD versus non AD dementia). The common causes of death in dementia are cardiovascular, cerebrovascular and pneumonia. VaD patients have higher mortality from cardiovascular disease than AD. Current management is based around early diagnosis, support, education and the use of cholinesterase inhibitors and a NMDA receptor antagonist.

Chapter 9 – Alzheimer's disease is a primary degenerating brain condition. Its etiology is unknown and it is characterized by the presence of neuropathological and neurochemical features. This condition generally starts slowly and in an insidious way and it progresses gradually along a period of time, normally years. The clinical symptoms include a progressive and total deterioration of the cognitive function which is often accompanied by personality and behavior changes. This leads to a reduction of the capacity to carry out activities of daily living (ADL) by the person affected. Currently, Alzheimer's disease is the most common type of dementia. The consequences of this condition are devastating. The patient will have his cognitive function affected, his normal behavior altered and he will progressively need help to perform the ADL. These consequences also extend to the family who also suffer the impact of the effects of dementia. The family will be absolutely essential in order to provide the care needed by the patient during the time of the condition and its progression. Nowadays, there are studies that have analyzed and compared the effectiveness of different rehabilitation approaches. These techniques have shown improvements of the ADL performance and the quality of life of the patients diagnosed with Alzheimer's disease. From the rehabilitation approach of Occupational Therapy, the objective is to maintain as long as possible the independence of the person to perform ADL. Slowing down the progression of the disability and improving the quality of life of the person and his family is of crucial importance. This can only be achieved with a holistic approach that allows the management of the complexity of Alzheimer's disease from the psychological., physical and social view, including as well the environment as all these factors have an influence on the performance of ADL. Considering the reported benefits of rehabilitation on the quality of life of these patients, the objective of this chapter was to analyse the results obtained by different authors in relation to the effects that rehabilitation, with a special focus on Occupational Therapy, has on subjects diagnosed with Alzheimer's disease. The results obtained showed that there is scientific literature that indicates that Occupational Therapy has a positive effect on persons with this condition. The main improvements were seen in behavior and emotional aspects, in carer burden, in the quality of life, independence, cognitive function and the institutionalisation of the subjects.

Chapter 10 – Idiopathic normal pressure hydrocephalus (INPH) is characterized by progressive gait apraxia, cognitive dysfunction and urinary incontinence (Hakim-Adams syndrome). INPH is associated with communicating hydrocephalus (as demonstrated by brain CT or MRI) and cerebrospinal fluid (CSF) pressure within the normal range (7-24 cm H2O). The clinical triad of Hakim-Adams syndrome is present in approximately 50% of cases; however, only one or a combination of two symptoms should be considered for diagnostic investigation. It is a differential diagnosis for most of the dementia syndromes and occurs mainly in elderly populations and it is one of the causes of potentially reversible dementia. Treatment of INPH is based in three pillars: conservative, ventriculoperitoneal shunt (VPS) and endoscopic third ventriculostomy (ETV). Conclusion: Appropriate and well designed high-level evidence studies are still lacking, but the current gold standard treatment of INPH is performed with VPS.

Chapter 11 – Basal ganglia calcifications (BGC) may be present in various medical conditions, such as infections, metabolic, psychiatric and neurological diseases, associated with different etiologies and clinical outcomes, including parkinsonism, psychosis, mood swings and dementia. A literature review was performed highlighting main neuropsychological findings of BGC, with particular attention to clinical reports of cognitive decline. Neuroimaging studies combined with neuropsychological analysis show that some patients present progressive disturbances of selective attention, declarative memory and verbal perseveration. Therefore, the calcification process might represent a putative cause for demential syndromes, suggesting a probable link between calcinosis, the aging process and eventually with neuronal death. The increasing number of reports available will foster a necessary discussion about cerebral calcinosis and its role in determining symptomatology in demential patients.

Chapter 12 – Background: Spatial disorientation (SD) is a severe and persistent impairment of spatial navigation in familiar as well as new environments and a trait marker of dementia (DA). Virtual reality (VR) provides a tool for the assessment and improvement of SD. In VR training program different degrees of motor control over navigation may be implemented (i.e., more passive spatial navigation vs. more active). Increasing demands of active motor control may overload those failing visuo-spatial resources necessary for learning spatial orientation and navigation. In the present study the authors used a VR-based verbally-guided passive navigation training program to improve general spatial abilities in DA patients with spatial disorientation.

Methods: Forty DA patients which showed deficits in spatial orientation, as well as 20 healthy controls performed a route finding training in a virtual environment. Participants learned and recalled different routes for navigation in a virtual city over nine training sessions. Before and after VR training, general spatial abilities were assessed with standardized neuropsychological tests.

Results: Route finding ability in the VR task increased over the ten training sessions. Moreover, both groups improved different aspects of spatial abilities after VR training in comparison to the spatial performance before VR training.

Conclusions: Verbally-guided passive navigation training in VR enhances general spatial cognition in DA patients with spatial disorientation as well as in healthy controls and can therefore be useful in the rehabilitation of spatial deficits associated with SD.

Chapter 13 – Changes in sleep organization are a hallmark of the normal aging process. Sleep macro- and micro-structure changes are more evident in the context of dementia. The "Sleep and neurodegeneration and/or dementia" issue contains a causality dilemma; in the context of neurodegeneration, sleep-wake promoting neurons may be affected, while in many of the neurodegenerative disorders, central respiratory drive and autonomic neurons are also degenerated and may cause primary sleep disorders. Conversely, several recent studies suggest that common sleep disorders (i.e., insomnia, daytime sleepiness and generally decreased amplitude and robustness of sleep-wake cycle), which are mostly prevalent among the cognitively impaired people, may precede clinical symptoms of dementia and may be risk factors for cognitive decline and dementia.

Here, sleep, its alteration and sleep disorders in the context not only of dementia but also in pre-dementia stages (i.e., the mild cognitive impairment - MCI) are reviewed. Moreover, the complex interactions between sleep and dementia and the previously-mentioned causality dilemma are addressed by also reviewing the existing management strategies and evidence of the impact of therapeutic approaches on sleep disorders in dementia.

In: Dementia
Editor: Pamela Tanner

ISBN: 978-1-63321-928-1

Chapter 1

Genetic Risk Factors for Alzheimer's Disease

Christiane Reitz, M.D., Ph.D.*

The Taub Institute for Research on Alzheimer's Disease and the Aging Brain,
The Gertrude H. Sergievsky Center, The Department of Neurology,
The Dept. of Epidemiology, Columbia University, New York,
New York, US

Abstract

Over the past five years, studies exploiting high-throughput genome technologies have significantly advanced the knowledge on the genomic underpinnings of Alzheimer's disease (AD) by identifying more than 20 disease-associated loci. The cumulative population attributable fraction (PAR) associated with these genetic variants amounts to ~80%. High throughput sequencing studies have started to map specific causative variants in these genes and have provided instrumental evidence for an involvement of rare variants in AD overturning the common-disease-common variant hypothesis. The ongoing translational studies and next generation whole genome or whole exome sequencing efforts hold the promise to map the specific causative variants in these genes, to identify several additional risk variants and to identify novel targets for genetic testing, prevention and treatment.

Introduction

Late-onset Alzheimer disease (AD) is the most common form of dementia leading to a considerable healthcare burden. It is estimated that 24 million people worldwide have AD. [1] In the US alone, five million people are affected leading to a direct estimated health-care cost of $215 billion dollars per year. [1, 2]

* Phone: 212-305-0865, Fax: 212-305-2518, E-mail: cr2101@columbia.edu.

The annual incidence rate increases from 1% among people aged 65 years to approximately 8% for people aged 85 years and older. The longevity of those born in the post-World War II era suggests that these numbers will triple by the year 2050 resulting in an increase of nearly 80% in total societal costs per adult. [2]

Diagnosis of AD

AD typically begins with the onset of symptoms after age 60 and evolves slowly from mildly impaired memory function to severe cognitive loss, terminating inevitably in complete incapacity and death. Although in recent years there have been significant advances in biomarkers (plasma Abeta, CSF Abeta and tau, amyloid imaging) [3-5] for the disease and prediction in cognitive decline, to date, there are no definitive diagnostic tests or biological markers of the disease. The diagnosis during life is based on a clinical examination. The pathological key hallmarks in brain include deposits of extracellular β-amyloid protein (Aβ) in diffuse plaques and plaques containing elements of degenerating neurons ("neuritic plaques"). Intracellular changes include deposits of abnormally hyperphosphorylated tau protein, a microtubule assembly protein, in the form of neurofibrillary tangles. In addition, activation of microglia and loss of neurons and synapses is widespread.

Genetic Epidemiology of AD

Efforts to limit the prevalence and incidence of AD are being held up by the lack of success of experimental drugs, which is attributable to incomplete characterization of the basic pathologic mechanisms. It is clear that there is a significant genetic component with a heritability of 58% to 79%. [6-8] Determining which genes and gene networks contribute to AD risk would reveal the major basic pathogenic mechanisms and highlight key proteins/pathways for drug development ("druggable targets"). In addition, identification of underlying genetic variants would inform the development of genetic testing methods for identifying those at greatest risk for AD when preventive measures become available.

Consistent with the role of a significant genetic contribution, the heritability of AD is 58% to 79%, and a positive family history is the strongest risk factor. [9, 10] Families multiply affected by AD are at increased risk for dementia, but the distribution of secondary cases is not consistent with Mendelian inheritance. AD is more frequent among monozygotic than dizygotic twins, [8, 9, 11] and first-degree relatives of patients with AD have approximately twice the expected lifetime risk of developing the disease. Studies of numerous large pedigrees with early-onset AD (onset age: 30-50 years) led to the discovery of autosomal dominant mutations in the amyloid precursor protein (*APP*), presenilin 1 (*PSEN1*), and presenilin 2 (*PSEN2*) genes. [12-14] These studies suggested a common pathogenic mechanism involving enhanced generation and aggregation of Aβ. According to this "amyloid hypothesis", β-secretase cleaves APP near the N terminus of the Aβ peptide; then, the membrane-bound C-terminal APP fragment is cleaved by γ-secretase leading to accumulation of Aβ40 and Aβ42.

Role of rare and common variants in AD. For several decades, the main hypothesis advocated for complex diseases was the "common disease-common variant hypothesis' suggesting that the genetic factors underlying common diseases will be alleles that are themselves quite common in the population at large. [15] In line with this notion, over the past several years, the most common strategy for finding novel AD gene candidates has been the genome-wide association study (GWAS), in which as many as several million genetic markers (single nucleotide polymorphisms, SNPs) are tested for genetic association with disease risk and/or phenotypic endophenotypes such as age-of-onset, biomarkers, imaging results, and neuropathological endpoints.

These studies, however, have identified loci accounting for only part of the heritability of most complex diseases. Although some of this 'missing heritability' may be ascribed to a large number of SNPs with weak effect, it is now clear that there is a substantial contribution from rare variants with large effect that are not readily identifiable by SNP-based methods [16, 17] unless very large sample sizes (for example, >250,000 unselected individuals) are assessed. [18] Thus, in recent work resequencing of known risk loci and whole genome (WGS) and whole exome (WES) sequencing has been pursued to reveal rare point mutations that may have an appreciable impact on disease risk or severity and explain part of this "missing heritability".

Apolipoprotein E (APOE) region. For more than a decade, only one genetic risk factor, the *APOE*ε4 allele, located on chromosome 19q13, was an unequivocally established "susceptibility" gene in non-Hispanic Whites of European ancestry. APOE is a lipid-binding protein and is expressed in humans as three common isoforms coded for by three alleles, APOEε2, ε3, and ε4. A single *APOE-ε4* allele is associated with a 2- to 3-fold increased risk, having two copies is associated with a five-fold or more increase. [19] In addition, each inherited APOEε4 allele lowers the age-at-onset by 6-7 years. [20-27] APOEε4 is also associated with lower cognitive performance, in particular the memory domain, is associated with mild cognitive impairment (MCI) [28-31] and with progression from MCI to dementia [28-38]. While the population attributable risk for APOEε4 is estimated at 20-50%, [39] the presence of ε4 is neither necessary nor sufficient for developing the disease [40]. In ethnic groups other than non-Hispanic Whites the association between *APOE* and LOAD is largely inconsistent across studies.

Findings from candidate gene and GWA studies. Due to a paucity of data in other ethnic groups, most genetic association studies have restricted their efforts to non-Hispanic white populations. In addition, there are differences in linkage disequilibrium (LD) and allele frequencies between ethnic groups, which can lead to genetic background noise and the likelihood of false-positive findings due to confounding in combined analyses. Consequently, the largest GWAS to date which included up to 75,000 subjects were performed in individuals of European ancestry and identified *CR1, BIN1, CD2AP, EPHA1, CLU, MS4A6A, PICALM, ABCA7, HLA-DRB5/HLA-DRB1, PTK2B, SORL1, SLC24A4/RIN3, INPP5D, MEF2C, NME8, ZCWPW1, CELF1, FERMT2, CASS4, CD33* and *EPHA1* as AD susceptibility loci. [41-45] The majority of these genes cluster into three pathways: inflammation and immune response, lipid metabolism, and endocytosis/intracellular trafficking. The *SORL1* (sortilin-related receptor, L(DLR class) 1) gene had previously been demonstrated to modulate intracellular trafficking and processing of APP in a candidate gene approach. [46, 47] CLU, also known as apolipoprotein J (ApoJ), is a lipoprotein highly expressed in both the periphery and the brain. [48] Like ApoE, it is involved in lipid transport. [49] CLU is also hypothesized to act as an extracellular chaperone that influences Aβ-aggregation and receptor-mediated Aβ clearance by endocytosis. [48] Unlike APOE, there are no known coding variants that account for the observed genetic association to CLU, suggesting that genetic variation in expression levels may be responsible for the altered risk for LOAD. [50] *BIN1* (amphiphysin II) is a member of the Bin1/amphiphysin/RVS167 (BAR) family of genes that are involved in diverse cellular processes, including actin dynamics, membrane trafficking and clathrin-mediated endocytosis [51] which affect APP processing and Aβ production or Aβ clearance from brain. PICALM is also involved in clathrin-mediated endocytosis and recruits clathrin and adaptor protein complex 2 to sites of vesicle assembly [52]. CR1 is a cell-surface receptor that is part of the complement system. It has binding sites for complement factors C3b and C4b and is involved in clearing immune-complexes containing these two proteins. Since Aβ oligomers can bind C3b, CR1 may participate in the clearance of Aβ. CR1 may also play a role in neuroinflammation, which is a prominent feature in AD. [53] Interestingly, CLU may play a role in this process as an inhibitor [54]. The *CD33* gene encodes a protein that is a member of a family of cell surface immune receptors that bind extracellular sialylated glycans and signal via a cytoplasmic domain called the immunoreceptor tyrosine inhibitory motif. [55, 56] CD33 has primarily been studied in the peripheral immune system where it is expressed on myeloid progenitors and monocytes and also in the brain. In the periphery, CD33 appears to inhibit proliferation of myeloid cells. [57] The *MS4A4A/MS4A4E/MS4A6E* locus is part of a cluster of 15 *MS4A* genes on chromosome 11 and encodes proteins with multiple membrane-spanning domains that were initially identified by their homology to CD20, a B-lymphocyte cell surface molecule. Little is known about the function of MS4A4A gene products; however, like CD33, MS4A4A is expressed on myeloid cells and monocytes and likely has an immune-related function. *EPHA1* encodes a member of the ephrin family of cell surface receptors which interact with ephrin ligands on adjacent cells to modulate cell adhesion, migration, and axon guidance and synapse formation and plasticity. While there is a substantial body of research on the function of ephrin receptors in general., little is known about the EPHA1 gene product. Like other ephrin receptors, it regulates cell morphology and motility [58] and early work implicated this receptor in regulating vascular morphogenesis and angiogenesis. [59] Knocking out the EPHA1 gene in mice results in abnormal tail and reproductive tract development, [60] but no effects on the brain. Consistent with this notion, in mice, expression is restricted to epithelial tissue. In humans, EPHA1 is expressed by CD4-positive T lymphocytes [61], monocytes, [62] intestinal epithelium, and colon. Combined with the lack of evidence for brain expression this may suggest that, like CD33, CR1, and MS4A4/MS4A6E, the role of the *EPHA1* gene product in AD may be mediated though the immune system. The CD2 associated protein gene (CD2AP) encodes a scaffolding protein that binds directly to actin [63], nephrin and other proteins involved in cytoskeletal organization. In the immune system, CD2AP is required for synapse formation [64] in a process that involves clathrin-dependent actin polymerization. *ABCA7* is an integral transmembrane ATP-binding cassette transporter belonging to the ABC family proteins that mediate the biogenesis of high-density lipoprotein with cellular lipid and helical apolipoproteins. [65] It binds APOA-I and functions in apolipoprotein-mediated phospholipid and cholesterol efflux from cells. [66] In addition, *ABCA7* affects the transport of other important proteins, including amyloid precursor protein, [66] through the cell membrane and is involved in host defense through effects on phagocytosis by macrophages of apoptotic cells. [65] The results on the additional genes further suggest the existence of additional pathways such as hippocampal synaptic function (*MEF2C, PTK2B*), cytoskeletal function and axonal transport (*CELF1, NME8, CASS4*), regulation of gene expression and post-translational modification of proteins, and microglial and myeloid cell function (*INPPD5*).

Consistent with the notion of a genetically complex disorder, the ORs of all disease-associated loci other than the APOEε4 allele range from 1.1 to 1.3. Examining the genetic effect attributable to all the associated loci, the most strongly associated SNPs at each locus other than *APOE* shows population-attributable fractions (PAFs) or preventive fractions between 1.0–8.0%. [45] The cumulative population attributable fraction has been estimated at 89.4%.[45] In addition, the largest of these GWAS identified 13 suggestive loci with association p-values <10-6 (an intergenic locus at chr1q31.2, *HS3ST1, SQSTM1, TREML2, NDUFAF6, ECHDC3, AP2A2, ADAMTS20, IGH, SPPL2A, TRIP4, SCIMP, ACE*).

Few studies were performed in minority groups. In the largest GWAS performed to date in Caribbean Hispanics, [67] associations in *CLU, PICALM*, and *BIN1* were replicated and several additional loci on 2p25.1, 3q25.2, 7p21.1 and 10q23.1 - which could be replicated in an independent cohort of non-Hispanic Whites of European ancestry from the National Institute on Aging Late-Onset Alzheimer's Disease Family Study (NIA-LOAD) - were observed. In the largest GWAS of African Americans performed, Reitz et al. [68] identified *ABCA7* as a major susceptibility locus in this ethnic group. In addition, this study replicated *CR1*, *BIN1*, *EPHA1*, and *CD33*. A large-scale GWAS study in Asian (Japanese and Korean) populations identified SORL1 as a susceptibility gene, [69] candidate gene studies performed in Asian populations confirmed *MS4A6A, CD33, PICALM, CR1,* and *CLU*. [70-75] The effect of the APOEε4 allele was universally observed in all GWAS performed across ethnic groups. These findings suggest that there is at least to some degree overlap in causative genetic loci across different ethnic groups although the causative variants within the disease-associated genes and the variant-associated effect sizes may differ.

Rare variants in LOAD. Several loci containing rare, causative sequencing variants have been identified, some of which overlap with the abovementioned common variant loci identified by GWAS. In large multiplex pedigrees with late-onset AD, targeted exome sequencing of *APP*, *PSEN1*, *PSEN2*, *APOE, GRN* and *MAPT* has identified 33 missense, nonsense and splice-site variants in 60 families (13.7%), 18 of which were novel. [76] A recent study of whole-genome sequence data from 1,795 Icelanders identified a rare, coding mutation (A673T) in the APP gene protecting against LOAD and cognitive decline in the elderly without cognitive impairment [77]. A673T is adjacent to the aspartyl protease β-site in APP, and results in an approximately 40% reduction in the formation of amyloidogenic peptides in vitro. This strong protective effect of the A673T substitution against LOAD provides proof of principle for the hypothesis that reducing the β-cleavage of APP may protect against the disease. The *TREM2/TREML2* locus associated with LOAD in case-control GWAS had previously been reported by two independent multi-stage studies that combined sequencing analyses followed by a meta-analysis of independent imputed datasets (see below), with additional direct genotyping in other independent samples and functional analyses. These studies identified a rare exonic variant (R47H) associated with a 3-4 fold increased risk of developing AD. [78, 79]

An exon sequencing study of PICALM in 48 AD cases and 48 controls identified an exonic splicing enhancer variation in exon 5 in LD with GWAS SNP rs3851179. [80] Other genes with rare variants for late-onset AD include *SORL1*, [81] *ADAM10,* [82] and *PLD3* [83]. PLD3 is a poorly characterized member of the PLD superfamily of phospholipases, but seems to affect APP processing. [76]

Conclusion

Over the past five years, studies capitalizing on high-throughput genome technologies have significantly advanced the knowledge on the genetic underpinnings of AD by identifying more than 20 AD genes implicating a specific set of pathophysiological mechanisms besides APP metabolism, including innate immune response and inflammation, lipid metabolism, endocytosis, cell migration, tau pathology, hippocampal synaptic function and axonal transport, regulation of gene expression and post-translational modification of proteins, and microglial and myeloid cell function. As described above, the cumulative population attributable fraction of the common GWAS loci has been estimated at 89.4%. [45] Considering the possibility that that part of this estimation may be explained by the winner's curse (ie. an overestimation of genetic effect size in initial studies) the true attributable fraction of the common GWAS loci might be somewhat lower. Consistent with this notion, high throughput sequencing studies have started to map additional causative rare variants in these genes providing invaluable evidence for an involvement of rare variants and non-coding RNA in this complex disease. [84] While the human genome contains about 20,000 protein-coding genes, 98.8% consists of non-protein-coding DNA sequence. [84] The majority of these sequences are dynamically transcribed, mainly into non-protein-coding RNAs, with tens if not hundreds of thousands that show specific expression patterns and subcellular locations, as well as many classes of small regulatory RNAs. The emerging evidence indicates that these RNAs control the epigenetic states that underpin development, and that many are dysregulated in cancer and other complex diseases including AD. [84] In addition, there is evidence that animals, particularly primates, have evolved plasticity in these RNA regulatory systems, especially in the brain. Thus, it appears that what was dismissed as 'junk' because it was not understood may hold a significant part of the key to understanding human evolution, development, and cognition.

Elucidating the genetic underpinnings of AD is invaluable for the development of therapeutic targets. The ongoing large-scale next generation sequencing approaches such as the Alzheimer's disease Sequencing Project (ADSP), major collaborate whole exome and whole genome sequencing effort by the NIH, have been designed to identify a large part of the missing heritability dueto rare causative and structural variants. However, before novel genomic information can be used in clinical settings and safely considered for pharmaceutical intervention, functional studies extensive functional studies will be needed to the clarify pathogenic pathways and interacting factors. are needed to identify the specific causative variants and the specific factors with which they interact.

Acknowledgment

Dr. Reitz was supported by a Paul B. Beeson Career Development Award (K23AG034550).

References

[1] Hurd M. D., Martorell P., Delavande A., Mullen K. J., Langa K. M. Monetary costs of dementia in the United States. *N. Engl. J. Med.*, 2013; 368: 1326-1334.

[2] 2010 Alzheimer's disease facts and figures. *Alzheimers Dement.*, 2010; 6: 158-194.

[3] Roe C. M., Fagan A. M., Grant E. A., Holtzman D. M., Morris J. C. CSF biomarkers of Alzheimer disease: "noncognitive" outcomes. *Neurology,* 2013; 81: 2028-2031.

[4] Rowe C. C., Bourgeat P., Ellis K. A., Brown B., Lim Y. Y., Mulligan R., Jones G., Maruff P., Woodward M., Price R., Robins P., Tochon-Danguy H., O'Keefe G., Pike K. E., Yates P., Szoeke C., Salvado O., Macaulay S. L., O'Meara T., Head R., Cobiac L., Savage G., Martins R., Masters C. L., Ames D., Villemagne V. L. Predicting Alzheimer disease with beta-amyloid imaging: results from the Australian imaging, biomarkers, and lifestyle study of ageing. *Ann. Neurol.*, 2013; 74: 905-913.

[5] Laske C. Blood-based biomarkers in Alzheimer disease: where are we now and where have we to go? *JAMA Neurol.*, 2013; 70:133.

[6] Alsop D. C., Detre J. A. Reduced transit-time sensitivity in noninvasive magnetic resonance imaging of human cerebral blood flow. *J. Cereb. Blood Flow Metab.*, 1996; 16: 1236-1249.

[7] Gatz M., Pedersen N. L., Berg S., Johansson B., Johansson K., Mortimer J. A., Posner S. F., Viitanen M., Winblad B., Ahlbom A. Heritability for Alzheimer's disease: the study of dementia in Swedish twins. *J. Gerontol. A Biol. Sci. Med. Sci.*, 1997; 52: M117-125.

[8] Gatz M., Reynolds C. A., Fratiglioni L., Johansson B., Mortimer J. A., Berg S., Fiske A., Pedersen N. L. Role of genes and environments for explaining Alzheimer disease. *Arch. Gen. Psychiatry,* 2006; 63: 168-174.

[9] Lautenschlager N. T., Cupples L. A., Rao V. S., Auerbach S. A., Becker R., Burke J., Chui H., Duara R., Foley E. J., Glatt S. L., Green R. C., Jones R., Karlinsky H., Kukull W. A., Kurz A., Larson E. B., Martelli K., Sadovnick A. D., Volicer L., Waring S. C., Growdon J. H., Farrer L. A. Risk of dementia among relatives of Alzheimer's disease patients in the MIRAGE study: What is in store for the oldest old? *Neurology,* 1996;46: 641-650.

[10] Mayeux R., Sano M., Chen J., Tatemichi T., Stern Y. Risk of dementia in first-degree relatives of patients with Alzheimer's disease and related disorders. *Arch. Neurol.*, 1991;48: 269-273.

[11] Bergem A. L., Lannfelt L. Apolipoprotein E type epsilon4 allele, heritability and age at onset in twins with Alzheimer disease and vascular dementia. *Clin. Genet.*, 1997;52: 408-413.

[12] Goate A., Chartier-Harlin M. C., Mullan M., Brown J., Crawford F., Fidani L., Giuffra L., Haynes A., Irving N., James L., et al. Segregation of a missense mutation in the

amyloid precursor protein gene with familial Alzheimer's disease. *Nature,* 1991;349: 704-706.

[13] Levy-Lahad E., Wasco W., Poorkaj P., Romano D. M., Oshima J., Pettingell W. H., Yu C. E., Jondro P. D., Schmidt S. D., Wang K., et al. Candidate gene for the chromosome 1 familial Alzheimer's disease locus. *Science,* 1995; 269: 973-977.

[14] Sherrington R., Rogaev E. I., Liang Y., Rogaeva E. A., Levesque G., Ikeda M., Chi H., Lin C., Li G., Holman K., Tsuda T., Mar L., Foncin J. F., Bruni A. C., Montesi M. P., Sorbi S., Rainero I., Pinessi L., Nee L., Chumakov I., Pollen D., Brookes A., Sanseau P., Polinsky R. J., Wasco W., Da Silva H. A., Haines J. L., Perkicak-Vance M. A., Tanzi R. E., Roses A. D., Fraser P. E., Rommens J. M., St George-Hyslop P. H. Cloning of a gene bearing missense mutations in early-onset familial Alzheimer's disease. *Nature,* 1995; 375: 754-760.

[15] Lander E. S. The new genomics: global views of biology. *Science,* 1996; 274: 536-539.

[16] Pritchard J. K. Are rare variants responsible for susceptibility to complex diseases? *Am. J. Hum. Genet.*, 2001; 69: 124-137.

[17] Manolio T. A., Collins F. S., Cox N. J., Goldstein D. B., Hindorff L. A., Hunter D. J., McCarthy M. I., Ramos E. M., Cardon L. R., Chakravarti A., Cho J. H., Guttmacher A. E., Kong A., Kruglyak L., Mardis E., Rotimi C. N., Slatkin M., Valle D., Whittemore A. S., Boehnke M., Clark A. G., Eichler E. E., Gibson G., Haines J. L., Mackay T. F., McCarroll S. A., Visscher P. M. Finding the missing heritability of complex diseases. *Nature,* 2009; 461: 747-753.

[18] Agarwala V., Flannick J., Sunyaev S., Altshuler D. Evaluating empirical bounds on complex disease genetic architecture. *Nat. Genet.*, 2013; 45: 1418-1427.

[19] Kuusisto J., Koivisto K., Kervinen K., Mykkanen L., Helkala E. L., Vanhanen M., Hanninen T., Pyorala K., Kesaniemi Y. A., Riekkinen P., et al. Association of apolipoprotein E phenotypes with late onset Alzheimer's disease: population based study. *BMJ,* 1994; 309: 636-638.

[20] Breitner J. C., Wyse B. W., Anthony J. C., Welsh-Bohmer K. A., Steffens D. C., Norton M. C., Tschanz J. T., Plassman B. L., Meyer M. R., Skoog I., Khachaturian A. APOE-epsilon4 count predicts age when prevalence of AD increases, then declines: the Cache County Study. *Neurology,* 1999; 53: 321-331.

[21] Corder E. H., Saunders A. M., Strittmatter W. J., Schmechel D. E., Gaskell P. C., Small G. W., Roses A. D., Haines J. L., Pericak-Vance M. A. Gene dose of apolipoprotein E type 4 allele and the risk of Alzheimer's disease in late onset families. *Science,* 1993;261:921-923.

[22] Gomez-Isla T., West H. L., Rebeck G. W., Harr S. D., Growdon J. H., Locascio J. J., Perls T. T., Lipsitz L. A., Hyman B. T. Clinical and pathological correlates of apolipoprotein E epsilon 4 in Alzheimer's disease. *Ann. Neurol.*, 1996; 39: 62-70.

[23] Holmes C., Levy R., McLoughlin D. M., Powell J. F., Lovestone S. Apolipoprotein E: non-cognitive symptoms and cognitive decline in late onset Alzheimer's disease. *J. Neurol. Neurosurg. Psychiatry,* 1996; 61: 580-583.

[24] Kurz A., Altland K., Lautenschlager N., Zimmer R., Busch R., Gerundt I., Lauter H., Muller U. Apolipoprotein E type 4 allele and Alzheimer's disease: effect on age at onset and relative risk in different age groups. *J. Neurol.*, 1996; 243: 452-456.

[25] Murman D. L., Foster N. L., Kilgore S. P., McDonagh C. A., Fink J. K. Apolipoprotein E and Alzheimer's disease: strength of association is related to age at onset. *Dementia,* 1996; 7: 251-255.

[26] Poirier J., Davignon J., Bouthillier D., Kogan S., Bertrand P., Gauthier S. Apolipoprotein E polymorphism and Alzheimer's disease. *Lancet,* 1993;342:697-699.

[27] Roses A. D. Alzheimer's disease: the genetics of risk. *Hosp. Pract. (Minneap),* 1997;32: 51-55, 58-63, 67-59.

[28] Barabash A., Marcos A., Ancin I., Vazquez-Alvarez B., de Ugarte C., Gil P., Fernandez C., Encinas M., Lopez-Ibor J. J., Cabranes J. A. APOE, ACT and CHRNA7 genes in the conversion from amnestic mild cognitive impairment to Alzheimer's disease. *Neurobiol. Aging,* 2007.

[29] Petersen R. C., Smith G. E., Ivnik R. J., Tangalos E. G., Schaid D. J., Thibodeau S. N., Kokmen E., Waring S. C., Kurland L. T. Apolipoprotein E status as a predictor of the development of Alzheimer's disease in memory-impaired individuals. *Jama,* 1995;273:1274-1278.

[30] Sasaki M., Kodama C., Hidaka S., Yamashita F., Kinoshita T., Nemoto K., Ikejima C., Asada T. Prevalence of four subtypes of mild cognitive impairment and APOE in a Japanese community. *Int. J. Geriatr. Psychiatry,* 2009.

[31] Tyas S. L., Salazar J. C., Snowdon D. A., Desrosiers M. F., Riley K. P., Mendiondo M. S., Kryscio R. J. Transitions to mild cognitive impairments, dementia, and death: findings from the Nun Study. *Am. J. Epidemiol.*, 2007; 165: 1231-1238.

[32] Blom E. S., Giedraitis V., Zetterberg H., Fukumoto H., Blennow K., Hyman B. T., Irizarry M. C., Wahlund L. O., Lannfelt L., Ingelsson M. Rapid progression from mild cognitive impairment to Alzheimer's disease in subjects with elevated levels of tau in cerebrospinal fluid and the APOE epsilon4/epsilon4 genotype. *Dement. Geriatr. Cogn. Disord.*, 2009;27:458-464.

[33] Devanand D. P., Pelton G. H., Zamora D., Liu X., Tabert M. H., Goodkind M., Scarmeas N., Braun I., Stern Y., Mayeux R. Predictive utility of apolipoprotein E genotype for Alzheimer disease in outpatients with mild cognitive impairment. *Arch. Neurol.*, 2005;62:975-980.

[34] Hamalainen A., Grau-Olivares M., Tervo S., Niskanen E., Pennanen C., Huuskonen J., Kivipelto M., Hanninen T., Tapiola M., Vanhanen M., Hallikainen M., Helkala E. L., Nissinen A., Vanninen R. L., Soininen H. Apolipoprotein E epsilon 4 allele is associated with increased atrophy in progressive mild cognitive impairment: a voxel-based morphometric study. *Neurodegener. Dis.*, 2008;5:186-189.

[35] Hsiung G. Y., Sadovnick A. D., Feldman H. Apolipoprotein E epsilon4 genotype as a risk factor for cognitive decline and dementia: data from the Canadian Study of Health and Aging. *Cmaj.*, 2004;171:863-867.

[36] Jack C. R., Jr., Petersen R. C., Xu Y. C., O'Brien P. C., Smith G. E., Ivnik R. J., Boeve B. F., Waring S. C., Tangalos E. G., Kokmen E. Prediction of AD with MRI-based hippocampal volume in mild cognitive impairment. *Neurology,* 1999; 52: 1397-1403.

[37] Ramakers I. H., Visser P. J., Aalten P., Bekers O., Sleegers K., van Broeckhoven C. L., Jolles J., Verhey F. R. The association between APOE genotype and memory dysfunction in subjects with mild cognitive impairment is related to age and Alzheimer pathology. *Dement. Geriatr. Cogn. Disord.*, 2008;26:101-108.

[38] Tierney M. C., Szalai J. P., Snow W. G., Fisher R. H., Tsuda T., Chi H., McLachlan D. R., St George-Hyslop P. H. A prospective study of the clinical utility of ApoE genotype in the prediction of outcome in patients with memory impairment. *Neurology,* 1996;46:149-154.

[39] Slooter A. J., Cruts M., Kalmijn S., Hofman A., Breteler M. M., Van Broeckhoven C., van Duijn C. M. Risk estimates of dementia by apolipoprotein E genotypes from a population-based incidence study: the Rotterdam Study. *Arch. Neurol.*, 1998;55:964-968.

[40] Myers R. H., Schaefer E. J., Wilson P. W., D'Agostino R., Ordovas J. M., Espino A., Au R., White R. F., Knoefel J. E., Cobb J. L., McNulty K. A., Beiser A., Wolf P. A. Apolipoprotein E epsilon4 association with dementia in a population-based study: The Framingham study. *Neurology,* 1996;46:673-677.

[41] Harold D., Abraham R., Hollingworth P., Sims R., Gerrish A., Hamshere M. L., Pahwa J. S., Moskvina V., Dowzell K., Williams A., Jones N., Thomas C., Stretton A., Morgan A. R., Lovestone S., Powell J., Proitsi P., Lupton M. K., Brayne C., Rubinsztein D. C., Gill M., Lawlor B., Lynch A., Morgan K., Brown K. S., Passmore P. A., Craig D., McGuinness B., Todd S., Holmes C., Mann D., Smith A. D., Love S., Kehoe P. G., Hardy J., Mead S., Fox N., Rossor M., Collinge J., Maier W., Jessen F., Schurmann B., van den Bussche H., Heuser I., Kornhuber J., Wiltfang J., Dichgans M., Frolich L., Hampel H., Hull M., Rujescu D., Goate A. M., Kauwe J. S., Cruchaga C., Nowotny P., Morris J. C., Mayo K., Sleegers K., Bettens K., Engelborghs S., De Deyn P. P., Van Broeckhoven C., Livingston G., Bass N. J., Gurling H., McQuillin A., Gwilliam R., Deloukas P., Al-Chalabi A., Shaw C. E., Tsolaki M., Singleton A. B., Guerreiro R., Muhleisen T. W., Nothen M. M., Moebus S., Jockel K. H., Klopp N., Wichmann H. E., Carrasquillo M. M., Pankratz V. S., Younkin S. G., Holmans P. A., O'Donovan M., Owen M. J., Williams J. Genome-wide association study identifies variants at CLU and PICALM associated with Alzheimer's disease. *Nat. Genet.*, 2009; 41: 1088-1093.

[42] Naj A. C., Jun G., Beecham G. W., Wang L. S., Vardarajan B. N., Buros J., Gallins P. J., Buxbaum J. D., Jarvik G. P., Crane P. K., Larson E. B., Bird T. D., Boeve B. F., Graff-Radford N. R., De Jager P. L., Evans D., Schneider J. A., Carrasquillo M. M., Ertekin-Taner N., Younkin S. G., Cruchaga C., Kauwe J. S., Nowotny P., Kramer P., Hardy J., Huentelman M. J., Myers A. J., Barmada M. M., Demirci F. Y., Baldwin C. T., Green R. C., Rogaeva E., St George-Hyslop P., Arnold S. E., Barber R., Beach T., Bigio E. H., Bowen J. D., Boxer A., Burke J. R., Cairns N. J., Carlson C. S., Carney R. M., Carroll S. L., Chui H. C., Clark D. G., Corneveaux J., Cotman C. W., Cummings J. L., DeCarli C., DeKosky S. T., Diaz-Arrastia R., Dick M., Dickson D. W., Ellis W. G., Faber K. M., Fallon K. B., Farlow M. R., Ferris S., Frosch M. P., Galasko D. R., Ganguli M., Gearing M., Geschwind D. H., Ghetti B., Gilbert J. R., Gilman S., Giordani B., Glass J. D., Growdon J. H., Hamilton R. L., Harrell L. E., Head E., Honig L. S., Hulette C. M., Hyman B. T., Jicha G. A., Jin L. W. Johnson N., Karlawish J., Karydas A., Kaye J. A., Kim R., Koo E. H., Kowall N. W., Lah J. J., Levey A. I., Lieberman A. P., Lopez O. L., Mack W. J., Marson D. C., Martiniuk F., Mash D. C., Masliah E., McCormick W. C., McCurry S. M., McDavid A. N., McKee A. C., Mesulam M., Miller B. L., Miller C. A., Miller J. W., Parisi J. E., Perl D. P., Peskind E., Petersen R. C., Poon W. W., Quinn J. F., Rajbhandary R. A., Raskind M., Reisberg B., Ringman J. M., Roberson E. D., Rosenberg R. N., Sano M., Schneider L. S., Seeley W.,

Shelanski M. L., Slifer M. A., Smith C. D., Sonnen J. A., Spina S., Stern R. A., Tanzi R. E., Trojanowski J. Q., Troncoso J. C., Van Deerlin V. M., Vinters H. V., Vonsattel J. P., Weintraub S., Welsh-Bohmer K. A., Williamson J., Woltjer R. L., Cantwell L. B., Dombroski B. A., Beekly D., Lunetta K. L., Martin E. R., Kamboh M. I., Saykin A. J., Reiman E. M., Bennett D. A., Morris J. C., Montine T. J., Goate A. M., Blacker D., Tsuang D. W., Hakonarson H., Kukull W. A., Foroud T. M., Haines J. L., Mayeux R., Pericak-Vance M. A., Farrer L. A., Schellenberg G. D. Common variants at MS4A4/MS4A6E, CD2AP, CD33 and EPHA1 are associated with late-onset Alzheimer's disease. *Nat. Genet.*, 2011;43:436-441.

[43] Seshadri S., Fitzpatrick A. L., Ikram M. A., DeStefano A. L., Gudnason V., Boada M., Bis J. C., Smith A. V., Carassquillo M. M., Lambert J. C., Harold D., Schrijvers E. M., Ramirez-Lorca R., Debette S., Longstreth W. T., Jr., Janssens A. C., Pankratz V. S., Dartigues J. F., Hollingworth P., Aspelund T., Hernandez I., Beiser A., Kuller L. H., Koudstaal P. J., Dickson D. W., Tzourio C., Abraham R., Antunez C., Du Y., Rotter J. I., Aulchenko Y. S., Harris T. B., Petersen R. C., Berr C., Owen M. J., Lopez-Arrieta J., Varadarajan B. N., Becker J. T., Rivadeneira F., Nalls M. A., Graff-Radford N. R., Campion D., Auerbach S., Rice K., Hofman A., Jonsson P. V., Schmidt H., Lathrop M., Mosley T. H., Au R., Psaty B. M., Uitterlinden A. G., Farrer L. A., Lumley T., Ruiz A., Williams J., Amouyel P., Younkin S. G., Wolf P. A., Launer L. J., Lopez O. L., van Duijn C. M., Breteler M. M. Genome-wide analysis of genetic loci associated with Alzheimer disease. *JAMA,* 2010;303:1832-1840.

[44] Lambert J. C., Heath S., Even G., Campion D., Sleegers K., Hiltunen M., Combarros O., Zelenika D., Bullido M. J., Tavernier B., Letenneur L., Bettens K., Berr C., Pasquier F., Fievet N., Barberger-Gateau P., Engelborghs S., De Deyn P., Mateo I., Franck A., Helisalmi S., Porcellini E., Hanon O., de Pancorbo M. M., Lendon C., Dufouil C., Jaillard C., Leveillard T., Alvarez V., Bosco P., Mancuso M., Panza F., Nacmias B., Bossu P., Piccardi P., Annoni G., Seripa D., Galimberti D., Hannequin D., Licastro F., Soininen H., Ritchie K., Blanche H., Dartigues J. F., Tzourio C., Gut I., Van Broeckhoven C., Alperovitch A., Lathrop M., Amouyel P. Genome-wide association study identifies variants at CLU and CR1 associated with Alzheimer's disease. *Nat. Genet.*, 2009;41:1094-1099.

[45] Lambert J. C., Ibrahim-Verbaas C. A., Harold D., Naj A. C., Sims R., Bellenguez C., Jun G., Destefano A. L., Bis J. C., Beecham G. W., Grenier-Boley B., Russo G., Thornton-Wells T. A., Jones N., Smith A. V., Chouraki V., Thomas C., Ikram M. A., Zelenika D., Vardarajan B. N., Kamatani Y., Lin C. F., Gerrish A., Schmidt H., Kunkle B., Dunstan M. L., Ruiz A., Bihoreau M. T., Choi S. H., Reitz C., Pasquier F., Hollingworth P., Ramirez A., Hanon O., Fitzpatrick A. L., Buxbaum J. D., Campion D., Crane P. K., Baldwin C., Becker T., Gudnason V., Cruchaga C., Craig D., Amin N., Berr C., Lopez O. L., De Jager P. L., Deramecourt V., Johnston J. A., Evans D., Lovestone S., Letenneur L., Moron F. J., Rubinsztein D. C., Eiriksdottir G., Sleegers K., Goate A. M., Fievet N., Huentelman M. J., Gill M., Brown K., Kamboh M. I., Keller L., Barberger-Gateau P., McGuinness B., Larson E. B., Green R., Myers A. J., Dufouil C., Todd S., Wallon D., Love S., Rogaeva E., Gallacher J., St George-Hyslop P., Clarimon J., Lleo A., Bayer A., Tsuang D. W., Yu L., Tsolaki M., Bossu P., Spalletta G., Proitsi P., Collinge J., Sorbi S., Sanchez-Garcia F., Fox N. C., Hardy J., Naranjo M. C., Bosco P., Clarke R., Brayne C., Galimberti D., Mancuso M., Matthews

F., Moebus S., Mecocci P., Del Zompo M., Maier W., Hampel H., Pilotto A., Bullido M., Panza F., Caffarra P., Nacmias B., Gilbert J. R., Mayhaus M., Lannfelt L., Hakonarson H., Pichler S., Carrasquillo M. M., Ingelsson M., Beekly D., Alvarez V., Zou F., Valladares O., Younkin S. G., Coto E., Hamilton-Nelson K. L., Gu W., Razquin C., Pastor P., Mateo I., Owen M. J., Faber K. M., Jonsson P. V., Combarros O., O'Donovan M. C., Cantwell L. B., Soininen H., Blacker D., Mead S., Mosley T. H., Jr., Bennett D. A., Harris T. B., Fratiglioni L., Holmes C., de Bruijn R. F., Passmore P., Montine T. J., Bettens K., Rotter J. I., Brice A., Morgan K., Foroud T. M., Kukull W. A., Hannequin D., Powell J. F., Nalls M. A., Ritchie K., Lunetta K. L., Kauwe J. S., Boerwinkle E., Riemenschneider M., Boada M., Hiltunen M., Martin E. R., Schmidt R., Rujescu D., Wang L. S., Dartigues J. F., Mayeux R., Tzourio C., Hofman A., Nothen M. M., Graff C., Psaty B. M., Jones L., Haines J. L., Holmans P. A., Lathrop M., Pericak-Vance M. A., Launer L. J., Farrer L. A., van Duijn C. M., Van Broeckhoven C., Moskvina V., Seshadri S., Williams J., Schellenberg G. D., Amouyel P. Meta-analysis of 74,046 individuals identifies 11 new susceptibility loci for Alzheimer's disease. *Nat. Genet.*, 2013.

[46] Rogaeva E., Meng Y., Lee J. H., Gu Y., Kawarai T., Zou F., Katayama T., Baldwin C. T., Cheng R., Hasegawa H., Chen F., Shibata N., Lunetta K. L., Pardossi-Piquard R., Bohm C., Wakutani Y., Cupples L. A., Cuenco K. T., Green R. C., Pinessi L., Rainero I., Sorbi S., Bruni A., Duara R., Friedland R. P., Inzelberg R., Hampe W., Bujo H., Song Y. Q., Andersen O. M., Willnow T. E., Graff-Radford N., Petersen R. C., Dickson D., Der S. D., Fraser P. E., Schmitt-Ulms G., Younkin S., Mayeux R., Farrer L. A., St George-Hyslop P. The neuronal sortilin-related receptor SORL1 is genetically associated with Alzheimer disease. *Nat. Genet.*, 2007;39:168-177.

[47] Reitz C., Cheng R., Rogaeva E., Lee J., Tokuhiro S., Zou F., Bettens K., Sleegers K., Tan E. K., Kimura R., Shibata N., Arai H., Kamboh M. I., Prince J., Maier W., Riemenschneider M., Owen M., Harold D., Hollingworth P., Cellini E., Sorbi S., Nacmias B., Takeda M., Pericak-Vance M. A., Younkin S., Williams J., Van Broeckhoven C., Farrer L., St. George-Hyslop P., Mayeux R. Meta-analysis of the association between variants in SORL1 and Alzheimer's disease *Arch. Neurol.*, 2010;In press.

[48] Nuutinen T., Suuronen T., Kauppinen A., Salminen A. Clusterin: a forgotten player in Alzheimer's disease. *Brain Res. Rev.*, 2009;61:89-104.

[49] Wollmer M. A., Sleegers K., Ingelsson M., Zekanowski C., Brouwers N., Maruszak A., Brunner F., Huynh K. D., Kilander L., Brundin R. M., Hedlund M., Giedraitis V., Glaser A., Engelborghs S., De Deyn P. P., Kapaki E., Tsolaki M., Daniilidou M., Molyva D., Paraskevas G. P., Thal D. R., Barcikowska M., Kuznicki J., Lannfelt L., Van Broeckhoven C., Nitsch R. M., Hock C., Papassotiropoulos A. Association study of cholesterol-related genes in Alzheimer's disease. *Neurogenetics,* 2007; 8: 179-188.

[50] DeMattos R. B., Cirrito J. R., Parsadanian M., May P. C., O'Dell M. A., Taylor J. W., Harmony J. A., Aronow B. J., Bales K. R., Paul S. M., Holtzman D. M. ApoE and clusterin cooperatively suppress Abeta levels and deposition: evidence that ApoE regulates extracellular Abeta metabolism in vivo. *Neuron,* 2004;41:193-202.

[51] Pant S., Sharma M., Patel K., Caplan S., Carr C. M., Grant B. D. AMPH-1/Amphiphysin/Bin1 functions with RME-1/Ehd1 in endocytic recycling. *Nat. Cell Biol.*, 2009;11:1399-1410.

[52] Tebar F., Bohlander S. K., Sorkin A. Clathrin assembly lymphoid myeloid leukemia (CALM) protein: localization in endocytic-coated pits, interactions with clathrin, and the impact of overexpression on clathrin-mediated traffic. *Mol. Biol. Cell,* 1999;10:2687-2702.

[53] Crehan H., Holton P., Wray S., Pocock J., Guerreiro R., Hardy J. Complement receptor 1 (CR1) and Alzheimer's disease. *Immunobiology,* 2012;217:244-250.

[54] McGeer P. L., Rogers J. Anti-inflammatory agents as a therapeutic approach to Alzheimer's disease. *Neurology,* 1992;42:447-449.

[55] Cao H., Crocker P. R. Evolution of CD33-related siglecs: regulating host immune functions and escaping pathogen exploitation? *Immunology,* 2011;132:18-26.

[56] von Gunten S., Bochner B. S. Basic and clinical immunology of Siglecs. *Ann. N Y Acad. Sci.*, 2008;1143:61-82.

[57] Vitale C., Romagnani C., Falco M., Ponte M., Vitale M., Moretta A., Bacigalupo A., Moretta L., Mingari M. C. Engagement of p75/AIRM1 or CD33 inhibits the proliferation of normal or leukemic myeloid cells. *Proc. Natl. Acad. Sci. U S A,* 1999; 96: 15091-15096.

[58] Yamazaki T., Masuda J., Omori T., Usui R., Akiyama H., Maru Y. EphA1 interacts with integrin-linked kinase and regulates cell morphology and motility. *J. Cell Sci.*, 2009;122:243-255.

[59] Adams R. H., Klein R. Eph receptors and ephrin ligands. essential mediators of vascular development. *Trends Cardiovasc. Med.*, 2000;10:183-188.

[60] Duffy S. L., Coulthard M. G., Spanevello M. D., Herath N. I., Yeadon T. M., McCarron J. K., Carter J. C., Tonks I. D., Kay G. F., Phillips G. E., Boyd A. W. Generation and characterization of EphA1 receptor tyrosine kinase reporter knockout mice. *Genesis,* 2008;46:553-561.

[61] Holen H. L., Nustad K., Aasheim H. C. Activation of EphA receptors on CD4+CD45RO+ memory cells stimulates migration. *J. Leukoc. Biol.*, 2010;87:1059-1068.

[62] Sakamoto A., Sugamoto Y., Tokunaga Y., Yoshimuta T., Hayashi K., Konno T., Kawashiri M. A., Takeda Y., Yamagishi M. Expression profiling of the ephrin (EFN) and Eph receptor (EPH) family of genes in atherosclerosis-related human cells. *J. Int. Med. Res.*, 2011;39:522-527.

[63] Lehtonen S., Zhao F., Lehtonen E. CD2-associated protein directly interacts with the actin cytoskeleton. *Am. J. Physiol. Renal. Physiol.*, 2002; 283: F734-743.

[64] Dustin M. L., Olszowy M. W., Holdorf A. D., Li J., Bromley S., Desai N., Widder P., Rosenberger F., van der Merwe P. A., Allen P. M., Shaw A. S. A novel adaptor protein orchestrates receptor patterning and cytoskeletal polarity in T-cell contacts. *Cell,* 1998;94:667-677.

[65] Tanaka N., Abe-Dohmae S., Iwamoto N., Yokoyama S. Roles of ATP-binding cassette transporter A7 in cholesterol homeostasis and host defense system. *J. Atheroscler. Thromb.*, 2011;18:274-281.

[66] Chan S. L., Kim W. S., Kwok J. B., Hill A. F., Cappai R., Rye K. A., Garner B. ATP-binding cassette transporter A7 regulates processing of amyloid precursor protein in vitro. *J. Neurochem.*, 2008;106:793-804.

[67] Lee J. H., Cheng R., Barral S., Reitz C., Medrano M., Lantigua R., Jimenez-Velazquez I. Z., Rogaeva E., St George-Hyslop P. H., Mayeux R. Identification of novel loci for

Alzheimer disease and replication of CLU, PICALM, and BIN1 in Caribbean Hispanic individuals. *Arch. Neurol.*, 2011;68:320-328.

[68] Reitz C., Jun G., Naj A., Rajbhandary R., Vardarajan B. N., Wang L. S., Valladares O., Lin C. F., Larson E. B., Graff-Radford N. R., Evans D., De Jager P. L., Crane P. K., Buxbaum J. D., Murrell J. R., Raj T., Ertekin-Taner N., Logue M., Baldwin C. T., Green R. C., Barnes L. L., Cantwell L. B., Fallin M. D., Go R. C., Griffith P., Obisesan T. O., Manly J. J., Lunetta K. L., Kamboh M. I., Lopez O. L., Bennett D. A., Hendrie H., Hall K. S., Goate A. M., Byrd G. S., Kukull W. A., Foroud T. M., Haines J. L., Farrer L. A., Pericak-Vance M. A., Schellenberg G. D., Mayeux R. Variants in the ATP-binding cassette transporter (ABCA7), apolipoprotein E 4,and the risk of late-onset Alzheimer disease in African Americans. *JAMA,* 2013; 309: 1483-1492.

[69] Miyashita A., Koike A., Jun G., Wang L. S., Takahashi S., Matsubara E., Kawarabayashi T., Shoji M., Tomita N., Arai H., Asada T., Harigaya Y., Ikeda M., Amari M., Hanyu H., Higuchi S., Ikeuchi T., Nishizawa M., Suga M., Kawase Y., Akatsu H., Kosaka K., Yamamoto T., Imagawa M., Hamaguchi T., Yamada M., Moriaha T., Takeda M., Takao T., Nakata K., Fujisawa Y., Sasaki K., Watanabe K., Nakashima K., Urakami K., Ooya T., Takahashi M., Yuzuriha T., Serikawa K., Yoshimoto S., Nakagawa R., Kim J. W., Ki C. S., Won H. H., Na D. L., Seo S. W., Mook-Jung I., St. George-Hyslop P., Mayeux R., Haines J. L., Pericak-Vance M. A., Yoshida M., Nishida N., Tokunaga K., Yamamoto K., Tsuji S., Kanazawa I., Ihara Y., Schellenberg G. D., Farrer L. A., Kuwano R. SORL1 is genetically associated with late-onset Alzheimer's disease in Japanese, Koreans and Caucasians. *PLoS One,* 2013;8:e58618.

[70] Chen L. H., Kao P. Y., Fan Y. H., Ho D. T., Chan C. S., Yik P. Y., Ha J. C., Chu L. W., Song Y. Q. Polymorphisms of CR1, CLU and PICALM confer susceptibility of Alzheimer's disease in a southern Chinese population. *Neurobiol. Aging,* 2012;33:210 e211-217.

[71] Chung S. J., Lee J. H., Kim S. Y., You S., Kim M. J., Lee J. Y., Koh J. Association of GWAS top hits with late-onset Alzheimer disease in Korean population. *Alzheimer Dis. Assoc. Disord.*, 2013;27:250-257.

[72] Tan L., Yu J. T., Zhang W., Wu Z. C., Zhang Q., Liu Q. Y., Wang W., Wang H. F., Ma X. Y., Cui W. Z. Association of GWAS-linked loci with late-onset Alzheimer's disease in a northern Han Chinese population. *Alzheimers Dement.*, 2013;9:546-553.

[73] Yuan Q., Chu C., Jia J. Association studies of 19 candidate SNPs with sporadic Alzheimer's disease in the North Chinese Han population. *Neurol. Sci.*, 2012;33:1021-1028.

[74] Li H. L., Shi S. S., Guo Q. H., Ni W., Dong Y., Liu Y., Sun Y. M., Bei W., Lu S. J., Hong Z., Wu Z. Y. PICALM and CR1 variants are not associated with sporadic Alzheimer's disease in Chinese patients. *J. Alzheimers Dis.*, 2011;25:111-117.

[75] Yu J. T., Song J. H., Ma T., Zhang W., Yu N. N., Xuan S. Y., Tan L. Genetic association of PICALM polymorphisms with Alzheimer's disease in Han Chinese. *J. Neurol. Sci.*, 2011;300:78-80.

[76] Cruchaga C., Haller G., Chakraverty S., Mayo K., Vallania F. L., Mitra R. D., Faber K., Williamson J., Bird T., Diaz-Arrastia R., Foroud T. M., Boeve B. F., Graff-Radford N. R., St. Jean P., Lawson M., Ehm M. G., Mayeux R., Goate A. M., Consortium N-LNFS.

Rare variants in APP, PSEN1 and PSEN2 increase risk for AD in late-onset Alzheimer's disease families. *PLoS One,* 2012;7:e31039.

[77] Jonsson T., Atwal J. K., Steinberg S., Snaedal J., Jonsson P. V., Bjornsson S., Stefansson H., Sulem P., Gudbjartsson D., Maloney J., Hoyte K., Gustafson A., Liu Y., Lu Y., Bhangale T., Graham R. R., Huttenlocher J., Bjornsdottir G., Andreassen O. A., Jonsson E. G., Palotie A., Behrens T. W., Magnusson O. T., Kong A., Thorsteinsdottir U., Watts R. J., Stefansson K. A mutation in APP protects against Alzheimer's disease and age-related cognitive decline. *Nature,* 2012;488:96-99.

[78] Guerreiro R., Wojtas A., Bras J., Carrasquillo M., Rogaeva E., Majounie E., Cruchaga C., Sassi C., Kauwe J. S., Younkin S., Hazrati L., Collinge J., Pocock J., Lashley T., Williams J., Lambert J. C., Amouyel P., Goate A., Rademakers R., Morgan K., Powell J., St. George-Hyslop P., Singleton A., Hardy J. TREM2 variants in Alzheimer's disease. *N. Engl. J. Med.*, 2013;368:117-127.

[79] Jonsson T., Stefansson H., Steinberg S., Jonsdottir I., Jonsson P. V., Snaedal J., Bjornsson S., Huttenlocher J., Levey A. I., Lah J. J., Rujescu D., Hampel H., Giegling I., Andreassen O. A., Engedal K., Ulstein I., Djurovic S., Ibrahim-Verbaas C., Hofman A., Ikram M. A., van Duijn C. M., Thorsteinsdottir U., Kong A., Stefansson K. Variant of TREM2 associated with the risk of Alzheimer's disease. *N. Engl. J. Med.*, 2013; 368: 107-116.

[80] Schnetz-Boutaud N. C., Hoffman J., Coe J. E., Murdock D. G., Pericak-Vance M. A., Haines J. L. Identification and confirmation of an exonic splicing enhancer variation in exon 5 of the Alzheimer disease associated PICALM gene. *Ann. Hum. Genet.*, 2012; 76: 448-453.

[81] Pottier C., Hannequin D., Coutant S., Rovelet-Lecrux A., Wallon D., Rousseau S., Legallic S., Paquet C., Bombois S., Pariente J., Thomas-Anterion C., Michon A., Croisile B., Etcharry-Bouyx F., Berr C., Dartigues J. F., Amouyel P., Dauchel H., Boutoleau-Bretonniere C., Thauvin C., Frebourg T., Lambert J. C., Campion D., Collaborators P. G. High frequency of potentially pathogenic SORL1 mutations in autosomal dominant early-onset Alzheimer disease. *Mol. Psychiatry,* 2012; 17: 875-879.

[82] Kim M., Suh J., Romano D., Truong M. H., Mullin K., Hooli B., Norton D., Tesco G., Elliott K., Wagner S. L., Moir R. D., Becker K. D., Tanzi R. E. Potential late-onset Alzheimer's disease-associated mutations in the ADAM10 gene attenuate {alpha}-secretase activity. *Hum. Mol. Genet.*, 2009; 18: 3987-3996.

[83] Cruchaga C., Karch C. M., Jin S. C., Benitez B. A., Cai Y., Guerreiro R., Harari O., Norton J., Budde J., Bertelsen S., Jeng A. T., Cooper B., Skorupa T., Carrell D., Levitch D., Hsu S., Choi J., Ryten M., Hardy J., Trabzuni D., Weale M. E., Ramasamy A., Smith C., Sassi C., Bras J., Gibbs J. R., Hernandez D. G., Lupton M. K., Powell J., Forabosco P., Ridge P. G., Corcoran C. D., Tschanz J. T., Norton M. C., Munger R. G., Schmutz C., Leary M., Demirci F. Y., Bamne M. N., Wang X., Lopez O. L., Ganguli M., Medway C., Turton J., Lord J., Braae A., Barber I., Brown K., Passmore P., Craig D., Johnston J., McGuinness B., Todd S., Heun R., Kolsch H., Kehoe P. G., Hooper N. M., Vardy E. R., Mann D. M., Pickering-Brown S., Kalsheker N., Lowe J., Morgan K., David Smith A., Wilcock G., Warden D., Holmes C., Pastor P., Lorenzo-Betancor O., Brkanac Z., Scott E., Topol E., Rogaeva E., Singleton A. B., Kamboh M. I., St. George-Hyslop P., Cairns N., Morris J. C., Kauwe J. S., Goate A. M. Rare coding variants in

the phospholipase D3 gene confer risk for Alzheimer's disease. *Nature,* 2014; 505: 550-554.

[84] Mattick J. S. The central role of RNA in human development and cognition. *FEBS Lett.*, 2011; 585: 1600-1616.

In: Dementia
Editor: Pamela Tanner

ISBN: 978-1-63321-928-1

Chapter 2

Veterans Affairs Dementia Care Strategies As a Model

Katherine Luci and Kye Y. Kim*
Department of Psychiatry and Behavioral Medicine
Virginia Tech Carilion School of Medicine, Virginia, US

Abstract

Dementia is a distressing, progressively disabling, financially burdening, and, most of all, self-erasing illness. The nature of the disease presents patients, families, and care providers from multiple domains with numerous, multi-faceted challenges. As a rule, these challenges morph into new and distinctive challenges as patients move through various stages of the disease. In general., the service needs of the patient with dementia tend to intensify as severity of the disease increases. Due to the fact that most patients with dementia receive care and support from multiple providers, the risk of fragmentation in care provision is very real. Providers are called to search for better ways to ensure a continuum of care as the patient with dementia moves from living in the home to a long-term care facility. Also, end-of-life (EOL) care presents its own unique set of challenges and should be considered a key phase in planning for care continuum. Additionally, providing adequate and appropriate care and support to caregivers should be considered a central element of treatment planning. Similar to the patients themselves, caregivers require different forms of support, in varying degrees, as time and the disease progress. As the number of veterans being diagnosed with this complex medical issue increases, the Veterans Health Administration (VHA) looks to its Office of Geriatrics and Extended Care, a central body that provides policy direction for the development, coordination, and integration of geriatrics and long-term care clinical programs, and for the advancement of geriatrics and long-term care through research, education and evaluation of clinical models. A myriad of important programs and services exist within the Office of Geriatrics and Extended Care, including 20 "GRECCS" (Geriatric Research, Education and Clinical Centers), institutional care programs, non-institutional care programs, inpatient dementia units, and outpatient dementia clinics. This chapter will first present

* Corresponding author: Kye Y. Kim, M.D. (kykim@carilionclinic or kyekim726@gmail.com).

the many facets of dementia care, highlighting the complex nature of the illness as it occurs across disease stages. The chapter will subsequently reveal past and current efforts of the largest medical system in the United States as it works to provide comprehensive, coordinated care for veterans with dementia.

Introduction

Caring for persons with dementia represents one of the most challenging medical issues of the 21st century. A sense of urgency related to the problem of dementia has recently intensified, as the number of patients receiving a new dementia diagnosis is rapidly on the rise (Alzheimer's Association, 2014). This number is expected to escalate rapidly with the baby boomer generation, and as the number of Americans living into their 80s and 90s is expected to rise dramatically in the years to come. Currently, more than 5 million Americans are living with Alzheimer's disease (AD), the most common type of dementia. By 2050, the number of people age 65 and older with Alzheimer's disease may nearly triple, from 5 million to as many as 16 million, barring the development of medical breakthroughs to prevent, slow or stop the disease

The United States Department of Veterans Affairs (VA) is the nation's largest healthcare system, which is operated by the Veterans Health Administration (VHA). VHA faces similarly rapid increases in the number of veterans with dementia; that number is projected to increase to 218,000 by 2017, a 42% increase from 2006 (Spotswood, 2007). The VHA must also factor into its planning for future dementia care the recent discovery that dementia occurs approximately twice as often in individuals with posttraumatic stress disorder (PTSD) (Yaffe et al., 2010), a disorder common amongst veterans. With so many veterans developing dementia, the VHA will likely be looked to as an important model for comprehensive dementia care within a large medical system.

Dementia is a distressing, progressively disabling, financially burdening, and, most of all, self-erasing illness. The nature of the disease presents patients, families, and care providers from multiple domains with numerous, multi-faceted challenges. As a rule, these challenges morph into new and distinctive challenges as patients move through various stages of the disease. In general., the service needs of the patient with dementia tend to intensify as severity of the disease increases. Due to the fact that most patients with dementia receive care and support from multiple providers, the risk of fragmentation in care provision is very real. Providers are called to search for better ways to ensure a continuum of care as the patient with dementia moves from living in the home to a long-term care facility. Also, end-of-life (EOL) care presents its own unique set of challenges and should be considered a key phase in planning for care continuum. Additionally, providing adequate and appropriate care and support to caregivers should be considered a central element of treatment planning. Similar to the patients themselves, caregivers require different forms of support, in varying degrees, as time and the disease progress.

As the number of veterans being diagnosed with this complex medical issue increases, the VHA looks to its Office of Geriatrics and Extended Care, a central body that provides "policy direction for the development, coordination, and integration of geriatrics and long-term care clinical programs, and for the advancement of geriatrics and long-term care through research, education and evaluation of clinical models" (Department of Veterans Affairs,

2010). A myriad of important programs and services exist within the Office of Geriatrics and Extended Care, including 20 GRECCS (Geriatric Research, Education and Clinical Centers), institutional care programs (e.g., Community Living Centers), non-institutional care programs (e.g., Home Based Primary Care), inpatient dementia units, and outpatient dementia clinics.

This chapter will first present the many facets of dementia care, highlighting the complex nature of the illness as it occurs across disease stages. The article will subsequently reveal past and current efforts of the largest healthcare system in the United States as it works to provide comprehensive, coordinated care for veterans with dementia.

Disease Staging/Milestones

In discussing approaches to dementia care, Rabheru (2007) suggests that the concepts of clinical milestones and disease staging help capture the complexity of AD as it affects multiple domains. Cognition, function, behavior, caregiver burden (CB), quality of life (QOL), and cost (by stage) represent some of the more common domains studied by AD researchers. Of these domains, cognition and global functioning have higher predictive power than the other domains mentioned, and they have been used by the American Psychiatric Association in developing research criteria. Nevertheless, Rabheru emphasizes the importance of including milestones from multiple domains, stating that even cognition is inadequate as an independent screening factor for a person with AD at any stage. Several neuropsychiatric symptoms, for instance, have been associated with different disease stages and can be helpful in targeting treatment according to disease stage. For example, depression, anxiety, and agitation are common in early AD. Similarly, hallucinations have potential as useful clinical markers in late dementia. Knowing that neuropsychiatric disturbances and declining patient functioning lead to increased CB informs treatment planning. CB is, in turn, predictive of death or institutionalization of the patient. Additionally, QOL milestones (including confinement to home, lack of activity, and lack of positive affect) and cost of care (which increases dramatically with increasing disease severity) serve to help target therapy and services. Rabheru also highlights the potential usefulness of biological markers, stating that as advances are made in this line of AD research, they may potentially become the more objective, reliable, specific, and sensitive method for tracking disease progression.

Dementia Diagnosis and Care in Primary Care

Dementia is frequently under-recognized and under-diagnosed by physicians. Chodosh and colleagues (2004) discovered that physicians fail to recognize cognitive impairment in 40% of their cognitively impaired patients. In another study by Boustani and colleagues (2005), only 19% of primary care patients who were found to have dementia by an expert panel of investigators had documentation of dementia in their medical record. A meta-analysis of the literature revealed that 50-66% of dementia cases in primary care samples across multiple studies had not received a dementia diagnosis (Boustani, 2003). One of the barriers to dementia diagnosis is that a positive screening test alone is not sufficient for making an accurate diagnosis. Ashford and colleagues (2007) emphasize the importance of proceeding through the "standard of care diagnostic procedures for dementia diagnosis", rather than simply diagnosing Alzheimer's Disease based solely on the results of a dementia screening test. However, older adults frequently refuse further diagnostic assessment for dementia after receiving positive results on dementia screening tests, and many are unwilling to undergo routine screening for memory problems (Kansagara & Freeman, 2010).

The above brief overview of some of the challenges related to dementia screening in primary care demonstrates the complicated, multi-faceted nature of this issue. Multiple medical comorbid conditions further complicate the role of primary care physicians in the care of patients with dementia. Schubert and colleagues (2006) found that primary care patients with dementia have 2.4 chronic conditions on average and receive 5.1 medications. Alarmingly, 50% of dementia patients were found to be exposed to at least one anticholinergic medication, despite the patients' already existing cholinergic deficit. Such exposure to anticholinergic medications puts patients with dementia at higher risk of anticholinergic adverse effects (e.g., delirium, falls, increased cognitive deficits). Also complicating the care of patients with dementia in primary care is their decreased ability to recall recent symptoms, and language deficits impair the patient's ability to report symptoms or drug side effects.

One study (Callahan, Hendrie, and Tierney, 1995) revealed that cognitive impairment is associated with increased utilization of health services; that is, patients with cognitive impairment were more likely to be hospitalized and visit the emergency department. They were also found to be less likely to visit ambulatory clinics. By contrast, health service utilization rates decreased when a geriatric psychiatrist was involved in patient care (Aupperle, Mac Phee, Coyne, Blume, & Sanchez, 2003). Specifically, institutionalization rates were significantly lower in patients receiving care from a geriatric psychiatrist (4.6%) compared to those who were being seen only by their primary care physicians (30.0%). On a related note, a Canadian study by Yaffe, Orzeck, and Barylak (2008) found that family doctors wanted more education on AD. Also, these physicians expressed concerns regarding limited access to consultation with specialists (e.g., neurology, geriatrics). In addition, the study revealed that physicians were "generally unaware" of community resources available for patients and their caregivers; and, unfortunately, they indicated that they were not interested in learning more about such community resources.

Callahan and colleagues (2006) present "collaborative care" as one strategy for improving the care of patients with dementia in a primary care environment. In this model of care, patients with AD receive care from an interdisciplinary team led by an advanced practice nurse. Patients in this study were, at minimum, recommended for treatment with cholinesterase inhibitors and received education by the care manager (a geriatric nurse practitioner). Care managers also worked with caregivers; they met with the patients and their caregivers in the primary care clinic bimonthly initially, then monthly for a period of 1 year. In addition to education, individualized recommendations regarding how to manage the patient's behavioral symptoms were provided. Another important component of the collaborative care model was that the care manager met weekly with a support team (including a geriatrician, geriatric psychiatrist, and a psychologist) and communicated both the patients' and caregiver's current clinical status to the entire care team via a web-based longitudinal tracking system. Finally, caregivers were invited to participate in a support session led by a psychologist. Patients who received this intervention demonstrated significantly fewer behavioral and psychological symptoms of dementia, and their caregivers reported significant improvements in caregiver distress.

Caregivers of Dementia Patients

The caregiver plays a key role in determining the course of treatment for a dementia patient. Mittelman, Haley, Clay, and Roth (2006) found that by addressing caregiver burden thru counseling and other supportive interventions, the rate of nursing home placement was reduced by 28.3%. Along a similar vein, Spitznagel, Tremont, Duncan Davis, and Foster (2006) revealed that higher levels of caregiver burden were associated with a caregiver's desire to institutionalize the dementia patient. The caregiver's desire to institutionalize was also higher for those caring for patients who exhibited more frontal systems behavior problems, and for those experiencing a decrease in independence in activities of daily living (ADLs).

Additionally, overall family functioning and social support were shown to affect desire for institutionalization (Spitznagel, Tremont, Duncan Davis, & Foster 2006). Tremont, Duncan Davis, and Bishop (2006) found that poorer family functioning (in terms of communication and roles) is associated with higher levels of caregiver burden, regardless of the caregiver's relationship to the patient (i.e., spouse or child). Tremont and colleagues assert that caregiver interventions that include a family systems component have potential usefulness in addressing burden in these individuals. Indeed, Mittelman, Roth, Coon, and Haley (2004) found that a caregiver intervention that included individual and family counseling, as well as participation in a caregiver support group, produced sustained benefits in reducing depressive symptoms in spouse-caregivers. Caregivers who received this intervention, which provided caregivers the opportunity to learn new skills and develop psychosocial coping resources useful over the long course of caring for a patient with Alzheimer's disease, demonstrated fewer depressive symptoms more than three years after enrollment in the program. In addition, a study by Gaugler, Roth, Haley, and Mittelman (2008) suggests that an intervention consisting of individual and family counseling may provide benefits to caregivers during the transition to institutionalization. While institutionalization alone appears to reduce both caregiver burden and depressive symptoms, burden and depressive symptoms were decreased significantly further in caregivers who received counseling both at the time of and after the transition to institutionalization.

Prevalence and Economic Impacts of AD

The prevalence of AD in the U.S. is striking. In 2014, approximately 5.2 million Americans aged 65 and older had AD (Alzheimer's Association, 2014). Put another way, 1in 8 Americans over age 65, or 13 percent, have AD. Every 67 seconds, someone in the U.S. develops AD. Accordingly, the economic impact of this disease is daunting. The total payments for health care and long-term care services for people aged 65 and older with AD and other dementias in the year 2014 was estimated at $214 billion. Additionally, the value of unpaid care for persons with Alzheimer's and other dementias, as provided by almost 11 million Americans (i.e., family members and friends), was estimated to reach $144 billion (in 2009).

The number of veterans in the U.S. with AD and other dementias is similarly large. Krishnan and colleagues (2005) found that between 1997 and 2001, 2.4 million veterans aged 65 and older who were seen in the VA carried a dementia diagnosis. That is, 7.3% of veterans aged 65 and older had been diagnosed with dementia. More specifically, across individual VISNs, the prevalence ranged from 5.8 to 9.4%. Regional differences in prevalence were notable; with the highest prevalence in VISNs located in Maryland, Virginia, West Virginia, Kentucky, Tennessee, North Carolina, South Carolina, Georgia, Alabama, Mississippi, Louisiana, Arkansas, Texas, and Oklahoma (i.e., many of the states representing what has been termed the "stroke belt"). Not surprisingly, Alzheimer's disease was the most common type of dementia (44.6%) in veterans nationwide.

Statistics compiled by the VA parallel Krishnan et al.'s findings. Spotswood (2007) reports that, among the veterans registered as patients of the VA in 2004, 155,000 had been diagnosed with dementia (including dementia due to Parkinson's disease). However, it is estimated that approximately 261,000 likely had dementia at that time. The number of veterans receiving VA care who have a diagnosis of dementia is expected to peak in 2017 at roughly 218,000; this would be a 42 per cent increase from the year 2006. In 2006, half of the VA's patient workload—2.4 million veterans—were 65 and older. Also, the VA counted 1.1 million veterans aged 85 and older in 2006, and 1 out of every 2 veterans in that age group (the "oldest old") are likely to suffer from some form of dementia.

Veterans As a Special Population

In discussing dementia within a specific population, it is important to consider the unique characteristics of that population. Morgan, Teal., Reddy, Ford, and Ashton (2005) describe several distinctive characteristics of the U.S. veteran population. For instance, veterans as a group are predominantly male, though this is projected to decline significantly (i.e., by approximately 27 percent) from 2005-2020 (Morgan et al. citing U.S. Department of Veterans Affairs, 2000). Accordingly, the number of female veterans is growing rapidly and is expected to increase by 12 percent over the same time period. In terms of age, the median age of all veterans is 55, with the majority of veterans having served during World War II, the Korean War, and the Vietnam War. Veterans account for 60 percent of all white males over the age of 65 living in the U.S.; while veterans account for only 45 percent of African-American and 35 percent of Hispanic males in the same age group. Overall, veterans have higher levels of education and are better off financially than the general U.S. male population (Morgan et al. citing Klein, 2001; Klein and Stockford, 2001). However, veterans who utilize VA Health Administration (VHA) services are distinct from veterans as a larger group; patients of the VA tend to be "poorer, older, less well educated, more likely to be unemployed or underemployed, more likely to be African American, and more likely to report poorer physical and mental health and more chronic health conditions" than veterans who do not use VA services or the general U.S. population (Morgan et al. citing Kazis, Miller, and Clark, 1998; Agha, Lofgren and Van Ruiswyk, 2000).

The Veterans Health Administration (VHA): An Overview

The Veterans Administration was established in 1930 and expanded significantly following the Servicemen's Readjustment Act of 1944 (also known as the "GI Bill of Rights"), which provided additional resources for social services to veterans (Perlin, Kolodner, and Roswell, 2004). In 1989, the Veterans Administration was assigned Cabinet status and transformed into The Department of Veterans Affairs. The Department of Veterans Affairs includes three divisions: Veterans Health Administration (VHA), Veterans Benefits Administration, and the National Cemetery System.

As a result of the Veterans Health Care Eligibility Reform Act created in 1996, the VHA was restructured from a hospital system to an integrated health care system; it now represents the largest health system in the United States (Perlin, Kolodner, and Roswell, 2004). Structural changes involved the creation of 22 geographically defined Veterans Integrated Services Networks, (or VISNs). Concurrent with this reorganization, came a shift from a hospital environment to ambulatory-care facilities and increased home care services. Furthermore, the VA enhanced its original information system (veterans health information systems and technology architecture or "VistA") with the addition of the computerized patient record system (CPRS). CPRS provides a more user-friendly graphical interface for healthcare providers to review patients' medical records and to place orders (e.g., for medications, procedures). CPRS also supports performance improvement-- it provides computerized provider order entry (with a real-time order-checking system), critical alerts, access to remote data from other VA facilities, and a clinical reminder system that allows providers to track preventive healthcare and disease treatment.

In recent years, the VHA's mission to provide patient-centered care coordination has received much emphasis. Such care "extends the focus of disease management to better and more efficiently integrate every patient's disease-specific and general health needs with the resources of the health system" (Perlin, Kolodner, and Roswell, 2004). Technology, from simple supportive technologies (e.g., daily voice or text queries assessing the patient's status) to electronic scales attached to computers or phones, is central to this form of patient-centered care; it extends the environment of care beyond the hospital and provides safe, effective, and convenient care coordination to veterans.

Geriatric Research, Education, and Clinical Center (GRECC)

GRECCs were established by the VHA in the 1970s to meet the anticipated challenges that were to be presented by the aging World War II veteran population (Department of Veterans Affairs, 2011). Each of the 20 GRECCs nationwide is a center of excellence and contains three components: research, education, and clinical. Thus GRECCs were intentionally designed to attract researchers and health science students to the field of geriatrics; they foster the development of a basic knowledge of aging, help transmit this knowledge to health care providers, and contribute to the overall quality of care provided to older adults. Currently, six GRECCs focus much of their research efforts on Alzheimer's disease-related topics.

The Office of Geriatrics and Extended Care

The Office of Geriatrics and Extended Care provides "policy direction for the development, coordination, and integration of geriatrics and long-term care clinical programs, and for the advancement of geriatrics and long-term care through research, education and evaluation of clinical models (Department of Veterans Affairs, 2010). The Office of Geriatrics and Extended Care works with institutional programs, including VA Community Living Centers or CLCs, which are nursing homes located within or near VA medical centers, state veterans homes, and hospice and palliative care. It also provides policy direction for non-institutional programs, including home-based primary care, adult day healthcare, home respite care, purchased skilled home care, homemaker and home health aide services, home hospice care, and community residential care. Geriatric programs include specialized Alzheimer's and dementia care (e.g., outpatient dementia clinics, inpatient dementia units), the Geriatric Evaluation and Management program (an interdisciplinary team approach to assessment and treatment planning), geriatric primary care (a coordinated, interdisciplinary team approach to care management by the primary care provider and support team), and geriatric research (GRECC). In 2006, the VHA's Office of Geriatrics and Extended Care has implemented the Dementia Steering Committee to enhance dementia care continually through the provision of comprehensive, coordinated, evidence-based dementia care throughout the VHA healthcare (Cooley, Asthana, 2010).

Dementia Care (American Association for Geriatric Psychiatry)

The American Association for Geriatric Psychiatry has developed a care model ("Dementia Care") for the treatment of patients with AD (American Association for Geriatric Psychiatry, 2006). The stated aims of this model are to "delay disease progression, delay functional decline, improve quality of life, support dignity, control symptoms, and provide comfort at all stages of AD". While this is conceptualized as an evolving model due to the limited amount of scientific evidence of beneficial outcomes on which it is based, AAGP's model for dementia care maintains that there does currently exist a minimal set of care principles for this patient population and their caregivers. The set of care principles defined in AAGP's model of care address disease therapies based on current pathophysiological understanding of the disease, symptomatic therapies for cognitive and neuropsychiatric symptoms, and interventions to support patients and their caregivers.

In terms of comprehensive, coordinated care, the VHA dementia steering committee focused on the following models in their review of the literature: Partners in Dementia Care, Care Management using Dementia Practice Guidelines, Collaborative Care Model, VA Office of Care Coordination (based on the Wagner Chronic Care Model), and Dementia Demonstration Project (based on a milestones model).

Partners in Dementia Care (PDC)

Developed by VISN 2 of the VHA as part of the national demonstration project "Chronic Care Networks for Alzheimer's Disease" (CCN/AD), Partners in Dementia Care (PDC) was co-sponsored by the National Chronic Care Consortium and the Alzheimer's Association (Alzheimer's Association, 2005). Designed as an intervention encompassing care coordination and support services for veterans with dementia and their family caregivers, PDC created a partnership between the VISN 2 health care network and four Alzheimer's Association chapters located in the same region.

The PDC model of care addressed four problems common across VA and non-VA health care settings: 1) under-identification of dementia, 2) inadequate diagnostic assessments, 3) a lack of coordination between healthcare providers and community services, and 4) a lack of information and support for family caregivers. PDC aimed to improve care for individual veterans and their families and to change the system of care for all veterans with dementia. As a key component of this care model, a Dementia Care Coordinator (DCC) was placed within each of VISN 2's five medical centers. The DCCs were delegated the tasks of planning, training (a major focus of PDC), enrollment of veterans into the program, and ongoing care coordination within the VA and between VA and Alzheimer's Association (AA) chapters. Program evaluation revealed several positive findings, including that almost all veterans enrolled in PDC completed the recommended diagnostic assessment. Additionally, veterans and caregivers who accessed AA chapter services were more likely to report having received sufficient information or help in areas such as treatment options, family concerns, daily living tasks, and legal/financial issues. Those who reported having received sufficient information in these areas reported higher levels of satisfaction; lower levels of depression; as well as less physical., emotional., and relationship strain

Care Management using Dementia Practice Guidelines

Vickrey and colleagues (2006) conducted a randomized controlled trial study to explore whether or not a care management program based on dementia practice guidelines could enhance adherence to guideline recommendations. In this disease management program, health care organization-based dementia care managers (primarily social workers) worked with patient and caregiver dyads in generating a prioritized problem list and recommendations (based on in-home assessements). Results revealed that adherence to guideline recommendations was significantly higher in the intervention group than in the usual care group. In addition, substantial improvement in quality of life for patients with dementia, and improvements in social support and caregiving quality were demonstrated for those who received the intervention. The results from another randomized controlled study (Chodosh et al., 2006) which implemented a comprehensive dementia care management model did not reveal clear benefits in terms of provider knowledge or attitudes favorable to dementia care.

Collaborative Care Model

The collaborative care model utilizes an interdisciplinary team approach. A controlled clinical study by Callahan and colleagues (2006) found that patients who received 1 year of care management by an interdisciplinary team (including a geriatric nurse practitioner and a primary care physician) were more likely to receive cholinesterase inhibitors and antidepressants, and to have significantly fewer behavioral and psychological symptoms of dementia. Caregivers who received the intervention experienced significant improvements in distress and symptoms of depression. Austrom, Hartwell, Moore, Boustani, Hendrie, and Callahan (2005) describe key components of a collaborative care model to include, "1) a comprehensive screening and diagnosis protocol; 2) a multidisciplinary team approach coordinated by a geriatric advance practice nurse; and 3) a proactive longitudinal tracking system". The latter is used to track both pharmacological and non-pharmacological interventions. Non-pharmacological interventions include the provision of general education about Alzheimer's disease, protocols for the treatment of behavioral disturbances, and a psychoeducational support group for caregivers (including, e.g., education on communication skills, coping skills, legal and financial issues) (Austrom et al., 2004).

VA Office of Telehealth Services

The VA Office of Telehealth Services has incorporated lessons from Edward Wagner's Chronic Care Model (Wagner, Austin, Davis, Hindmarsh, Schaefer, & Bonomi, 2001) to meet patients' needs effectively. The Chronic Care Model was developed as a guide for chronic care improvement, and it holds as one of its major tenets the notion that high-quality chronic illness care depends on productive interactions between the treatment team and the patient. Such interactions must consistently provide "the assessments, support for self-management, optimization of therapy, and follow-up" that have consistently been found to be associated with good outcomes in the management of chronic illness. There exists an abundance of evidence documenting the effectiveness of computer or telephone technologies towards such an end.

The VA's use of telehealth services ensures that veterans "get the right care in the right place at the right time" (Department of Veterans Affairs, n.d.). The Care Coordination/Home Telehealth (CCHT) program is now embedded in many VA services and clinics, and is widely employed in the provision of routine chronic care management services to patients with diabetes mellitus, congestive heart failure, hypertension, posttraumatic stress disorder, chronic obstructive pulmonary disease, and depression (Darkins et al., 2008). CCHT helps patients avoid unscheduled acute care visits through regular communication with primary care and other specialy care providers as needed. With a significant increase in the patient census for CCHT (i.e., from 2,000 to 31,570 patients over a 4-year period), Darkins and colleagues documented an associated reduction in hospital admissions and a reduction in bed days of care (BDOC). Importantly, home telehealth models have been successfully implemented in both medical and mental health care coordination.

Dementia Demonstration Project

The Dementia Demonstration Project, a project led by the Geriatric Research, Education and Clinic Center (GRECC) at the Minneapolis Veterans Affairs Medical Center, was based on a disease milestones model, such as that described by Rabheru (2007). A major component of the Dementia Demonstration Project was its use of a Dementia Care Coordinator, an Advanced Practice Registered Nurse who led a dementia care team within a primary care clinic at each of seven VA Medical Centers participating in the project. The dementia care team met with primary care patients (and their family caregivers) who failed a three-item memory test, to discuss diagnosis and treatment recommendations. Interventions were designed to promote patient participation, and they were based on the severity of dementia and on the needs of the patients and their caregivers. The dementia care team provided informational materials to caregivers and provided support regarding movement from home to an assisted living facility (ALF) or a skilled nursing facility (SNF) for patients in the later stages of dementia.

Caregiver Support

Mary Mittelman (2005) asserts that any comprehensive care model for patients with chronic illness should include family caregiver interventions. Her review of numerous studies related to the outcome of caregiver interventions reveals that long-term, psychosocial interventions are most efficacious. While psychoeducational interventions are used most frequently and do demonstrate improved knowledge, supportive interventions have greater impact on the emotional and psychological well-being of both the patient and the caregiver. Mittelman discusses the stress-process model as a theoretical framework for understanding why psychosocial interventions are so effective. A major component of this model is the hypothesis that social support does not necessarily alter the stress of caregiving; rather, social support alters the caregiver's appraisal of stress and contributes to psychological well-being.

Two large-scale research programs investigating the effectiveness of different forms of caregiver interventions include the Resources for Enhancing Alzheimer's Caregiver Health (REACH) project and the NYU ADRC program. REACH was created by the National Institute on Aging (NIA) and the National Institute of Nursing Research (NINR) to develop and empirically test caregiver interventions aimed at enhancing caregiving skills and generally helping families to manage the stress of caring for people with Alzheimer's disease and other dementias (Schulz et al., 2003). The REACH initiative funded six research projects at six sites; each project evaluated various multicomponent interventions such as individual support strategies, group support and family systems therapy, psychoeducation, skill-based training, etc., REACH projects were culturally tailored to meet the needs of both ethnic majority and minority caregivers; also, the experience of REACH revealed the need for caregiver interventions to be tailored to meet the specific needs of the individual. A major focus of the ensuing REACH II program was to utilize a risk appraisal approach to help prioritize the amount of emphasis that should be placed on each of the treatment components (i.e., safety, self-care, social support, emotional well-being, and problem behaviors).

From 1987 to 2005, New York University's Spouse-Caregiver Intervention Study (at NYU's Aging and Dementia Research Center), examined the impact that a counseling and support intervention for spousal caregivers had on the patient (i.e., by delaying nursing home placement) and on depressive symptoms in the caregiver (Mittelman, Haley, Clay, & Roth, 2006; Mittelman, Roth, Coon, & Haley, 2004; Mittelman, 2003; Mittelman, Ferris, Shulman, Steinberg, & Levin, 1996). The intervention consisted of six sessions of individual and family counseling sessions, ad hoc telephone counseling, and monthly support group attendance. For patients with dementia, this psychosocial intervention delayed their placement in a nursing home by a median time of 557 days (Mittelman, Haley, Clay, & Roth, 2006). For caregivers, improvement in depressive symptoms was significant and was sustained for 3.1 years following baseline (Mittelman, Roth, Coon, & Haley, 2004).

Palliative Care

End-of-life care needs to be proactively integrated into the longitudinal care of dementia, regardless of the care venue. The Veterans Affairs Hospice and Palliative initiative provides comfort-oriented, supportive care services in the home; or in community, outpatient, or inpatient settings (Department of Veterans Affairs). Hospice and Palliative care services aim to minimize not only physical suffering, but also psychological., social., and spiritual suffering. Additionally, optimizing the patient's quality of life is a strategic goal of Hospice and Palliative Care (Department of Veterans Affairs, 1999). Some VA medical centers offer various complementary therapies, including music therapy, art therapy, massage, relaxation/visualization, and life review therapy. Spiritual care is also provided, with chaplains serving as key members of the interdisciplinary palliative care team. Many VA hospice and palliative care programs also offer bereavement support for families.

Dementia Special Care Units

Presently, a national policy on dementia care units in the VA healthcare system does not exist. Studies investigating the treatment effectiveness of special care units (SCUs) conducted by the National Institute on Aging (NIA) (Maslow & Ory, 2001) have demonstrated that while placement in an SCU is not generally effective for patients with dementia in terms of improvement in cognition or physical functional performance, SCUs are modestly effective in improving certain processes of care (including increased engagement and sociability, and increased display of pleasure). Within the VA, a dementia-specific care unit is best provided in the form of a sub-unit of the Community Living Center (CLC, formerly "Nursing Home Care Units" or NHCU), or as a separate dementia unit within the CLC. Dementia care units should provide security to reduce the exiting of patients, as well as specific therapeutic activity programming. Also, a dementia care unit's nursing team must be trained for dementia-specific clinical issues.

Medical Foster Homes

One of the VA's most recent innovations in dementia care is the Medical Foster Home. The Medical Foster Home is a community-based home "chosen" by the veteran who is unable to live independently, as a preferred means to receive family-style living with room, board, and personal care. The Medical Foster Home is a cost-effective alternative for veterans who prefer a non-institutional setting for their long-term care. This model of care forms a unique partnership between privately owned and operated adult foster homes and Home Based Primary Care (HBPC) services as provided by the VA. Independent living in a medical foster home is promoted through the support of assistive devices and home care services. An interdisciplinary HBPC team provides home assessment, caregiver education, and comprehensive patient care within the foster home.

Conclusion

Just as the number of Americans ages 65 and older with dementia is projected to increase significantly during the coming decades, the number of veterans with dementia will also rise at a dramatic pace. The VHA's Office of Geriatrics and Extended Care has implemented the Dementia Steering Committee to enhance dementia care continually through the provision of comprehensive, coordinated, evidence-based dementia care throughout the VHA healthcare system. With an emphasis on collaborative work between the VA and community based programs and on the use of telehealth treatment approaches, the VA aims to provide comprehensive care to veterans when and where they can most readily access it. Caregiver support is also being included as a major component of the VA's comprehensive care approach for veterans with dementia. Looking forward, the VA faces a major challenge in the provision of ongoing education and training for its staff as these practices are implemented in its medical centers nationwide. Also of great importance is the interdisciplinary approach required in the provision of this type of comprehensive care; the VA is now tasked with developing coordinated interdisciplinary treatment teams who can effectively serve the many older veterans with dementia who require their long-term support and care.

References

Alzheimer's Association (2010). *Facts and Figures.* Retrieved December 1, 2010, from http://www.alz.org/documents_custom/report_alzfactsfigures2010.pdf

Alzheimer's Association (2005). *Partners in dementia care: A chronic care network for Alzheimer's disease (CCN/AD) project.* Retrieved May 23, 2011, from http://www.alz.org/national/documents/Partners_in_Dementia_Care_Final_Report.pdf

American Association for Geriatric Psychiatry (2006). *AAGP position statement: Principles of care for patients with dementia resulting from Alzheimer disease.* Retrieved May 6, 2011, from http://www.aagponline.org/prof/position_caredmnalz.asp

Ashford, J. W., Borson, S., O'Hara, R., Dash, P., Frank, L., Robert, P., Shankle, W. R., Tierney, M. C., Brodaty, H., Schmitt, F. A., Kraemer, H. C., Buschke, H. & Fillit, H. (2007). Should older adults be screened for dementia? It is important to screen for evidence of dementia! *Alzheimer's & Dementia*, *3*, 75-80.

Aupperle, P. M., MacPhee, E. R., Coyne, A. C., Blume, J. & Sanchez, B. (2003). Health service utilization by Alzheimer's disease patients: a 2-year follow-up of primary versus subspecialty care. *Journal of Geriatric Psychiatry and Neurology*, *16*(1), 15-17.

Boustani, M., Callahan, C. M., Unverzagt, F. W., Austrom, M. G., Perkins, A. J., Fultz, B. A., Hui, S. L. & Hendrie, H. C. (2005). Implementing a screening and diagnosis program for dementia in primary care. *Journal of General Internal Medicine*, *20*, 572-577.

Boustani, M., Peterson, B., Hanson, L., Harris, R. & Lohr, K. (2003). Screening for dementia in primary care: A summary of the evidence for the U.S. Preventive Services Task Force. *Annals of Internal Medicine*, *138*(11), 927-937.

Callahan, C. M., Boustani, M. A., Unverzagt, F. W., Austrom, M. G., Damush, T. M., Perkins, A. J., Fultz, B. A., Hui, S. L., Counsell, S. R. & Hendrie, H. C. (2006). Effectiveness of collaborative care for older adults with Alzheimer disease in primary care. *Journal of the American Medical Association*, *295*(18), 2148-2157.

Callahan, C. M., Hendrie, H. C. & Tierney, W. M. (1995). Documentation and evaluation of cognitive impairment in elderly primary care patients. *Annals of Internal Medicine*, *122*, 422-429.

Chodosh, J., Petitti, D. B., Elliott, M., Hays, R. D., Crooks, V. C., Reuben, D. B., Galen Buckwalter, J. &Wenger, N. (2004). Physician recognition of cognitive impairment: evaluating the need for improvement. *Journal of the American Geriatrics Society*, *52*(7), 1051-1059.

Cooley, S. G. & Asthana S. (2010). Dementia care for veterans: enhancing comprehensive coordinated services. *Generations*, *34* (2), 57 – 63,

Darkins, A., Ryan, P., Kobb, R., Foster, L., Edmonson, E., Wakefield, B. & Lancaster, A. E. (2008). Care Coordination/Home Telehealth: The systematic implementation of health informatics, home telehealth, and disease management to support the care of veteran patients with chronic conditions. *Telemedicine and e-Health*, *14*(10), 1118-1126.

Department of Veterans Affairs. (1999). *Statement of Thomas Holohan, M.D., and Judith A. Salerno, M.D., on improving care at the end of life with complementary medicine before the Committee On Government Reform U.S. House of Representatives.* Washington, D.C.: Author.

Department of Veterans Affairs. (2010). *Geriatrics and Extended Care: About us.* Retrieved December 1, 2010, from http://www1.va.gov/GERIATRICS/About_Us.asp

Department of Veterans Affairs. (2011). *Geriatric Research Education and Clinical Centers.* Retrieved April 35, 2011, from http://www.va.gov/grecc/

Department of Veterans Affairs. (n.d.). *Hospice and Palliative Care.* Retrieved June 13, 2011, from http://www.va.gov/GERIATRICS/Hospice_Palliative_Care2.asp

Department of Veterans Affairs. (n.d.). *Medical Foster Home.* Retrieved June 13, 2011, from http://www.va.gov/GERIATRICS/Medical_Foster_Home.asp

Department of Veterans Affairs. (n.d.). *VHA Office of Telehealth Services.* Retrieved June 13, 2011, from http://www.telehealth.va.gov/index.asp

Gaugler, J. E., Roth, D. L., Haley, W. E. & Mittelman, M. S. (2008). Can counseling and support reduce Alzheimer's caregivers‘ burden and depressive symptoms during the transition to institutionalization? Results from the NYU Caregiver Intervention Study. *Journal of the American Geriatrics Society*, *56*(3), 421-428.

Improving Chronic Illness Care. (n.d.). *The chronic care model: Model elements.* Retrieved June 3, 2011, from http://www.improvingchroniccare.org/index.php?p=Model_Elements&s=18

Krishnan, L. L., Petersen, N. J., Snow, A. L., Cully, J. A., Schulz, P. E., Graham, D. P., Morgan, R. O., Braun, U., Moffett, M. L., Yu, H.-J. & Kunik, M. E. (2005). Prevalence of dementia among Veterans Affairs Medical Care System users. *Dementia and Geriatric Cognitive Disorders*, *20*, 245-253.

Maslow, K. & Ory, M. (2001). Dementia special care unit research: Lessons learned and future directions. *Alzheimer's Care Quarterly*, *2*(3), 10-16.

Mittelman, M. (2005). Taking care of the caregivers. *Current Opinion in Psychiatry*, *18*, 633-639.

Mittelman, M. S. (2003). Psychosocial intervention for dementia caregivers: What can it accomplish? *International psychogeriatrics*, *15*(1), 247-249.

Mittelman, M. S., Ferris, S. H., Shulman, E., Steinberg, G. & Levin, B. (1996). A family intervention to delay nursing home placement of patients with Alzheimer disease. *Journal of the American Medical Association*, *276*(21), 1725-1731.

Mittelman, M. S., Haley, W. E., Clay, O. J. & Roth, D. L. (2006). Improving caregiver well-being delays nursing home placement of patients with Alzheimer disease. *Neurology*, *67*, 1592-1599.

Mittleman, M. S., Roth, D. L., Coon, D. W. & Haley, W. E. (2004). Sustained benefit of supportive intervention for depressive symptoms in caregivers of patients with Alzheimer's disease. *American Journal of Psychiatry*, *161*(5), 850-856.

Morgan, R. O., Teal., C. R., Reddy, S. G., Ford, M. E. & Ashton, C. M. (2005). Measurement in Veterans Affairs health services research: Veterans as a special population. *Health Services Research*, *40*(5), 1573-1583.

Perlin, J. B., Kolodner, R. M. & Roswell, R. H. (2004). The Veterans Health Administration: Quality, value, accountability, and information as transforming strategies for patient-centered care. *The American Journal of Managed Care*, *10*(11), 828-836.

Rabheru, K. (2007). Disease staging and milestones. *The Canadian Journal of Neurological Sciences*, *34*(Suppl. 1), S62-66.

Schubert, C. C., Boustani, M., Callahan, C. M., Perkins, A. J., Carney, C. P., Fox, C., Unverzagt, F., Hui, S. & Hendrie, H. C. (2006). Comorbidity profile of dementia patients in primary care: Are they sicker? *Journal of the American Geriatrics Society*, *54*, 104-109.

Schulz, R., Burgio, L., Burns, R., Eisdorfer, C., Gallagher-Thompson, D., Gitlin, L. N., Feeney Mahoney, D. (2003). Resources for Enhancing Alzheimer's Caregiver Health (REACH): Overview, site-specific outcomes, and future directions. *Gerontologist*, *43*(4), 514-520.

Spitznagel, M. B., Tremont, G., Duncan Davis, J. & Foster, S. M. (2006). Psychosocial predictors of dementia caregiver desire to institutionalize: Caregiver, care recipient, and family relationship factors. *Journal of Geriatric Psychiatry and Neurology*, *19*(1), 16-20.

Spotswood, S. (2007). VA examines dementia care as number of cases rise. *U.S. Medicine*, 23-28.

Tremont, G., Duncan Davis, J. & Bishop, D. S. (2006). Unique contribution of family functioning in caregivers of patients with mild to moderate dementia. *Dementa and Geriatric Cognitive Disorders*, *21*(3), 170-174.

Wagner, E. H., Austin, B. T., Davis, C., Hindmarsh, M., Schaefer, J. & Bonomi, A. (2001). Improving chronic illness care: Translating evidence into action. *Health Affairs*, *20*(6), 64-78.

Yaffe, K., Vittinghoff, E., Lindquist, K., Barnes, D., Covinsky, K. E., Neylan, T., Kluse, M. & Marmar, C. (2010). Posttraumatic stress disorder and risk of dementia among US veterans. *Archives of General Psychiatry*, *67*(5), 608-613.

Yaffe, M. J., Orzeck, P. & Barylak, L. (2008). Family physicians' perspectives on care of dementia patients and family caregivers. *Canadian Family Physician*, *54*, 1008-1015.

In: Dementia
Editor: Pamela Tanner

ISBN: 978-1-63321-928-1

Chapter 3

Research in Advance Dementia: Lessons Learned from the Community

Sweta Tewary*[*,1], Ph.D., MSW, Nicole Cook[2], Ph.D., MPA,
Cecilia Rokusek[2], Ed.D., R.D.,
Naushira Pandya[3], M.D., CMD, FACP,
and Susan McCurry[4], Ph.D.

[1]Diabetes and Interprofessional Research, Department of Geriatrics,
Florida Coastal Geriatric Resources, Education and Training Center (GREAT GEC),
Nova Southeastern University, College of Osteopathic Medicine,
Ft. Lauderdale, Florida, US

[2]Public Health Program, College of Osteopathic Medicine,
Florida Coastal Geriatric Resources, Education and Training Center (GREAT GEC),
Nova Southeastern University, College of Osteopathic Medicine,
Ft. Lauderdale, Florida, US

[3]Florida Coastal Geriatric Resources, Education and Training Center (GREAT GEC)
Public of Health Program, College of Osteopathic Medicine,
Nova Southeastern University, Nova Southeastern University,
College of Osteopathic Medicine, Ft. Lauderdale, Florida, US

[4]The Department of Psychosocial and Community Health,
University of Washington, Seattle, Washington, US

Abstract

Introduction: Florida has the second highest percentage of persons with advanced dementia in the United States. While sleep disturbances are common in older persons in general., sleep disturbances can be more pronounced for persons with dementia (PWD) and can be stressful for caregivers of PWDs. Sleep disturbances among PWD, including

[*] Corresponding and Main Author.

unsupervised wandering and pacing, can be dangerous for PWDs, and may increase the risk of physical and psychological morbidity for both the PWD and caregiver. This chapter covers a brief epidemiology of sleep in Alzheimer's disease and related disorders, describes the burden of sleep disturbances for PWDs and caregivers, and reviews non-pharmacologic interventions that have been developed to improve sleep for non-institutionalized PWDs. One such program is NITE-AD (Nighttime Insomnia, Treatment, and Education for Alzheimer's disease), a home based caregiver training program that includes light exposure, exercise, and sleep hygiene education to improve sleep among PWD. We describe a six-week community–informed group delivery modification of NITE-AD conducted with caregivers of PWD attending adult-day care programs. The results will be outlined and discussed.

Introduction

The Patient's Story

Cynthia, 75 years of age, had been living with her 83 year old partner George for 30 years. She was the primary caregiver for George, who has moderate dementia. Cynthia was willing to make numerous attempts to help her partner deal with daily challenges of dementia. According to Cynthia, George experienced numerous sleep disturbances including nighttime wandering and pacing, multiple awakenings, and difficulty falling asleep. Cynthia enrolled in the sleep study program in order to learn strategies to help reduce George's sleep disturbances. Typical of many caregivers, pre-testing of caregiver burden and depression suggests that Cynthia was significantly burdened by her caregiving role and may be suffering from major depression (Center of Epidemiologic Studies Depression Scale= 36; Zarit burden interview score =46. Unfortunately, before starting the study, Cynthia called the study team and withdrew her participation in the study. The night before, George, under the influence of alcohol, had grabbed her by the neck and attempted to choke her. Cynthia was able to save herself by distracting George, throwing a nearby flower vase, running outside the house, and calling for the police. George was hospitalized. He begged for forgiveness; however, Cynthia could not continue to risk her life by living with her partner, even though she loves him tremendously.

Stories like above have informed us about the challenges of caregivers of persons with dementia and have provided important insights into designing community based programs for PWDs and caregivers of PWDs. Lessons learned are discussed in the chapter below.

Background

Alzheimer's and Dementing Illness Epidemiology

Currently, it is estimated that 5.2 million Americans have Alzheimer's disease (AD), most of whom are age 65 and older. [1-3] Approximately 360,000 people age 65 and older have other dementing illnesses including vascular dementia, Parkinson's or Lewy body disease, front temporal dementia, corticobasal degeneration, and other dementing illnesses.

[4] As the United States' population ages, the proportion of people with AD and other dementias will continue to grow rapidly. Between 1999 to 2008, AD related mortality among individuals 85 years and older surpassed diabetes related mortality (1096.6 verses 1006.5 per 100,000, respectively.) [5] It is estimated that by 2050, 13.8 million people will have some form of dementing illness [6] and 43% of deaths occurring among individuals 65 years and older will have a comorbidity of AD. [7] Age is the primary risk factor for dementia onset. Other factors associated with an increased likelihood of dementia include non-white race, female gender, and having lower educational attainment and income levels. [8]

In 2010, Florida was home to an estimated 450,000 patients with AD, making it the second highest state in the nation for the number of patients with AD (California is first with 480,000.) In Florida, it is expected that the number of older Americans aged 65 and older with AD will increase by 64% from 360,000 in 2000 to 590,000 in 2025. [9, 10]

Informal Caregivers of People with Dementia

Simultaneous to the growth in patients with AD and other dementias is the number of informal caregivers. An estimated 43.5 million adults provide care to adults over age 50. [11] Unpaid caregivers comprise nearly 90% of the total in-home caregiving needed by adults. [11-13] An estimated 23% (over 10 million) of these unpaid caregivers provide care to someone with AD or another form of Alzheimer's, dementia or cognitive impairment. [13]

More than 80% of in-home caregiving for persons with dementia (PWDs) is provided by family caregivers. [12, 13] Informal caregivers provided an estimated 17 million hours of unpaid care in 2010, [10] including robust support with activities of daily living (e.g., bathing, dressing, assistance with personal hygiene) as well as coordinating care with outside government agencies, service providers, and community agencies [10]. A recent cohort study estimated the per person societal cost of dementia at $56,290 annually per patient, with informal caregiving contributing 49% of the total cost. [8]

Burden of Caregiving

Caregiver burden is a multidimensional construct, incorporating not only financial, physical., and social inputs, but also the emotional and psychological impact of caregiving. [11, 14-16] Among family caregivers of PWD, 61% rate the emotional stress of caregiving as high or very high. [10] The burden of caregiving varies by context. Caregiver risk factors associated with increased burden include gender (females are more likely to be burdened than males), increased age, depression, income level, and hours involved in care. [11, 15, 17] Care-recipient risk factors include medical co-morbidities, cognitive impairment (including dementia,) behavioral problems, activities of daily living impairments, incontinence, and decreased mobility. [15] Increased stress and burden among caregivers of PWD has been shown to lead to increased caregiver sleep disturbances, depression, [18, 19] [20-24] caregiver sleep disturbances, [23, 24] lower ratings of self-reported health [25] and increased mortality [26] among caregivers. [27-29]

Sleep Disturbances and Dementia

Sleep patterns change throughout a person's lifespan. [30, 31] The prevalence of sleep disturbances among older adults is widespread, [30, 32, 33] with estimates up to 60% of adults indicating a chronic sleep problem. [34] Sleep disturbances are often comorbid with other medical and psychiatric conditions, [30] including depression. [35] Clinically, sleep behavior changes as people age are associated with increased time to sleep onset, frequent awakenings, reduction in stage 3 and stage 4 deep sleep time, as well as decreased slow wave and rapid eye movement sleep on polysomnography, the gold standard for studying sleep behavior. [36]

The prevalence of sleep disturbances among AD patients has been estimated to range between 25-71%. [37-41] While sleep problems are increased in older persons in general., sleep problems among PWD may be exacerbated by daytime napping, sundowning and side effects of medication. [34, 42, 43] Sleep disturbances in PWDs can result in increased frequency and length of nighttime awakenings, as well as an increased frequency of daytime napping. Nighttime awakenings can result in unsupervised wandering, pacing, or engaging in other inappropriate nighttime behaviors which are disruptive for family caregivers trying to themselves sleep, and also potentially dangerous for the PWD. [44]

Nighttime wandering by PWD and other nocturnal behaviors that awaken caregivers at night greatly increase caregiver burden, which may result in an exacerbation of depressive symptoms and reduced quality of life. [15, 45-49] Caregivers of PWD rate sleep problems as one of the most troublesome aspects of caring for a person with the disease, [50] contributing heavily to caregiver decisions to institutionalize loved ones. [45, 51] These may include falls, fatigue, worsening cognition and daytime somnolence. Reducing sleep disturbances among PWDs, however, is an ongoing challenge. Pharmacotherapies are available, but there is no good evidence regarding drug efficacy and adverse effects are common. [52-54] Non-pharmacologic therapies, including light therapy and exercise, have shown promise, but evidence, while growing, remains limited. [55] A paucity in evidence is particularly glaring with regards to community-based interventions, verses studies conducted in institutions and hospitals. [55]

Nighttime Insomnia, Treatment, and Education for Alzheimer's Disease (NITE-AD) is a community-based program aimed at training caregivers to implement good sleep hygiene with persons with AD. NITE-AD feasibility has been empirically tested in two randomized-control trials. [55, 56] Recognizing the wide spectrum of differences among caregivers and patients with AD, NITE-AD uses an individualized approach to set feasible, tailored goals related to improving sleep, including identifying environmental and dietary "triggers" for nocturnal awakenings; stabilizing bed- and rise-time routines; reducing daytime inactivity and increasing physical exercise; and increasing daytime exposure to light/reducing ambient light at night.

In the original 2005 study, caregivers in the NITE-AD intervention group significantly ($P<.05$) changed sleep practices, including consistent bedtimes, consistent rising times, nap restriction, and improved adherence to walking routines of AD patients compared to control group subjects. [57] Care-receivers in NITE-AD had significant improvements in total night sleep, percentage of time asleep, number of awakenings, and duration of time awake compared to educational contact controls. [57] NITE-AD participants also had significantly lower levels of depression than control subjects. Over six months, the program was effective in increasing AD patient time awake and reducing the number and duration of night time awakenings (p<.05). Results were later replicated in a larger trial that compared NITE-AD to walking and light exposure alone; all active treatments were superior to the contact control condition at post-test, but no one treatment was superior to another, and improvements were attenuated at 6-month follow-up. [58]

The authors hypothesized that this decrease in sustained treatment improvements was in part due to reduced adherence over time to treatment recommendations and challenges with proxy observations/reports about sleep disturbances in PWDs. [59, 60] The original NITE-AD program was time-intensive, and the 2011 trial results suggested that more abbreviated variants of the full NITE-AD protocol could produce sleep benefits for persons with cognitive impairment. In a study conducted by a group of researchers in South Florida, a modified group delivery format version of NITE-AD for caregivers of PWD attending adult day care facilities was implemented. Feasibility, effectiveness, and costs were examined. The method for this study is outlined so that it can be replicated in the community.

Recruitment recommendations for the future if conducting community based sleep studies

1	Include incentives on flyer (but likely will not encourage more caregivers to participate).
2	Larger font. Add food (lunch) to flyer.
3	Clarify that there is no medical evaluation
4	Use referring agencies to help identify caregivers (to reduce loss to follow-up and ensure follow-through with program)
5	Create a short screening tool so people can self-select if they are eligible or not
6	Extend the study to additional sites including other adult day care centers and potentially assisted living facilities as well.
7	Concerns were raised about the inclusion and the exclusion criteria. Be clear about who can be included. For example if paid caregivers can be included or not. This can be important as daily and live- in caregivers may not have time for the study.
9	In addition, participants suggested ways to clarify the educational materials, including the sleep diary, by increasing the font size and condensing the materials to one page.
10	Reducing the number of questionnaires, due to the time commitment (>45 minutes) required to complete all the surveys

The community based study was designed to be completed in two phases. Phase 1 included two structured feedback sessions to gather community input on study materials and the program curriculum. The feedback sessions included twenty five older adults, age 55 and older, who were members of a continuing Lifelong Learning program where they attended daily classes. The structured feedback session was facilitated through a short presentation of program materials, followed by discussion from feedback session participants. Data collection was associated with feedback from the program participants on the draft program manual., reaction to length and type of questionnaires in the assessment packages, review of the sleep diary, incentives for participants, and content and language of the flyers used for recruitment purposes. Data was analyzed through digital notes during the two sessions.

Feedback received from older adults participating identified several programmatic opportunities that had not been considered by the project team. In particular, participant comments pointed towards the need to strengthen the mechanisms of data collection and study procedures. For example, when asked to comment on the potential sleep study handouts, focus group participants provided valuable feedback to clarify, simplify, and streamline the process for future study participants.

Implementing Sleep Study

Recruitment of participants and caregivers in a sleep study is an overarching challenge that is impacted by the strict restriction of Institution Review Boards (IRBs) and an overall lack of understanding about the complex variation in dementia. Considerations should be given to caregivers of dementia who have conflicting caregiving demands. These include

1	Acute illness of the caregiver, for example (HIV)
2	Patients becoming violent at home
3	PWD transfer to nursing home
4	Fear of caregiving time being compromised
5	Scheduling classes according to each participant date/time
6	Transportation to the venue of the sleep education classes
7	Conflicts with other personal., medical., and social commitments

Instruments Used

- The Sleep Disorder Inventory (SDI): The SDI describes the frequency, severity, and caregiver burden of sleep-disturbed behaviors during a period prior to its administration. The SDI consists of eight questions assessing the frequency, severity, and caregiver distress reported by the caregivers based on their observations with the patients. The scoring of the SDI is based on each symptom reported. If present, then the score is the product of the frequency and severity (i.e., frequency score 1-4 times the severity score 1-3) resulting in an approximate range of 1 to 12 for each item. If the item is absent then its scores is 0. The total SDI score is the sum of the symptom scores. For all eight symptoms together, there are potentially eight symptoms that are present and scored, the range of total scores from 0 to 96 are derived. [46]
- Cornell Scale of Depression (CSDD): The Cornell scale for depression is designed to assess signs and symptoms of major depression in patients with dementia. The CSDD obtains information through two semi-structured interviews; an interview with an

  Informant and an interview with the patient. Scoring for Cornell scale of depression varies with the items. The scores range from zero to 60, with the higher scores indicating the presence of more symptomatology. [61]
- Zarit Burden Interview: The Zarit Burden Interview was originally a 29 item questionnaire. The revised version used in the study contains 22 items. Each

individual item asks to endorse a 5 point scale- Options range from 0 (Never) to 4 (Nearly Always). The scores range from 0-88. Scores between 0-21 represent little or no burden, while scores 61-88 represent sever burden [16]

Examples of Research Implementation

Inclusion Criteria

- Family caregiver who is talking care of a PWD age 65 or above.
- Caregiver endorsing one or more PWD sleep behaviors on SDI as occurring several times a week or more often. If only a single SDI item was endorsed and that item was "Does your relative sleep excessively during the day," it was required that at least one additional item reflecting nighttime sleep disruptions also be endorsed as occurring several times a week or more often.

Exclusion Criteria

- Persons with medical conditions causing PWD night time awakenings, such as severe pain, alcoholism, and emphysema.
- Preexisting diagnosis of primary sleep disorders in patient (e.g., sleep apnea or nocturnal myoclonus)

Program Curriculum

As part of the program, the authors developed a six-week, group delivery format program curriculum manual to be used as a step-by-step guide for Phase 2 of the program. The curriculum was modeled after the original one-on-one NITE-AD intervention [57], and also incorporated elements of a sleep intervention program (*Treatment Manual for Cognitive Behavioral Therapy for Sleep Problems in Patients with Dementia*, a pilot manual developed by Drs. William Wohlgemuth & Raymond L Ownby at the Memory Disorder Clinic of the University of Miami Miller School of Medicine)

The intervention included three brief (one hour) group sessions that were provided at Adult Day Care settings where the PWDs were enrolled, at a convenient time for the caregivers. Three in-person group sessions were held over a 6 week period (in weeks 1, 3, and 4), with follow-up phone calls in weeks 2 and 5. Sessions were led by a Sleep Educator (ST). To reinforce the educational strategies discussed at each class, two phone calls were placed on alternating weeks to caregivers by the Sleep Educator. A brief outline of the curriculum is presented below.

A brief outline of the schedule is presented below.

Common behavior and sleep issues that identified were incontinence, multiple awakenings, wandering, clapping and singing in the night. Some of the issues raised from the research included the following

- "My mom stamped me several times in the car"
- "My mom has a breathing problem and I have to listen to that and it is frustrating "
- "My mom sings and claps in the night and I want this to stop".

Table 1. Program Schedule

Week 1: Education Class 1	Introductions, goal setting, circadian rhythm, sleep norms effect of aging and dementia on sleep
Week2:Phone Call 1	Discuss any issues with the program, group, or challenges in general
Week 3: Education Class 2	Impact of exercise, light & sleep
Week4: Education Class 3	Education Class 3: Obstacles/Review of proposed intervention
Week5: Phone Call2	Phone Call 2: Discuss any issues with the program, group, or challenges in general
Week6: Feedback and closing	Feedback and closing: Overall feedback of the program1

Many of these behaviors are observed in a PWD. Possible interventions might include identifying triggers for violent behavior and ignoring the nighttime clapping and singing especially if the PWD's sleep is not impacted by this, using earbuds, sleeping in a different room, consulting a doctor if the behavior is violent etc.,

Examples of novel ideas that helped the participants include

1	PWD sleeps better when liquid diet is not given at dinner.
2	Wearing night pajamas after coming from daycare prepares the PWD that he/she has to sleep in the next two hours and makes it easier for the PWD to go to bed at night.
3	Reassuring PWDs several times before bed to reduce anxiety so that the PWD sleeps peacefully.
4	PWD wearing extra Depends and thick night time clothes so that he/she is not bothered a lot by urinary incontinence or cold.
5	Playing music by the PWD's bedside
6	Keeping the room dark with a night light
7	Switching off TV early in the evening
8	Delaying bedtime at night but keeping it consistent

Conclusion and Lessons Learned for Continuing Research

Caring for older adults with multiple chronic conditions can be challenging. Dementia, in addition to other comorbidities, can add to the burden of care. Moreover, quality of caregiving can be compromised if the caregivers themselves are older, suffering from multiple comorbidities, and in need of geriatric care themselves. The substantial caregiving burden of PWD with sleep disturbances is well described in the literature. [5, 11, 14] Studies have also described non-pharmacological interventions to reduce sleep problems among PWD. [63] Moreover, existing literature discusses that support group forums are beneficial for caregivers of patients with dementia. [62]

There are few empirical studies testing the efficacy of non-pharmacologic interventions on reducing sleep problems and reducing caregiver burden in community-based settings. The NITE-AD curriculum is the only empirically tested program that uses behavioral strategies to improve PWD sleep among community-dwelling caregiver-PWD dyads in Washington. This chapter highlights the modified NITE-AD program for group delivery in adult day-care settings and subsequently implemented the program with seven caregiver-PWD dyads. Caregivers received sleep education strategies in a group format to help the PWD sleep better. Results suggest that the program is acceptable to caregivers, but help is required in terms of transportation, caregiving time, and scheduling convenience to facilitate participation.

Continued research is important as sleep problems among PWDs are difficult issues for caregivers of PWD. Few non-pharmacologic interventions exist that have proven successful at improving sleep among PWDs. Caregiver education programs delivered in a group format are more cost-effective and facilitate shared support and information that can alleviate ongoing caregiver stress. Engaging the community in developing and modifying evidence-based programs can strengthen program relevance, facilitate recruitment and implementation, and enrich evaluation efforts. Literature

One lesson learned from a review of programs is that while the group format is well---received, the group leader should provide caregivers support depending on the needs and resources available to the providers. Group-based interventions in a support group format offered peer support and the opportunity to share and get new ideas for other caregivers. In the NITE-AD intervention, individualized home visits were easier for caregivers to coordinate, but more expensive to deliver. The NITE-AD program also had more time to focus 1-on-1 on triggers of nocturnal awakenings/behaviors and develop carefully crafted behavioral plans. In the modified NITE-Ad program delivered in South Florida caregivers reported enjoying the group format model, however all caregivers who participated expressed some difficulty with maintaining a consistent attendance throughout the 6 weeks program. These are all tradeoffs that community based organizations should consider in designing interventions for PWDs and their caregivers.

Another lesson learned was that future programs should include institutions that have larger caregiver populations and that can provide assistance with transportation as well as respite services for the PWD during the group classes. Programmatic challenges such as the study being a research study including completion of several forms, assessments as well as a consenting process both for the PWD as well as the patient could have possibly limited the enrollment criteria. Enrollment in groups can be easier if the education sessions were just offered programmatically as part of support groups services or special classes offered for caregivers who need help for PWDs with sleep issues.

Acknowledgments

The authors would like to acknowledge The Retirement Research Foundation, for providing support for the community based project "Educating Caregivers to Help Improve Sleep In Patients with Dementia" (Grant # 333482)].

References

[1] Hebert LE, Scherr PA, Bienias JL, et al. Alzheimer disease in the US population: prevalence estimates using the 2000 census. *Arch Neurol.* 2003;60(8):1119-1122.
[2] Alzheimer's A. 2012 Alzheimer's disease facts and figures. Alzheimer's & dementia : *The journal of the Alzheimer's Association.* 2012;8(2):131-168.
[3] Thies W, Bleiler L, Alzheimer's A. 2013 Alzheimer's disease facts and figures. Alzheimer's & dementia : *The journal of the Alzheimer's Association.* 2013;9(2):208-245.
[4] Plassman BL, Langa KM, Fisher GG, et al. Prevalence of dementia in the United States: the aging, demographics, and memory study. *Neuroepidemiology.* 2007;29(1-2):125-132.
[5] Moschetti K, Cummings PL, Sorvillo F, et al. Burden of Alzheimer's disease-related mortality in the United States, 1999-2008. *Journal of the American Geriatrics Society.* 2012;60(8):1509-1514.
[6] Hebert LE, Weuve J, Scherr PA, et al. Alzheimer disease in the United States (2010-2050) estimated using the 2010 census. *Neurology.* 2013;80(19):1778-1783.
[7] Weuve J, Hebert LE, Scherr PA, et al. Deaths in the United States among persons with Alzheimer's disease (2010-2050). Alzheimer's & dementia : *The journal of the Alzheimer's Association.* 2014;10(2):e40-46.
[8] Hurd MD, Martorell P, Delavande A, et al. Monetary costs of dementia in the United States. *The New England journal of medicine.* 2013;368(14):1326-1334.
[9] Hebert LE, Scherr PA, Bienias JL, et al. State-specific projections through 2025 of Alzheimer disease prevalence. *Neurology.* 2004;62(9):1645.
[10] Alzheimer's A, Thies W, Bleiler L. 2011 Alzheimer's disease facts and figures. Alzheimer's & dementia : *The journal of the Alzheimer's Association.* 2011;7(2):208-244.
[11] Adelman RD, Tmanova LL, Delgado D, et al. Caregiver burden: a clinical review. JAMA : *The journal of the American Medical Association.* 2014;311(10):1052-1060.
[12] Institute of Medicine (U.S.). Committee on the Future Health Care Workforce for Older Americans. Retooling for an aging America : *Building the health care workforce.* Washington, D.C.: National Academies Press 2008.
[13] AARP NAfCat. Caregiving in the U.S. 2004.

[14] Shankar KN, Hirschman KB, Hanlon AL., et al. Burden in caregivers of cognitively impaired elderly adults at time of hospitalization: a cross-sectional analysis. *Journal of the American Geriatrics Society*. 2014;62(2):276-284.

[15] Richardson TJ, Lee SJ, Berg-Weger M, et al. Caregiver health: health of caregivers of Alzheimer's and other dementia patients. *Current psychiatry reports*. 2013;15(7):367.

[16] Zarit SH, Reever KE, Bach-Peterson J. Relatives of the impaired elderly: correlates of feelings of burden. *The Gerontologist*. 1980;20(6):649-655.

[17] Sansoni J, Anderson KH, Varona LM, et al. Caregivers of Alzheimer's patients and factors influencing institutionalization of loved ones: some considerations on existing literature. *Annali di igiene : medicina preventiva e di comunita*. 2013;25(3):235-246.

[18] Schulz R, O'Brien AT, Bookwala J, et al. Psychiatric and physical morbidity effects of dementia caregiving: prevalence, correlates, and causes. *The Gerontologist*. 1995;35(6):771-791.

[19] Joling KJ, van Hout HP, Schellevis FG, et al. Incidence of depression and anxiety in the spouses of patients with dementia: a naturalistic cohort study of recorded morbidity with a 6-year follow-up. *The American journal of geriatric psychiatry : Official journal of the American Association for Geriatric Psychiatry*. 2010;18(2):146-153.

[20] Epstein-Lubow G, Gaudiano B, Darling E, et al. Differences in depression severity in family caregivers of hospitalized individuals with dementia and family caregivers of outpatients with dementia. *The American journal of geriatric psychiatry : Official journal of the American Association for Geriatric Psychiatry*. 2012;20(9):815-819.

[21] Givens JL, Mezzacappa C, Heeren T, et al. Depressive symptoms among dementia caregivers: role of mediating factors. *The American journal of geriatric psychiatry : official journal of the American Association for Geriatric Psychiatry*. 2014;22(5):481-488.

[22] Alexopoulos GS, Abrams RC, Young RC, et al. Use of the Cornell scale in nondemented patients. *J Am Geriatr Soc*. 1988;36(3):230-236.

[23] McCurry SM, Logsdon RG, Teri L, et al. Sleep disturbances in caregivers of persons with dementia: contributing factors and treatment implications. *Sleep medicine reviews*. 2007;11(2):143-153.

[24] McCurry SM, Gibbons LE, Logsdon RG, et al. Insomnia In Caregivers Of Persons With Dementia: Who Is At Risk And What Can Be Done About It? *Sleep medicine clinics*. 2009;4(4):519-526.

[25] Vitaliano PP, Zhang J, Scanlan JM. Is caregiving hazardous to one's physical health? A meta-analysis. *Psychol Bull*. 2003;129(6):946-972.

[26] Schulz R, Beach SR. Caregiving as a risk factor for mortality: the Caregiver Health Effects Study. *JAMA : The journal of the American Medical Association*. 1999;282(23):2215-2219.

[27] Buhr GT, Kuchibhatla M, Clipp EC. Caregivers' reasons for nursing home placement: clues for improving discussions with families prior to the transition. *The Gerontologist*. 2006;46(1):52-61.

[28] Yaffe K, Fox P, Newcomer R, et al. Patient and caregiver characteristics and nursing home placement in patients with dementia. *JAMA : The journal of the American Medical Association*. 2002;287(16):2090-2097.

[29] Taylor DH, Jr., Ezell M, Kuchibhatla M, et al. Identifying trajectories of depressive symptoms for women caring for their husbands with dementia. *Journal of the American Geriatrics Society*. 2008;56(2):322-327.

[30] Ancoli-Israel S, Ayalon L, Salzman C. Sleep in the elderly: normal variations and common sleep disorders. *Harvard review of psychiatry*. 2008;16(5):279-286.

[31] Dillon HR, Lichstein KL, Dautovich ND, et al. Variability in Self-Reported Normal Sleep Across the Adult Age Span. *The journals of gerontology Series B, Psychological sciences and social sciences*. 2014.

[32] Ohayon MM. Sleep and the elderly. J*ournal of psychosomatic research*. 2004;56(5):463-464.

[33] Crowley K. Sleep and sleep disorders in older adults. *Neuropsychol Rev*. 2011;21(1):41-53.

[34] McCurry SM, Vitiello, M. Sleep Disturbances in Alzheimer's Disease. *Continuing Medical Education,* CME course 1999.

[35] Campos Costa I, Nogueira Carvalho H, Fernandes L. Aging, circadian rhythms and depressive disorders: a review. *American journal of neurodegenerative disease*. 2013;2(4):228-246.

[36] Vitiello MV, Borson S. Sleep disturbances in patients with Alzheimer's disease: epidemiology, pathophysiology and treatment. *CNS Drugs*. 2001;15(10):777-796.

[37] Rose KM, Lorenz R. Sleep disturbances in dementia. Journal of gerontological nursing. 2010;36(5):9-14.

[38] Moran M, Lynch CA, Walsh C, et al. Sleep disturbance in mild to moderate Alzheimer's disease. *Sleep medicine*. 2005;6(4):347-352.

[39] Rongve A, Boeve BF, Aarsland D. Frequency and correlates of caregiver-reported sleep disturbances in a sample of persons with early dementia. *Journal of the American Geriatrics Society*. 2010;58(3):480-486.

[40] Ritchie K. *Behavioral disturbances of dementia in ambulatory care settings.* International psychogeriatrics / IPA. 1996;8 Suppl 3:439-442.

[41] Creese J, Bedard M, Brazil K, et al. Sleep disturbances in spousal caregivers of individuals with Alzheimer's disease. *International psychogeriatrics* / IPA. 2008;20(1):149-161.

[42] Bliwise DL. Sleep disorders in Alzheimer's disease and other dementias. *Clin Cornerstone*. 2004;6 Suppl 1A:S16-28.

[43] Rothman SM, Mattson MP. Sleep disturbances in Alzheimer's and Parkinson's diseases. *Neuromolecular Med*. 2012;14(3):194-204.

[44] Salami O, Lyketsos C, Rao V. Treatment of sleep disturbance in Alzheimer's dementia. *International journal of geriatric psychiatry*. 2011;26(8):771-782.

[45] Ancoli-Israel S, Vitiello MV. Sleep in dementia. The American journal of geriatric psychiatry : official journal of the American Association for Geriatric Psychiatry. 2006;14(2):91-94.

[46] Tractenberg RE, Singer CM, Cummings JL, et al. The Sleep Disorders Inventory: an instrument for studies of sleep disturbance in persons with Alzheimer's disease. *J Sleep Res*. 2003;12(4):331-337.

[47] Thomas P, Hazif-Thomas C, Pareault M, et al. [Sleep disturbances in home caregivers of persons with dementia]. *Encephale*. 2010;36(2):159-165.

[48] McCurry SM, Logsdon RG, Teri L, et al. Characteristics of sleep disturbance in community-dwelling Alzheimer's disease patients. *Journal of geriatric psychiatry and neurology*. 1999;12(2):53-59.

[49] Cupidi C, Realmuto S, Lo Coco G, et al. Sleep quality in caregivers of patients with Alzheimer's disease and Parkinson's disease and its relationship to quality of life. *International psychogeriatrics / IPA*. 2012;24(11):1827-1835.

[50] Donaldson C, Tarrier N, Burns A. Determinants of carer stress in Alzheimer's disease. *International journal of geriatric psychiatry*. 1998;13(4):248-256.

[51] Pollak CP, Perlick D. Sleep problems and institutionalization of the elderly. *Journal of geriatric psychiatry and neurology*. 1991;4(4):204-210.

[52] McCleery J, Cohen DA, Sharpley AL. Pharmacotherapies for sleep disturbances in Alzheimer's disease. *The Cochrane database of systematic reviews*. 2014;3:CD009178.

[53] Zhou QP, Jung L, Richards KC. The management of sleep and circadian disturbance in patients with dementia. *Current neurology and neuroscience reports*. 2012;12(2):193-204.

[54] McCleery J, Cohen, D.A., Sharpley, A.L. *Medicines for Sleep Problems in Alzheimer's Disease*. Cochrane Summaries 2014.

[55] Brown CA, Berry R, Tan MC, et al. A critique of the evidence base for non-pharmacological sleep interventions for persons with dementia. *Dementia*. 2013;12(2):210-237.

[56] McCurry SM, Pike KC, Vitiello MV, et al. Increasing walking and bright light exposure to improve sleep in community-dwelling persons with Alzheimer's disease: results of a randomized, controlled trial. *Journal of the American Geriatrics Society*. 2011;59(8):1393-1402.

[57] McCurry SM, Gibbons LE, Logsdon RG, et al. Nighttime insomnia treatment and education for Alzheimer's disease: a randomized, controlled trial. *Journal of the American Geriatrics Society*. 2005;53(5):793-802.

[58] McCurry SM, Pike KC, Vitiello MV, et al. Increasing walking and bright light exposure to improve sleep in community-dwelling persons with Alzheimer's disease: results of a randomized, controlled trial. *J Am Geriatr Soc*. 2011;59(8):1393-1402.

[59] McCurry SM, Pike KC, Logsdon RG, et al. Predictors of short- and long-term adherence to a daily walking program in persons with Alzheimer's disease. *American Journal of Alzheimer's Disease & Other Dementias*. 2010;25(6):505-512.

[60] McCurry SM, Vitiello, M. Best of sleep medicine 2012 : an annual collection of scientific literature. In Lee-Chiong T, (Ed). Best of sleep medicine 2012 : an annual collection of scientific literature. S.l.: *CreateSpace Independent Publishing Platform* 2012:210 p.

[61] Alexopoulos GS, Abrams RC, Young RC, et al. Cornell Scale for Depression in Dementia. *Biological psychiatry*. 1988;23(3):271-284.

[62] Chien LY, Chu H, Guo JL, et al. Caregiver support groups in patients with dementia: a meta-analysis. *Int J Geriatr Psychiatry*. 2011;26(10):1089-1098.

[63] Montgomery P, Dennis J. A systematic review of non-pharmacological therapies for sleep problems in later life. *Sleep medicine reviews*. 2004;8(1):47-62.

[64] Gitlin LN, Rose K. Factors associated with caregiver readiness to use nonpharmacologic strategies to manage dementia-related behavioral symptoms. *Int J Geriatr Psychiatry*. 2014;29(1):93-102.

In: Dementia
Editor: Pamela Tanner

ISBN: 978-1-63321-928-1

Chapter 4

Apathy in Dementia

Mamta Sapra, Nathan DeYoung and Kye Y. Kim [*]
Department of Psychiatry and Behavioral Medicine
Virginia Tech Carilion School of Medicine, Virginia, US

Abstract

Apathy is common across a variety of neurological disorders. However, apathy is one of the earliest and probably most persistent neuropsychiatric symptoms in patients with Alzheimer's disease and other dementing disorders. It affects approximately 70% of patients in the mild to moderate stages of Alzheimer's disease. It is defined as the absence or lack of feeling, emotion, interest, concern, and motivation and manifested by diminution of goal directed cognition and behavior relative to the individual's previous level of functioning. Apathy is linked with a faster progression of cognitive, functional., and emotional impairment. It is also associated with decreased insight. As a result, patients with apathy rely on caregivers to provide more care and it subsequently causes increased stress for caregivers. Neuropathological changes in Alzheimer's disease may result in apathy by affecting the orbitofrontal and anterior cingulate circuits. Although apathy is increasingly recognized in patients with neuropsychiatric symptoms, no official diagnostic classification systems offer a definition of apathy. In this chapter, treatment strategies of apathy in dementia patients are discussed along with a brief review of pathophysiological correlates, neuroimaging, and diagnosis.

Introduction

Apathy is defined as a state of primary motivational impairment. Different terms have been used for apathy including amotivation, avolition, loss of initiative/drive, withdrawal, and passivity. Marin proposed that apathy is a complex neuropsychiatric syndrome defined as the "lack of motivation, evidenced by diminished goal-directed overt behavior (as indicated by

[*] Corresponding author: Kye Y. Kim, MD (kykim@carilionclinic or kyekim726@gmail.com).

lack of effort, initiative, perseverance, and productivity), diminished goal-directed cognition (as indicated by diminished importance or value, lack of interest and concern about one's personal., health, or financial problems), and diminished emotional concomitants of goal-directed behavior (as indicated by unchanging affect, lack of emotional responsivity to positive or negative events, and absence of excitement)" (Marin, 1991). It can also be considered a symptom of another neurological or psychiatric syndrome if lack of motivation is attributable to intellectual impairment, emotional distress, or diminished level of consciousness. Furthermore, apathy is associated with different disorders including cerebrovascular disease, Alzheimer's disease, subcortical dementias, traumatic brain injuries, HIV, brain neoplasms, major depression and schizophrenia. The most common causes of clinically significant apathy are dementia and schizophrenia. Apathy is the most frequent neuropsychiatric symptom in Alzheimer's disease (AD) and in many other dementias and is present in different stages of neurodegenerative disease. In a European Alzheimer's disease consortium study, principal component analysis of cross sectional data from 2354 patients with AD, apathy syndrome was the most common occurring in almost 65% of patients out of four syndromes of hyperactivity, psychosis, affective symptoms and apathy (Aalten et al., 2007). The study also confirmed presence of apathy across several different neurodegenerative disorders including vascular dementia and frontotemporal dementia. Most studies report the prevalence of apathy in AD patients with the neuropsychiatric inventory to be between 32.1% to 93.2% (Srikanth et al., 2005). Studies using more specific scales like apathy evaluation scales have reported prevalence of apathy in AD outpatients between 24% and 86 % and in vascular dementia varying from 22.6% to 93.6% (Starkstein et al., 2006; Lykestos et al., 2000). Apathy is much more common in frontotemporal dementia with rates as high as 90-100% (Diehl-Schimd et al., 2006). In mild cognitive impairment, apathy has been reported between 11.1% and 39.8% of cases. A study of mild cognitive impairment patients by Robert et al. indicated that risk of conversion to AD was significantly higher for patients with lack of interest (Robert et al., 2008). The prevalence rate of apathy in dementia for patients living in nursing homes has varied from 23% -84 % (Margallo et al., 2001; Wood et al., 2000). Although literature indicates a wide range of reported prevalence in different dementias, apathy has been identified as a significant and frequently occurring behavioral syndrome that needs attention.

Apathy is one of the most disturbing neuropsychiatric symptoms for caregivers and has greatest impact on functional status and is associated with impaired activities of daily living in patients with Alzheimer's disease (Benoit et al., 2008; Stout et al., 2003). Deficits in motivation, along with progressive cognitive decline, create greater need of support from caregivers for patients with apathy, and consequently, it is associated with increased caregiver burden. In a study of patients with AD, presence of apathy contributed independently to 27% of the variance in functional status as measured by instrumental activities of daily living (Boyle et al., 2003). The symptoms associated with apathy decrease quality of life for both patients and caregivers. Families often are not able to recognize an apathetic state and misperceive the patient as lazy. Apathy is significantly related to reduced independence and poor outcomes in rehabilitation. Additionally, it was associated with deficits in nutritional status in Alzheimer's disease patients in a multicenter trial (Benoit et al., 2008). Apathy may also contribute to a lack of concern about one's own personal health and have an impact on self-care.

Diagnosis and Evaluation Scales

Making a reliable diagnosis of apathy is important prior to initiating treatment for apathy. The psychosocial history from the patient and informant is crucial to elicit the baseline level of motivation. The medical and neurological history and examination is an essential part of assessment which can give clues to differentiate the various neurodegenerative disorders. A complete neuropsychological assessment for cognitive function, with particular attention to frontal lobe function, is required. Marin first proposed the criteria for syndrome of apathy on the basis of 3 domains: diminished goal-directed overt behavior; diminished goal-directed cognition and diminished emotional interest (Marin, 1991). Since then, different conceptualizations of apathy have evolved, but all agree that lack of motivation is at the core of the disorder. Most recently, the European Alzheimer's Disease Consortium proposed diagnostic criteria for apathy in Alzheimer's disease and other neuropsychiatric disorders (Robert et al., 2009).

The most widely used and psychometrically robust measures for apathy are the Apathy Evaluation Scale and apathy subscale of Neuropsychiatric Inventory. The apathy evaluation scale (AES) was developed by Marin and has 3 versions: clinician administered, informant rated and self-rated (AES-C AES-I, AES-S0) and all have good reliability (Marin et al., 1991). AES-C has 18 core items that assess and quantify the affective, behavioral and cognitive domains of apathy. Each item is rated on a 4 point scale. Higher scores indicate more severe apathy. There is a 10-item shorter version of AES for demented nursing home residents whas has comparable reliability and validity for a nursing home setting (Lueken et al., 2007). The neuropsychiatric inventory (NPI) is a scale to assess and quantify neuropsychiatric disturbances in dementia, as well as, caregiver distress caused by these behaviors (Cummings et al., 1994). It is based on a structured interview with a caregiver, with apathy as one of the 10 domains assessed. Informants answer four main questions regarding apathetic symptoms of loss of interest, loss of motivation, poor engagement, and indifference. A positive endorsement of any of these questions triggers sub questions about frequency and severity of the symptom.

Neuropathophysiology and Imaging

Literature has increasingly supported that apathy may be associated with disruption of the frontal-subcortical circuit. This circuit initiates from the anterior cingulate cortex, to the ventral striatum, globus pallidus and thalamus, with final loop back to the anterior cingulate cortex. A Lesion anywhere in this circuit can result in apathy. Apathy has been related to disconnections of different brain circuitries, including amygdala, which is innervated by cholinergic projections from basal forebrain and thalamic nuclei. Recent data suggest that apathy originates in early AD from dysfunction in the orbitofrontal regions, with symptom progression corresponding with advancing disease to other adjacent areas of the brain (Holtoff et al., 2005). Robert et al. studied the differences in brain perfusion between AD patients with and without apathy as imaged by single-photon emission computed tomography (SPECT) (Robert et al., 2006). Decreased initiative and interest scores significantly correlated with decreased bilateral prefrontal cortex perfusion and right inferior temporal lobe perfusion.

The AD patients with apathy symptoms had reduced perfusion in the right anterior cortex compared with the AD patients without apathy symptoms. Marshall et al. correlated neurofibrillary tangles (NFT) and neuritic plaque counts of autopsied subjects' brains diagnosed with AD with the subjects' neuropsychiatric inventory (NPI) scores (Marshal et al., 2006). Chronic apathy and total NPI composite scores correlated with anterior cingulate NFT counts.

The authors proposed that chronic apathy in AD correlates with a greater anterior cingulate NFT burden. In a large study of 148 patients with a variety of dementias, the neuroanatomical correlates of behavioral abnormalities identified by NPI and quantified using voxel-based morphology were examined. Four of the 12 behaviors assessed with the NPI (apathy, disinhibition, eating disorders, and aberrant motor) were correlated with tissue loss. Apathy was independently associated with tissue loss in the right ventromedial superior frontal gyrus (Rosen et al., 2005).

Two neurotransmitters have been implicated in apathy in AD. AD is characterized by cortical cholinergic deficiency, most marked in the parietal., prefrontal and temporal cortices. Cummings, in 1998, proposed a cholinergic hypothesis of neuropsychiatric symptoms in AD suggesting that neuropsychiatric symptoms, including apathy in AD, are linked to cholinergic deficits, and improvement in cholinergic functioning can reduces these symptoms (Cummings and Back, 1998).

Nucleus basalis lesions disconnect the neocortex from a major source of limbic system input, leading to a reduction in emotional processing (Cummings and Kaufer, 1996). Alzheimer's dementia patients with apathy had lower perfusion in right orbitofrontal and left anterior cingulate cortex in SPECT study (Lanctot et al., 2007). The anterior cingulate has projections to the amygdala, ventral striatum and nucleus accumbens and this circuit is important for goal-directed motivated behavior. In a neuropathological study, anterior cingulate gyrus in AD showed significantly reduced cholinergic function (Davies and Verth, 1977). In systematic review, most randomized controlled trials of cholinesterase inhibitors reported small but significant improvement of apathetic symptoms (Drijgers et al., 2009).

Dopamine is known to mediate reward behavior and feelings of motivation and pleasure. Dopaminergic activity is separated into four major pathways in brain: nigrostriatal, mesolimbic, mesocortical., and tuberoinfundibular. Both mesocortical and mesolimbic pathways are involved in brain reward system and are implicated in feelings of motivation and apathy.

Several imaging studies have found correlates between pathophysiological changes to dopaminergic neurons containing brain reward system structures and feelings of apathy in AD patients. Anterior cingulate and orbitofrontal regions are important key areas of the brain reward system and hypoperfusion in these areas in patients has been linked to apathy in dementia patients. Evidence linking dopaminergic dysfunction to apathy is also provided by a destroamphetamine challenge (DAMPH) study. In this study apathetic AD patients demonstrated blunted behavioral response to dextroamphetamine challenge indicating dysfunction in the brain reward system (Lancot et al., 2008). Psychostimulants that target dopamine have been successful in treatment of apathy which further highlights the role of dopamine in apathy in dementia.

Comorbidity and Relationship to Depression

Both apathy and depression have been cited as the most frequently found neuropsychiatric symptoms in frontotemporal dementias, mild cognitive impairment, vascular dementia, Parkinson's disease, Huntington's disease, and AD. Apathy is often associated with epression, but half of AD patients with apathy have no comorbid
depression. Differentiating apathy from depression in dementia is difficult because the two often coexist and overlap in key symptoms such as loss of interest and motivation. However, the defining difference between the two symptoms is that the dysphoria present in depression is not evident in apathy. Apathy is often associated with disinihibition and depression is associated with anxiety, agitation and irritability. Despite this difference, the diagnosis of apathy may not be readily apparent in AD because it shares some characteristics with depression that may be found alone or in combination with apathy. Still some differences help distinguish between these two syndromes. Negative mood symptoms such as feeling sad, guilty, helpless and hopeless are common in depression but not in apathy. Self-criticism and negative thoughts about the future are common in depression but absent in apathetic individual who shows lack of concern. Patients with apathy are more impaired in their functional abilities to complete activities of daily living than in their cognitive status. Apathy appears to involve cholinergic deficits while depression is associated with serotonergic deficits or norepinephrine and dopamine deficits. Apathy can also result from treatment of depression, because serotonergic reuptake inhibitors affect dopaminergic system and can cause apathy.

Treatment

Despite the profound effects of this common syndrome, treatment of apathy has received little direct empirical investigation. Very few studies have used apathy as a primary outcome and most studies are open label. Successful treatment of apathy requires a multidisciplinary approach.

Pharmacological Treatments

Cholinesterase inhibitors

The "cholinergic hypothesis of Alzheimer's disease" proposes that degeneration of cholinergic neurons in the basal forebrain and the associated loss of cholinergic neurotransmission in the cerebral cortex and other areas contribute significantly to the deterioration in cognitive function seen in patients with AD (Bartus et al., 1982). Despite the loss of cholinergic neurons, postsynaptic cholinergic receptors remain intact in AD, and increasing levels of acetylcholine helps improve the cognitive function. Cholinesterase inhibitors inhibit enzyme acetyl cholinesterase leading to an increase in acetylcholine concentration in the central synapses which enhances cholinergic functioning.

Recent research has shown that cholinesterase inhibitors have beneficial effects on neuropsychiatric symptoms associated with dementia. The most studied cholinesterase inhibitor in treating apathy in dementia is donepezil. Multiple studies indicate significant improvement in apathy symptoms with use of donepezil (Mega et al., 1999; Weiner et al., 2000; Feldman et al., 2001; Tanaka et al., 2004; Rockwood et al., 2008). The studies have ranged from 8 weeks to 1 year long. Donepezil may be useful in treatment of apathy in Lewy body dementia (Lancot et al., 2000). Rivastigmine and galantamine have also been shown to have positive effects in improving apathy. There are no studies to support superior efficacy of one cholinesterase inhibitor over another.

Memantine

Memantine is an N-methyl-D-aspartate receptor antagonist that is FDA approved for moderate and severe stages of AD. It regulates the activity of glutamate and protects neurons from glutamatergic excitotoxicity. Two randomized double blind placebo controlled trials conducted in residential care settings in adults with diagnosis of AD and vascular dementia have shown significant improvement in apathy scores for the treatment group (Pantev et al., 1993; Winblad et al., 1999). A case series of three patients with frontotemporal dementia showed some improvement in apathy (Swanberg et al., 2007). The evidence for memantine in the treatment of apathy in dementia is not strong.

Psychostimulants

Current evidence suggests that apathy in AD is associated with a decrease in dopaminergic neurotransmission. Agents that increase dopamine have been explored as treatment options for apathy in AD. Stimulants like methylphenidate increase dopamine actions by blocking its reuptake and enhance the effects of dopamine in the dorsolateral prefrontal cortex that may improve attention, executive function and wakefulness. The Alzheimer's disease methylphenidate trial (ADMET) was a six week randomized double blind placebo controlled multicenter trial that assigned AD participants with apathy to take methylphenidate 20mg daily. Methylphenidate treatment was associated with significant apathy symptoms in Alzheimer's disease patients (Rosenburg et al., 2013). In another 12 week open label study using apathy as primary outcome, significant improvement was noted in patients with AD who were treated with methylphenidate (Padala et al., 2010).

Antidepressants

Antidepressants have failed to provide any improvement in apathy in dementia patients. Trials of antidepressants to treat apathy have primarily been negative. Serotonergic agents may increase apathy and reduce engagement with the environment.

Non-Pharmacological Treatments

The diagnostic criteria for apathy include clear psychosocial factors that can serve as points of intervention for nonpharmacological treatments (NPTs). Using NPTs to target the changes in behavior (i.e., decreased responsiveness to stimulation), cognition (i.e., loss of spontaneous ideas), and emotion (i.e., blunted affect) that occur when apathy is present can produce significant and meaningful symptom relief. While providers have traditionally relied upon pharmacological treatments to manage these changes, NPTs represent an alternative treatment modality that can be used independently, and in conjunction with medications, to decrease apathy symptoms.

Psychological., social., environmental., and neuropathophysiology factors can all contribute to increased levels of apathy (Treusch, 2011), and these factors are likely to interact as part of a dynamic system. The social and environmental disruptions that occur over the course of dementia can significantly impact each of the three symptom domains which define apathy. Studies suggest that individuals with dementia who move to a higher level of care frequently experience increased avoidance, passivity and apathy (Holthe, Thorsen, & Josephsson, 2007). This coupled with other psychosocial factors, such as depression, and the neurocognitive impairments of dementia, can make it difficult for individuals to adapt successfully to the changes and demands of life. NPTs can influence both the neurobiological and psychosocial mechanisms that contribute to apathy in individuals with dementia (Treusch, 2011), and should be considered as part of a multidisciplinary intervention for individuals experiencing apathy.

Psychosocial NPTs possess several benefits. As discussed earlier, pharmacological treatment of apathy in patients with dementia can be complicated by several factors including medical comorbidities, concurrent medications, and biological changes that occur with age. NPTs can be used for individuals when pharmacological interventions are contraindicated or not preferred and can be used to supplement treatment to reduce prescription dosages and enhance effectiveness. These treatments can often be administered in group formats by health professionals from a wide range of fields to help ensure that patients have access to effective interventions. Many NPTs are deliberate about tailoring interventions to fit the specific needs, symptoms, and abilities of an extremely heterogeneous group of individuals. Overall, nonpharmacological approaches can be an important tool to promote effective treatment of apathy for dementia patients with this symptom.

Conceptually, NPTs for apathy can broadly be broken down into prosthetic, behavioral/stimulation, emotional., or cognitive interventions (Rabins and McIntyre, 2010). As expected, nonpharmacological interventions map closely onto the domains that define apathy. However, before engaging interventions designed to target behavioral., emotional., or cognitive symptoms, it is important to ensure that an individual's apathy is not exacerbated by perceptual difficulties including vision, hearing, and mobility issues. Treatment of these conditions with assistive prosthetic devices such as hearing aids, glasses, magnifying glasses, wheelchairs, walkers, etc., can allow for other interventions (both non and pharmacological alike) to be more efficacious. Behaviorally orientated approaches use classical and operant conditioning principles in order to decrease apathy, often by observing patients to better understand antecedents and environmental factors that lead to apathy in order to anticipate and change those situations. This approach also includes interventions that attempt to increase goal directed behaviors through stimulating activities such as art therapy, music therapy, and other recreational/therapeutic approaches. Cognitive approaches capitalize on remaining cognitive functioning through training in order to minimize apathy while emotional oriented approaches attempt to increase well-being, self-worth, and reduce stress. NPTs that use validation and reminiscence techniques to improve overall emotional well-being fall into this category. Other positive mood induction interventions such as multi-sensory stimulation and interpersonal contact also typically fall into this category. Importantly, specific interventions that are being developed and implemented often draw from multiple approaches and fit well into multiple categories. Multi-Sensory Stimulation/Snoezelen therapy is designed to impact patient mood and apathy through both behavioral and emotional processes. It is also frequently necessary to tailor to the needs of each individual patient in order to address the progression of their dementia, current level of functioning, and their specific apathy symptoms.

Several NPTs continue to garner empirical support for being effective treatments for apathy; however, the current consensus continues to be that there remains a substantial lack of research demonstrating which NPTs best improve apathy symptoms in individuals with dementia. A 2005 review by Verkaik, van Weert and Francke cited only 2 high quality randomized controlled studies that supported the use of Multi-Sensory Stimulation/Snoezelen therapy to significantly decrease apathy in individuals with dementia. A more recent review by Brodaty and Burns (2012) found that 5 of the 6 studies of various methodological qualities looking at Multi-Sensory Stimulation/Snoezelen therapy treatment produced significant reductions in apathy. Other NPTs also appear to have positive or partially positive effects on apathy (Brodaty and Burns, 2012). Music therapy, special care programming, therapeutic activates, and "miscellaneous therapies" all have at least some support for their effectiveness as NPTs for apathy. Studies looking at therapeutic activities tended to be of the highest quality methodologically, with 13 out of 15 studies reviewed having positive outcomes. However, interventions grouped into the therapeutic activities category represented a wide range of behavior-oriented interventions including "stimulation, creative activities, cooking, Montessori methods, and behavioral elements, often individually tailored" (Brodaty and Burns, 2012). Out of the 56 studies reviewed, 10 showed non-significant results for the NPT under investigation. One of the largest difficulties noted across all reviews is the heterogeneity of methods and interventions that have been investigated which makes synthesis of the results more difficult and less generalizable.

Support for effective NPTs for the treatment of apathy in dementia is continuing to grow. Early indications suggest that individually tailored treatments that focused on behavioral activation through activities can lead to significant improvements in apathy. There is still a clear need and demand for additional research of good methodological quality to help illuminate which NPTs are effective and under what circumstances. Furthermore, very little work to date has seriously investigated how NPTs can interact with other multidisciplinary interventions to produce the best possible patient outcomes.

Conclusion

A holistic approach to treating apathy is recommended (Gauthier et al., 2010). Successful treatment of apathy requires a multidisciplinary approach. Educating caregivers and involving them in treatment planning is crucial. Caregivers should know that apathy is not just a physiologic change associated with neurodegenerative disorders, but it is a pathological state that can be a source of significant morbidities and distress to the patient and caregiver. Patients' comorbid medical condition should be treated and any reversible causes of apathy due to medications should be managed. Additionally, sensory deficits should be corrected. Environmental modification (adaptive devices including wheelchair, adequate lighting, orientation interventions) to optimize level of stimulation and activities is also beneficial. All of these basic steps can help enhance motivation and decrease apathy. Indications and timing for initiating apathy treatment are unclear. Important factors that can be helpful when making this decision can be the level of disability, potential for improvement in quality of life, and distress or burden to caregivers (this depends on the expectations of caregivers and can vary with family dynamics as well as premorbid personality of patient). Family members are more distressed in seeing a premorbidly active person suffer from apathy. When considering treatment options, it can be helpful to monitor symptoms for up to one month before starting pharmacological therapy. Current guidelines recommend starting with non-pharmacological interventions prior to use of pharmacological options. However, in cases when patients are very distressed or at risk of harm to themselves or others, pharmacological therapy may need to be started sooner. Pharmacological therapy recommends trial of cholinesterase inhibitors first before trying other possible medications like stimulants. Of course, reviewing and reassessing symptoms at regular intervals and need of medications is important.

Apathy in dementia is common, under-recognized, undertreated, and associated with significant adverse outcomes. Treatment requires a multidisciplinary approach including biomedical., psychological and socio-environmental factors. Future research should include randomized controlled trials with apathy as a primary outcome measure to evaluate different treatment options.

References

Aalten, P; Verhey, FR; Boziki, M; Bullock, R; Byrne, EJ; Camus, V; Caputo, M; Collins, D; De, Deyn, PP; Elina, K; Frisoni, G; Girtler, N; Holmes, C; Hurt, C; Marriott, A; Mecocci, P; Nobili, F; Ousset, PJ; Reynish, E; Salmon, E, Tsolaki, M; Vellas, B; Robert, PH. Neuropsychiatric syndromes in dementia. Results from the European Alzheimer Disease Consortium: Part I. *Dement Geriatr Cogn Disord*, 2007, 24(6), 457-63.

Bartus, RT; Dean, RL, 3rd; Beer, B; Lippa, AS. The cholinergic hypothesis of geriatric memory dysfunction. Science, 1982 Jul 30, 217(4558), 408-14.

Benoit, M; Andrieu, S; Lechowski, L; Gillette-Guyonnet, S; Robert, PH; Vellas, B; REAL-FR group. Apathy and depression in Alzheimer's disease are associated with functional deficit and psychotropic prescription. *Int J Geriatr Psychiatry*, 2008 Apr, 23(4), 409-14.

Boyle, PA; Malloy, PF; Salloway, S; Cahn-Weiner, DA; Cohen, R; Cummings, JL. Executive dysfunction and apathy predict functional impairment in Alzheimer disease. *Am J Geriatr Psychiatry*, 2003 Mar-Apr, 11(2), 214-21.

Brodaty; Henry; Kim, Burns. "Nonpharmacological management of apathy in dementia: a systematic review." *The American Journal of Geriatric Psychiatry*, 20.7 (2012), 549-564.

Cummings, JL; Back, C; Am, J. Geriatr Psychiatry. The cholinergic hypothesis of neuropsychiatric symptoms in Alzheimer's disease, 1998 spring, 6(2 Suppl 1), S64-78.

Cummings, JL; Kaufer, D. Neuropsychiatric aspects of Alzheimer's disease: the cholinergic hypothesis revisited. *Neurology*, 1996 Oct, 47(4), 876-83.

Cummings, JL; Mega, M; Gray, K; Rosenberg-Thompson, S; Carusi, DA; Gornbein J. The Neuropsychiatric Inventory: comprehensive assessment of psychopathology in dementia. *Neurology*, 1994 Dec, 44(12), 2308-14.

Davies, P; Verth AH. Regional distribution of muscarinic acetylcholine receptor in normal and Alzheimer's-type dementia brains. *Brain Res.*, 1977 Dec 16, 138(2), 385-92.

Diehl-Schmid, J; Pohl, C; Perneczky, R; Förstl, H; Kurz, A. Behavioral disturbances in the course of frontotemporal dementia. *Dement Geriatr Cogn Disord*, 2006, 22(4), 352-7.

Drijgers, RL; Aalten, P; Winogrodzka, A; Verhey, FR; Leentjens, AF. Pharmacological treatment of apathy in neurodegenerative diseases: a systematic review. *Dement Geriatr Cogn Disord.* 2009, 28(1), 13-22.

Feldman, H; Gauthier, S; Hecker, J; Vellas, B; Subbiah, P; Whalen, E, Donepezil MSAD Study Investigators Group. A 24-week, randomized, double-blind study of donepezil in moderate to severe Alzheimer's disease. *Neurology*, 2001 Aug 28, 57(4), 613-20.

Gauthier, S; Cummings, J; Ballard, C; Brodaty, H; Grossberg, G; Robert, P; Lyketsos, C. Management of behavioral problems in Alzheimer's disease. *Int Psychogeriatr.*, 2010 May, 22(3), 346-72.

Holthe, Torhild; Kirsten, Thorsen; Staffan, Josephsson. "Occupational patterns of people with dementia in residential care: An ethnographic study." *Scandinavian journal of occupational therapy*, 14.2 (2007), 96-107.

Holthoff, VA; Beuthian-Baumann, B; Kalbe, E; et al. Regional cerebral metabolism in early Alzheimer's disease with clinically significant apathy or depression. *Biol Psychiatry*, 2005, 57, 412-421.

Lancot, KL; herrmann, N. Donepezil for behavioral disorders associated with Lewy Bodies. A case series. *Int J Geriatr Psychiatry*, 2000, 15:338-345.

Lanctôt, KL; Herrmann, N; Black, SE; Ryan, M; Rothenburg, LS; Liu, BA; Busto, UE. Apathy associated with Alzheimer disease: use of dextroamphetamine challenge. *Am J Geriatr Psychiatry*. 2008 Jul, 16(7), 551-7.

Lanctôt, KL; Moosa, S; Herrmann, N; Leibovitch, FS; Rothenburg, L; Cotter, A; Black, SE. A SPECT study of apathy in Alzheimer's disease. *Dement Geriatr Cogn Disord.*, 2007, 24(1), 65-72.

Landes, AM; Sperry, SD; Strauss, ME; Geldmacher, DS. Apathy in Alzheimer's disease *J Am Geriatr Soc*, 2001 Dec, 49(12), 1700-7.

Lueken, U; Seidl, U; Völker, L; Schweiger, E; Kruse, A; Schröder, J. Development of a short version of the Apathy Evaluation Scale specifically adapted for demented nursing home residents. *Am J Geriatr Psychiatry*, 2007 May, 15(5), 376-85.

Lyketsos, CG; Steinberg, M; Tschanz, JT; Norton, MC; Steffens, DC; Breitner, JC. Mental and behavioral disturbances in dementia: findings from the Cache County Study on Memory in Aging. *Am J Psychiatry*, 2000 May, 157(5), 708-14.

Marin, RS. Apathy: A neuropsychiatric syndrome, *J Neuropsychiatry Clin Neurosci*, 1991, 3, 243–254.

Margallo-Lana, M; Swann, A; O'Brien, J; Fairbairn, A; Reichelt, K; Potkins, D; Mynt, P; Ballard, C. Prevalence and pharmacological management of behavioral and psychological symptoms amongst dementia sufferers living in care environments. *Int J Geriatr Psychiatry*, 2001 Jan, 16(1), 39-44.

Marshall, GA; Fairbanks, LA; Tekin, S; Vinters, HV; Cummings, JL. Neuropathologic correlates of Alzheimer's disease. *Demen Geriatr Cogn Disord*, 2006, 21, 144-147.

Mega, MS; Masterman, DM; O'Connor, SM; Barclay, TR; Cummings, JL. The spectrum of behavioral responses to cholinesterase inhibitor therapy in Alzheimer disease. *Arch Neurol.*, 1999 Nov, 56(11), 1388-93.

Padala, PR; Burke, WJ; Shostrom, VK; Bhatia, SC; Wengel, SP; Potter, JF; Petty, F. Methylphenidate for apathy and functional status in dementia of the Alzheimer type. *Am J Geriatr Psychiatry*, 2010 Apr, 18(4), 371-4.

Pantev, M; Ritter, R; Gortelmeyer, R: Clinical and behavioral evaluation in long term care patients with mild to moderate dementia under memantine treatment. *Zeitschrt fur Gerontopsychologic Und-Pychiatric*, 1993, 6, S103-117.

Philippe, H., Robert; Claudine, Berr; Magali, Volteau,Christelle, Bertogliati-Fileau,,Michel, Benoit; Olivier, Guerin; Marie, Sarazin; Sylvie, Legrain; Bruno, Dubois. Importance of Lack of Interest in Patients with Mild Cognitive Impairment. *The American Journal of Geriatric Psychiatry*, Volume 16, Issue 9, September 2008, Pages 770–776.

Rabins; Peter, V; John, S. McIntyre. "Treatment of patients with Alzheimer's disease and other dementias." (2010).

Rockwood, K; Black, S; Bedard, MA; Tran, T; Lussier, I. TOPS Study Investigators Specific symptomatic changes following donepezil treatment of Alzheimer's disease: a multi-centre, primary care, open-label study. *Int J Geriatr Psychiatry*. 2007 Apr, 22(4), 312-9.

Robert, PH; Darcourt, G; Koulibaly, MP; et al. Lack of initiative and interest in Alzheimer's disease: a single photon emission computed tomography study. *Eur J Neurol.*, 2006, 13, 729-735.

Robert, S Marin; Ruth, C. Biedrzycki, Sekip Firinciogullar. Reliability and validity of the apathy evaluation scale. *Psychiatry Research*, Volume 38, Issue 2, August 1991, Pages 143–162.

Rosen, HJ; Allison, SC; Schauer, GF; Gorno-Tempini, ML; Weiner, MW; Miller BL. Neuroanatomical correlates of behavioral disorders in dementia. *Brain*, 2005, 128, 2612-2625.

Rosenberg, PB; Lanctôt, KL; Drye, LT; Herrmann, N; Scherer, RW; Bachman, DL; Mintzer, JE. ADMET Investigators. Safety and efficacy of methylphenidate for apathy in Alzheimer's disease: a randomized, placebo-controlled trial. *J Clin Psychiatry*, 2013 Aug, 74(8), 810-6.

Srikanth, S; Nagaraja, AV; Ratnavalli. E. Neuropsychiatric symptoms in dementia-frequency, relationship to dementia severity and comparison in Alzheimer's disease, vascular dementia and frontotemporal dementia. *Journal of the Neurological Sciences*, Volume 236, Issues 1–2, 15 September 2005, Pages 43–48.

Starkstein, SE; Jorge, R; Mizrahi, R; Robinson, RG. A prospective longitudinal study of apathy in Alzheimer's disease. *J Neurol Neurosurg Psychiatry,* 2006, 77, 8-11

Stout, JC[1]; Wyman, MF; Johnson, SA; Peavy, GM; Salmon DP. Frontal behavioral syndromes and functional status in probable Alzheimer disease. *Am J Geriatr Psychiatry*, 2003 Nov-Dec, 11(6), 683-6.

Swanberg, MM. Memantine for behavioral disturbances in frontotemporal dementia: a case series. *Alzheimer Dis Assoc Disord.*, 2007 Apr-Jun, 21(2), 164-6.

Tanaka, M; Namiki, C; Thuy, DH; Yoshida, H; Kawasaki, K; Hashikawa, K; Fukuyama, H; Kita T. Prediction of psychiatric response to donepezil in patients with mild to moderate Alzheimer's disease. *J Neurol Sci.*, 2004 Oct 15, 225(1-2), 135-41.

Treusch, Y; et al. "Apathy and its nonpharmacological treatment in dementia." *GeroPsych: The Journal of Gerontopsychology and Geriatric Psychiatry*, 24.3 (2011), 155.

Weiner, MF; Martin-Cook, K; Foster, BM; Saine, K; Fontaine, CS; Svetlik, DA. Effects of donepezil on emotional/behavioral symptoms in Alzheimer's disease patients. *J Clin Psychiatry*, 2000 Jul, 61(7), 487-92.

Winblad, B; Poritis N. Memantine in severe dementia: results of the 9M-Best Study (Benefit and efficacy in severely demented patients during treatment with memantine). *Int J Geriatr Psychiatry*, 1999 Feb, 14(2), 135-46.

Wood, S; Cummings, JL; Hsu, MA; Barclay, T; Wheatley, MV; Yarema, KT; Schnelle, JF. Use of the neuropsychiatric inventory in nursing home residents. Characterization and measurement. *Am J Geriatr Psychiatry*, 2000 winter, 8(1), 75-83.

Verkaik, Renate; Julia van Weert; Anneke, L. Francke. "The effects of psychosocial methods on depressed, aggressive and apathetic behaviors of people with dementia: a systematic review." *International Journal of Geriatric Psychiatry*, 20.4 (2005), 301-314.

In: Dementia
Editor: Pamela Tanner
ISBN: 978-1-63321-928-1

Chapter 5

Physical Activity and Cognitive Ability in Older Adults: A Psychosocial Approach

Jennifer Stock[1,2,*] and Eef Hogervorst[1]
[1]School of Sport, Exercise and Health Sciences, Loughborough University, UK
[2]Centre for Positive Ageing, University of Greenwich, UK

Abstract

With an ageing population worldwide, the incidence of dementia and associated care costs are rising. As there is currently no cure, identifying effective preventative lifestyle interventions has been the focus of much recent research to reduce risk and delay onset. Risk factors for dementia overlap with those for cardiovascular disease and the cardiovascular benefits of physical activity are well documented. Thus, the scope for physical activity to improve cognitive abilities and reduce the risk of dementia has been increasingly investigated. Physical activity is also a targetable behaviour for older adults as the majority do not meet the minimum level recommended for health benefits. Reviewing the literature is challenging due to the wide variety of ways that this relationship has been investigated, such as study design, specific components of exercise, cognitive outcome measures and participant characteristics. Previous reviews have identified components of exercise which appear to afford the largest cognitive improvements and also moderators of the effect. However, there are inconsistent findings across reviews and meta-analyses as to which aspects of cognitive performance demonstrate the largest effect with exercise. A biopsychosocial approach to dementia in this context is argued to be more appropriate than a traditional medical or disease model due to the evidence of the impact of the social environment on cognitive improvement or decline. Physical activity does not occur independently of the environment. However, psychosocial factors in the relationship between physical activity and cognitive ability in

* Corresponding author: J.Stock@greenwich.ac.uk.

older adults have largely been neglected despite evidence for their effect in non-physical activity contexts. It is suggested that future work should investigate the role of psychosocial factors to further understand their impact on cognitive outcomes in a physical activity context. A better understanding of this would assist with exercise intervention design to maximise cognitive benefits.

Ageing Population

The world population is ageing. In the United Kingdom (UK), it is estimated that the number of people aged 60 or over will rise by more than 50% in the next 25 years and will exceed 20 million by 2031 (Office for National Statistics, 2009). It is projected that the number of people aged 80 and above will more than double by mid-2037, and that the number of people aged 90 and above will more than triple. This equates to one in twelve of the population being 80 and above by mid-2037 (Office for National Statistics, 2013). Ageing is associated with an increased risk of a range of diseases and conditions, including cognitive impairment and dementia (Launer & Hofman, 1992; Solfrizzi et al., 2004).

Dementia Incidence

In the UK in 2010, there were estimated to be over 820,000 older adults afflicted with late onset dementia (Luengo-Fernandez, Leal., & Gray, 2010). This is expected to rise to one million by 2025 and to exceed 1.7 million by 2051 (Alzheimer's Society, 2007). Dementia affects one in six people over 80 years old and one in three over 95 years old. It is estimated that one in three people over 65 years old will die with a form of dementia (Alzheimer's Society, 2007).

The economic costs of dementia in the UK are estimated to be £23 billion per year, which is approximately twice as much as cancer (Luengo-Fernandez et al., 2010). This includes the cost of providing health and social care, as well the reduction or loss of income of people with dementia and their caregivers. There are estimated to be 600,000 individuals in the UK acting as the main carers for individuals with dementia (Age UK, 2012). Caring for someone with dementia can have a profound impact on the caregiver‘s health and wellbeing, as evidence has demonstrated that caregivers suffer from higher rates of depression and anxiety, and show negative immunological changes compared to controls (Kiecolt-Glaser, Dura, Speicher, Trask, & Glaser, 1991; Schulz, O'Brien, Bookwala, & Fleissner, 1995; Richard Schulz & Martire, 2004).

Dementia is also one of the main causes of disability in later life, ahead of some cancers, strokes, and cardiovascular disease (Department of Health, 2009). Older adults are more likely to have multiple health conditions, however, dementia has a disproportionate impact on individuals' capacity for independent living (Alzheimer's Society, 2007).

Cognitive Decline and Dementia

Three types of cognitive decline associated with ageing have been recognised from a clinical and investigational perspective: age associated memory impairment (AAMI), mild cognitive impairment (MCI) and *dementia.* Their definitions and the distinctions between them have been discussed (see Fillit et al., 2002). AAMI attempts to describe cognitive decline that would be expected to occur with "normal ageing" and has also been called age-related cognitive decline and cognitive impairment-no dementia. Generally, individuals experiencing AAMI have subjective memory complaints but have normal scores on objective cognitive tests for their age group (Crook, Bartus, & Ferris, 1986). Less than 1% go on to develop dementia. Individuals suffering from MCI also experience subjective memory complaints, but score lower than is expected for their age on some objective cognitive tests (1.5 standard deviations below age adjusted mean; Petersen, 1999). MCI can, in some cases, be a prodromal stage of dementia as between six and 31% of individuals with MCI develop dementia each year (Bruscoli & Lovestone, 2004). The reliability of these definitions of cognitive decline and their clinical use has been debated (Petersen, 2004; Petersen et al., 2001; Smith et al., 1991) and reflect recent changes to diagnostic classifications.

The most recent Diagnostic and Statistical Manual (DSM-V) reclassified dementia under 'Neurocognitive Disorders' to distinguish diseases, such as Alzheimer's disease from psychiatric disorders that display cognitive impairment as a symptom rather than a defining feature, such as schizophrenia or depression (American Psychiatric Association, 2013). The terms mild and major neurocognitive disorders have been introduced with a distinction between them. Mild neurocognitive disorder (more widely known as MCI) is indicated by decline in one or more cognitive domains, while the individual can maintain their independence. These cognitive domains include memory loss, attention, executive function, language, and visuospatial., visuoperceptual., or social cognition. Major neurocognitive disorder (more widely known as dementia) is indicated by decline in two or more cognitive domains, which impacts on an individual's capacity for independent living. Evidence of objective decline in memory or learning is required to assign a specific diagnosis of Alzheimer's disease.

There are several types of dementia, which vary in aetiologies, symptoms and progression. Some types of dementia can be halted or potentially reversed by addressing the cause. For example, alcoholism, vitamin deficiencies, endocrine disease, electrolyte imbalance, and lead intoxication (Ghosh, 2010). Other types of dementia cannot be reversed and are progressive, with sufferers showing cognitive decline until death. The most common type of dementia is Alzheimer's disease followed by vascular *dementia* which account for approximately 62% and 27% of all cases of dementia, respectively (Alzheimer's Society, 2007). Other less common forms of non-reversible dementia include Lewy Body dementia, Frontotemporal dementia, dementia with Parkinson's disease and Creutzfeldt-Jakob disease (Thies, Bleiler, & Alzheimer's Association, 2013).

By definition, dementia impacts on activities of daily living which can lead to disability and a loss of independence. Cognitive impairment can impact on activities of daily living before dementia is diagnosed (i.e., during a prodromal stage). Functional impairment at baseline was found to be predictive of dementia incidence 3 years later and an increase in level of dependence between baseline and 3-year follow-up was found to predict dementia incidence at 5-year follow-up (Barberger-Gateau, Fabrigoule, Helmer, Rouch, & Dartigues, 1999). Activities which were found to be correlated with cognitive impairment independent of age, sex, and education were: telephone use, use of means of transportation, responsibility for medication intake and handling finances (Barberger-Gateau et al., 1992). Worldwide projections estimate that if the onset of Alzheimer's disease specifically could be delayed by just one year, by 2050 there would be 9.2 million fewer cases. In the UK, delaying the onset of dementia by five years would reduce deaths directly attributable to dementia by 30,000 a year (Alzheimer's Society, 2007). Therefore, interventions which only modestly delay the onset would have a major impact on public health. For example, reducing the number of individuals needing a high level of care, such as residential placement (Brookmeyer, Johnson, Ziegler-Graham, & Arrighi, 2007).

Clare (2007) discussed different conceptual frameworks for understanding dementia. Traditionally, a medical or disease model (Roth 1994) had been used as the 'standard paradigm' for understanding dementia (Kitwood, 1997). This model focuses on causal mechanisms that lead to neuropathological changes that are associated with dementia. For example, changes associated with Alzheimer's disease include neuronal atrophy in the medial temporal lobe (an area of the brain thought to be associated with memory) and an increase in amyloid-β plaques and tau tangles (Dubois, Feldman, & Jacova, 2007). Investigating dementia using this model has resulted in important advances in our understanding. However, other findings have indicated that the causal mechanisms are not straightforward. For example, amyloid-β plaques and tau tangles have been found in individuals with no cognitive impairments and conversely, individuals displaying the cognitive symptoms of Alzheimer's disease were found to have no observable abnormal neuropathology at post mortem (Snowdon, 2003). There has been controversial debate about whether Amyloid-β plaques are a cause or consequence of Alzheimer's disease, especially as research into pharmacological treatments targeting these plaques have been relatively unsuccessful to date (Johnson & Johnson, 2012; Lilly, 2010). The genetic risk of developing Alzheimer's disease is also not straight forward. The Apolipoprotein E epsilon 4 allele (APOE ε4) has been identified as a major risk factor for Alzheimer's disease (Ahn Jo et al., 2006) and is associated with amyloid-β plaque formation (Carter, 2005). However, not all individuals who have this allele go on to develop Alzheimer's disease and not all individuals who develop Alzheimer's disease have this allele (Henderson et al., 1995).

Possible explanations for the inconsistencies in pathological causal mechanisms and cognitive outcomes have been discussed (Clare, 2007). For example, the "cognitive reserve hypothesis" (Stern, 2002) proposes that a higher level of education, a wider social network and being more physically and mentally active is protective against the effects of Alzheimer's disease pathology (Scarmeas & Stern, 2003). The traditional disease model of dementia also does not explain periods where cognitive ability improves or stabilises after social or environmental changes (Langer & Rodin, 1976; Rodin & Langer, 1977; Sixsmith, Stilwell, & Copeland, 1993) or when it rapidly declines following hospitalisation (Kitwood, 1996).

An alternative model was proposed incorporating a biopsychosocial approach (Figure 1; Clare, 2007; Kitwood, 1997). The emphasis is on the interactions between biological and psychosocial variables. Kitwood (1997) postulated that events or states experienced at the mind or psychological level are also brain events or states. In addition to brain structure affecting experience, psychological states can also affect the brain structure. The brain develops in reaction to experience and the environment throughout life and there is evidence for the potential for change in the brain (experience-dependent plasticity) of older adults (e.g., Cabeza, Anderson, Locantore, & McIntosh, 2002). This experience-dependent plasticity has been demonstrated in a randomised control trial (RCT) of exercise training in older adults, whereby the aerobic exercise group increased functional connectivity between brain networks central to dysfunction in ageing, compared to the non-aerobic control group (Voss et al., 2010). Thus, Kitwood suggested that the environment and the interactions and behaviours that it facilitates, can have positive or negative effects on cognitive ability and functional health. For example, Kitwood hypothesised that a benign social psychology together with an enriched environment could facilitate some regeneration or at least the maintenance of function. In contrast, a malignant social environment could contribute to excess disability and speed up decline.

Direct physiological mechanisms of improved cognitive ability after physical activity have been investigated. These have included a reduction in blood lipids and lowering of blood pressure (Leon & Sanchez, 2001), increased cerebral blood flow (Brown et al., 2010), improved vascular output and cerebral perfusion (Bonner & Cousins, 1996) and encouraging neurogenesis through increases in Insulin-Like Growth Factor-1 which induces Brain-Derived Neurotrophic Factor (Bothwell, 1995; Nakajima, Ohsawa, Ohta, Ohno, & Mikami, 2010; Van Praag, Kempermann, & Gage, 1999; Zhao, Deng, & Gage, 2008). However, the evidence of the beneficial effect of cognitive stimulation on cognitive ability and quality of life (Woods, Aguirre, Spector, & Orrell, 2012) suggests that these physiological mechanisms may not be necessary to bring about positive effects. In addition, the effect of physical activity on cognitive ability does not appear to follow the same dose-response pattern (Etnier, Nowell, Landers, & Sibley, 2006) that it does for physical health benefits which you might expect if only the physical exercise itself was driving the effect. This suggests that there are other contributing factors.

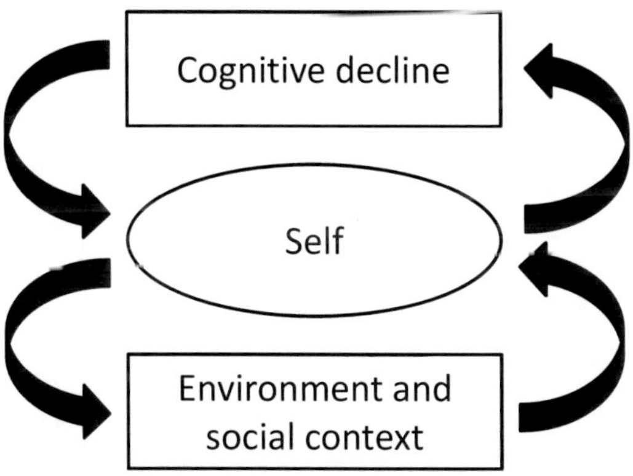

Adapted from Clare, 2007, based on Kitwood, 1997.

Figure 1. A biopsychosocial model of cognitive decline.

The evidence discussed thus far acknowledges that dementia involves changes and needs at the biological., psychological., and social levels and is also experienced within the social context with associated cultural beliefs and practices (Downs, Clare, & Anderson, 2008), therefore a biopsychosocial model for understanding dementia and the effectiveness of preventative strategies is appropriate (World Health Organization, 2001). The biopsychosocial model highlights the potential scope for the effectiveness of lifestyle interventions (such as physical activity) targeting modifiable risk factors for dementia. This evidence for physical activity as a preventative strategy is discussed further in the following sections.

Modifiable Risk Factors for Cognitive Decline: Physical Activity

As there is currently no cure for dementia, modifiable lifestyle behaviours, such as physical activity, have been investigated as a preventative strategy for delaying the onset of dementia and thus prolonging independent living (Angevaren, Aufdemkampe, Verhaar, Aleman, & Vanhees, 2008; Clifford, Bandelow, & Hogervorst, 2009; S. Colcombe & Kramer, 2003; Hogervorst, Clifford, Stock, Xin, & Bandelow, 2012; Lautenschlager, Cox, Cyarto, Gold, & Keller, 2012; Sofi et al., 2010). Physical activity can be defined as any movement of the body by skeletal muscles, which results in energy expenditure and which has a positive correlation with physical fitness (Biddle & Mutrie, 2007; Bouchard & Shephard, 1994; Caspersen, Powell, & Christenson, 1985). Exercise is a subcategory of physical activity which is distinct by its planned and structured nature and involves repetitive bodily movement. It is also highly positively correlated with physical fitness, as the main objective of exercise is to improve or maintain fitness, to improve performance or for health enhancement.

The health benefits of physical activity have been widely demonstrated, including reduced morbidity of numerous health conditions and mortality rates. For instance, moderately vigorous physical activity is associated with increased functional status, measured as the ability to carry out instrumental activities of daily living (Gu et al., 2009). The evidence for exercise and physical activity to improve cardiovascular health is well documented (Warburton, Nicol, & Bredin, 2006). Modifiable risk factors for cardiovascular disease overlap with those of dementia (Kivipelto et al., 2005), thus the scope for physical activity to act on cognitive ability has been the focus of much recent research (e.g., Angevaren, Aufdemkampe, Verhaar, Aleman, & Vanhees, 2008; Clifford, Bandelow, & Hogervorst, 2010; Hogervorst, Clifford, Stock, Xin, & Bandelow, 2012). Physical activity is accessible by almost everyone and is also low-cost and low-tech thus increasing the potential for widespread participation. Effective lifestyle behaviours for reducing dementia risk could be especially important in developing countries where access to healthcare may be limited. Furthermore, physical activity is a targetable risk factor in older adults as they are often inactive and spend much of their time engaging in sedentary behaviours, with the majority of older adults in the UK currently not meeting the minimum level of activity necessary to achieve health benefits (Age UK, 2012).

The physical activity guidelines in the UK recommend that older adults (65+ years old) should aim to be active every day (Bull & the Expert Working Groups, 2010; Nelson et al., 2007). This should add up to at least 150 minutes of moderate-intensity or 75 minutes vigorous-intensity aerobic activity every week. It is recommended that bouts of exercise are of at least 10 minutes, for example, 30 minutes on at least five days per week. Examples of moderate intensity activities include walking fast, pushing a lawn mower, ballroom dancing, and water aerobics. Examples of vigorous-intensity activities include jogging, swimming fast, playing singles tennis, and playing football. In addition, older adults should carry out muscle strengthening activities on two or more days a week that work all major muscle groups (hips, legs, back, abdomen, chest, arms and shoulders). Examples of these activities include carrying heavy groceries, heavy gardening like digging, yoga and lifting weights. Older adults are also recommended to minimise being sedentary for extended periods (e.g., sitting). Those at risk of falls should also carry out activities which improve balance and coordination on at least two days per week, for example, T'ai Chi and yoga. It is further recommended that these guidelines should be interpreted within individual physical and mental capabilities. Carrying out some physical activity is better than none, and higher levels of physical activity provide greater health benefits. It is estimated that only 19% of 65-74 year olds and 7% of those 75+ years in the UK report that they meet this level (Age UK, 2012).

The term physical fitness has occasionally been used of instead of physical activity in the context of improving cognitive abilities or delaying the onset of dementia. Physical fitness refers to a physiological state of wellbeing which represents an individual's capacity to meet the demands of daily living, or which provides the basis for performance in sport, or both. Health-related fitness relates to cardiovascular fitness, musculoskeletal fitness, body composition, and metabolism (Warburton et al., 2006). Physical fitness (assessed using objective measures) has been considered to capture physical activity more accurately than self-reports (Williams, 2001). However, the assessment of physical fitness is not practical in large population based investigations. Nonetheless, self-reports of physical activity are still strong predictors of mortality (Blair & Brodney, 1999) and provide irrefutable evidence for its preventative effect on numerous chronic diseases. These include cardiovascular disease, diabetes, hypertension, cancer, obesity, depression and osteoporosis (Warburton et al., 2006). Interestingly, physical activity related improvements in health status can occur without improvements in aerobic fitness (Nelson et al., 2007). There has been a shift in research focus to also include the health benefits of improving musculoskeletal fitness, which is associated with an improvement in overall health status and a reduction in chronic disease risk and disability (Warburton, Gledhill, & Quinney, 2001a, 2001b).

Levels of physical fitness (aerobic power, strength, flexibility and functional capacity) and physical activity both decline with age. The extent to which this is a biological process or due to physical inactivity has been discussed in the extant literature. For example, it was found that age related changes in the cardiovascular system can be exacerbated by physical inactivity but can also be reversed by increasing levels of physical activity (Taylor et al., 2004). Age-related muscle weakening was not found to be prevented by aerobic exercise (Harridge, Magnusson, & Saltin, 1997). However, regular resistance exercise was found to be effective in increasing muscle mass and strength, even in very old age (Rogers & Evans, 1993). This evidence demonstrates the positive effects of physical activity for maintaining and improving physical functioning into later life which would also help to prolong independent living. As cognitive decline also contributes substantially to risk of disability and dependence (Warburton et al., 2006), and due to the overlap in risk factors of cardiovascular disease and dementia, the scope for physical activity to reduce dementia risk has been investigated. However, this relationship is less clearly understood.

Evidence for the Effect of Physical Activity on Cognitive Ability and Dementia

Numerous systematic reviews and meta-analyses have been carried out to examine the effect of physical activity on cognitive ability or dementia incidence. It has been highlighted that in spite of the hundreds of studies that have been carried out to further our understanding of this relationship, reviewing the literature is challenging due to the variety of ways it has been investigated (Clifford et al., 2009; Etnier & Labban, 2012; Hogervorst et al., 2012). Variations include the study design, measurements of physical activity (objective and subjective), outcome measures (different cognitive tests across domains and dementia risk), specific components of exercise (types, intensity, frequency, and duration), and sample populations (different age groups, men or women or both sexes, with or without cognitive impairment). There is evidence to suggest that the effect of physical activity on cognitive ability may not be the same for everyone and that some individuals may benefit more than others. Such moderators include age, gender, genetic status, and baseline cognitive status. This chapter focuses on the chronic, rather than acute, effects of exercise and physical activity, as this reflects the potential for maintaining cognitive ability over time with increasing age, to delay the onset of dementia, and thus prolong independent living.

Study designs used to examine the evidence for physical activity‘s effect on cognitive ability vary from observational cross-sectional or prospective cohort data to acute or chronic exercise interventions, and the evidence from each type of study design is discussed in the following sections.

Cross-sectional Studies

Cross-sectional and observational studies tend to rely on self-report questionnaires of physical activity or exercise and an assessment of cognitive performance on a selection of tests or dementia diagnosis (frequently Alzheimer's disease or vascular dementia). Cross-sectional studies examine associations between physical activity and cognitive performance assessed at the same time. A systematic review revealed a variety of results from cross-sectional studies with cognitive performance as an outcome measure: seven studies found a beneficial effect of exercise across all cognitive tests administered, eight found a beneficial effect on some cognitive tests but not others, and one study with very healthy older adults found no beneficial effect (Clifford et al., 2009). No studies found an association between higher levels of physical activity and poorer cognitive abilities.

Prospective Studies

Prospective studies tend to measure baseline self-reported frequency of participation in specific physical activities (e.g., swimming or walking) of healthy middle-age to older adults and level of cognitive decline or dementia status between two to nine years later (Kramer & Erickson, 2007a). Dementia status is usually classified as cognitive impairment, Alzheimer's disease, vascular dementia or dementia as one group.

Overall the prospective evidence is consistent with a small and positive beneficial effect of physical activity on cognitive ability and risk of dementia in older adults. This evidence is based on numerous studies which often included large numbers of participants; for example, the Honolulu-Asia Ageing Study (N > 2000; Abbott, White, Ross, Masaki, & Petrovitch, 2004; Taaffe et al., 2008), the Nurse's Health Study (N > 16,000; Weuve et al., 2004), and the Whitehall II Study (N > 6000; Singh-Manoux, Hillsdon, Brunner, & Marmot, 2005). One review investigating the effect of physical activity on longitudinal cognitive decline found that older adults participating in physical activity showed less cognitive decline over two to ten-year follow up periods (Bherer, Erickson, & Liu-Ambrose, 2013). A meta-analysis of prospective studies investigating dementia risk found pooled relative reduction of risk of 0.72 for dementia and 0.55 for Alzheimer's disease for active individuals (Hamer & Chida, 2009) indicating a protective effect of physical activity. Another review looking at reduction of dementia risk found mixed results, with a reduction of 31% to 88% in dementia risk in those with higher levels of physical activity in five out of the 13 included studies (for Alzheimer's disease and vascular dementia). Four studies found a reduced risk in only certain types of dementia in individuals who exercised, while the remaining four studies found no reduction in risk of dementia (Clifford et al., 2009). This may be indicative of a selective effect of physical activity as protective against only some types of dementia. However, it was suggested that the lack of effect in some studies could be attributed to methodological limitations, for example, the small numbers of participants with vascular dementia and other less common types of dementia.

Physical Activity Measurement in Cross-sectional and Observational Studies

One methodological limitation of observational studies (both cross-sectional and prospective) is the reliance on self-report questionnaires to capture the level of physical activity that participants engage in. Self-report questionnaires are relatively cheap compared to objective measures of physical activity (e.g., pedometers or accelerometers), which allows data to be collected from a large number of participants. Unfortunately, this is at the expense of accuracy and reliability (Shephard, 2003). Self-report questionnaires rely on participants' ability to accurately estimate and recall levels of physical activity. Self-report in sample populations with cognitive decline is by definition unreliable (Clifford et al., 2009). There is a conceptual discrepancy when discussing the protective effect of physical activity on cognitive decline, as the specific types of physical activities are not standardised across studies. Some studies asked participants to self-report on a few specific physical activities, for example, only walking (e.g., Weuve et al., 2004; Yaffe, Barnes, Nevitt, Lui, & Covinsky, 2001) or only athletic activities (e.g., Lindwall, Rennemark, & Berggren, 2008), which do not represent individuals' overall level of physical activity. Some studies have tried to capture a range of physical activities, however what participants themselves consider "physical activities" is likely to vary. Exercise specifically may be considered a physical activity, but not housework or gardening, despite the prolonged standing periods and lifting heavy loads in the latter activities, as the bodily movements are incidental from the purpose of the activity. A questionnaire specifically designed to measure participation in exercise and physical training did not include gardening or household chores (Roth & Goode, 2003). The validity of physical activity measures for accurately capturing levels of physical activity is questionable and different measures used also makes comparisons between studies difficult. The small number of studies that captured a range of physical activities limits the recommendations for which specific physical activities are the most effective for reducing cognitive decline or risk of dementia. Additionally, limited reliability has been seen in the correlations on the same exercise questionnaire administered in the same group of participants on two separate occasions, which varied by 0.47 for light intensity exercise, 0.50 for moderate exercise, and 0.33 for vigorous exercise (Geda et al., 2010). In summary, there is disparity of definitions and variation in ways that frequency and intensity of physical activity has been captured and this makes comparison of findings between studies difficult (Miller, Taler, Davidson, & Messier, 2012).

Some studies assessed physical fitness, e.g., physical function or cardio-fitness in addition to (or instead of) level of physical activity, with the aim of capturing a reflection of physical fitness as a result of overall physical activity carried out by individuals. Varying levels of increased fitness between studies could result in different cognitive outcomes. The Honolulu Asia Aging study longitudinal cohort study (Abbott et al., 2004) demonstrated an association between physical activity and reduced risk of cognitive decline in physically fit elderly Hawaiian men of Japanese descent aged between 73 and 91 years of age. A much higher correlation was found between walking and lower cognitive decline than with physical function (balance assessment and time taken to walk 10 feet) suggesting that participation itself may be important (Taaffe et al., 2008). This suggests that other components of physical activity, such as mental stimulation or psychosocial factors, may play a part in the protective mechanisms of physical activity on cognitive decline (Miller et al., 2012).

The trajectory of decreases in physical activity rather than just physical activity at baseline can also give more insight into the relationship. In the European FINE study, 295 men gave self-report details of physical activity and were assessed using the Mini Mental State Examination (MMSE) at baseline and at a 10 year follow up. Duration of physical activity at baseline did not predict cognitive decline. However, there was 2.6 times more cognitive decline in those who decreased in physical activity (>60 min/day) over the 10 years compared to those who maintained it. Lowest intensity quartile physical activity at baseline was associated with a 1.8 times cognitive decline compared to other quartiles. However, a decrease in intensity over the 10 years was associated with a 3.6 times larger cognitive decline compared to those that maintained it (Van Gelder, Tijhuis, & Kalmijn, 2004). Although this study appears to suggest a causal direction of this relationship, it is still limited in its explanatory power. For example, lower levels of physical activity may be a consequence rather than a cause of cognitive decline due to the cognitive abilities (and perhaps personal confidence) required to participate in physical activity (Bielak, 2010). It may be that these individuals are experiencing prodromal cognitive changes which are affecting their participation in activities prior to detectable cognitive decline.

Limitations of Observational Studies

Physical activity is often related to other lifestyle choices and medical conditions, such as alcohol consumption, smoking, and obesity. For example, recent evidence suggests that those who are more physically active also tend to have completed a higher level of education and a higher household income (Farrell, Hollingsworth, Propper, & Shields, 2013). Therefore, these factors have often been included as covariates in observational studies together with demographic factors, such as socio-economic status, education, and age (Colcombe & Kramer, 2003). It has been suggested that observational studies can be biased through residual confounding as individuals who are physically active are likely to differ from sedentary participants in other unmeasured ways (Barnes et al., 2013). Potential inherent biases can be minimised through conducting intervention studies and allocating participants to groups using blinded randomisation procedures.

Observational studies which focus only on the physical components of physical activity neglect the potential impact of social interaction and mental stimulation. There is evidence for the protective effect of an engaged lifestyle with a larger social network and mentally stimulating leisure activities against cognitive decline (Fratiglioni, Paillard-borg, & Winblad, 2004; Paillard-Borg, Fratiglioni, Xu, Winblad, & Wang, 2012; Wang, Karp, Winblad, & Fratiglioni, 2002). Physical activities themselves can involve a substantial amount of social interaction and mental stimulation. A prospective study which rated the level of mental., physical and social components in leisure activities found that they contributed equally in reducing risk of dementia. Across a broad spectrum of activities, protective effects for risk of dementia were found for leisure activities involving two or more of these components (Karp et al., 2006). It is difficult to isolate the effects of physical activity carried out as part of daily life from social or mental components in observational studies, thus more recent studies have utilised an experimental design.

Randomised Controlled Trials with Healthy Older Adults

Although observational studies were initially useful in identifying the relationship between physical activity and cognitive ability or risk of dementia, they cannot offer explanations of cause and effect. A smaller but growing number of studies have investigated the relationship between physical activity and cognitive ability using exercise interventions. RCTs have the advantage over observational studies of being able to examine the cause and effect through isolation of physical activity as the variable of interest and by random allocation of participants to exercise and control groups. The majority of trials to date have used aerobic exercise and participants have tended to be aged 60 years and older and relatively sedentary prior to enrolment (Kramer & Erickson, 2007a). Exercise is usually carried out for between 30 minutes to one hour on several days of the week for several months to a year or more. The evidence from RCTs have generally failed to replicate the same magnitude of effect sizes compared to observational studies (e.g., Etnier et al., 1997a) and have also demonstrated mixed findings (Angevaren, Aufdemkampe, Verhaar, Aleman, & Vanhees, 2008; Clifford et al., 2010; Kramer & Erickson, 2007b). Even meta-analyses with very similar hypothesis have failed to find comparable effects (Angevaren et al., 2008). However, no RCTs have demonstrated a negative effect of exercise interventions on cognitive performance. A meta-analysis examining the dose-response relationship between aerobic fitness and cognitive performance did not find a significant relationship (Etnier, Nowell, Landers, & Sibley, 2006). Thus, a suggested explanation for the mixed findings could be that the positive effects of engagement in physical activities is driven by psychological mechanisms or physiological mechanisms other than aerobic fitness (Etnier, Nowell, Landers, & Sibley, 2006).

There is substantial variability in participant and experimental characteristics across studies. Explanations for the mixed findings in reviews and meta-analyses have included the wide range of cognitive outcome measures, the large variations in specific components of exercise interventions, and also participant characteristic moderators, such as, age, gender, genetic status, and baseline cognitive ability. The evidence for potential moderators identified in the existing exercise intervention literature are discussed in the following sections.

Moderators: Specific Components of Exercise Interventions

Specific components of exercise interventions vary in terms of the type and intensity of exercise, duration and frequency of sessions, and duration of the intervention. The majority of studies have implemented aerobic exercise interventions and found positive effects (Clifford et al., 2009). More recently a growing number of RCTs have investigated the effects of other types of exercise, for example, resistance or strength training and flexibility or toning exercises. There is promising results for the effect of resistance training (Cassilhas et al., 2007; T Liu-Ambrose & Donaldson, 2009; Teresa Liu-Ambrose et al., 2011; Nagamatsu, Handy, Hsu, Voss, & Liu-Ambrose, 2012). Additionally, larger effects have been found for interventions which combined aerobic exercise with strength and flexibility training compared to aerobic exercise alone (Colcombe & Kramer, 2003). Many studies have failed to find effects for toning and stretching exercises by themselves (Cassilhas et al., 2007; Colcombe et al., 2004; Kramer et al., 2001; Madden, Blumenthal., Allen, & Emery, 1989; Moul, Goldman, & Warren, 1995; Smiley-Oyen, Lowry, Francois, Kohut, & Ekkekakis, 2008).

When studies experimentally isolate physical activity as a variable in RCTs, the most appropriate control group is not entirely known (Miller et al., 2012). Some intervention studies have used a no-intervention or wait-list control group but as exercise does not occur independently of its environment, this does not isolate physical activity from social interaction and mental stimulation. Due to the positive effects of mental stimulation and social interaction on cognitive performance in non-exercise related contexts, these are potentially confounding variables (Stock, Clifford, & Hogervorst, 2012). An increasing number of studies have utilised flexibility or stretching exercise interventions as a pseudo control group (Cassilhas et al., 2007; Colcombe et al., 2004; Kramer et al., 2001; Madden, Blumenthal., Allen, & Emery, 1989; Moul, Goldman, & Warren, 1995; Smiley-Oyen, Lowry, Francois, Kohut, & Ekkekakis, 2008) which can help to control for these confounding factors. This can control for the mental stimulation from following instructions of a new type of exercise and the social engagement of interacting with experimenters and potentially exercise instructors and other participants if exercise is carried out in groups. In addition, these pseudo-control groups may help to control for some of the psychological benefits of carrying out exercise, such as sense of achievement. Other pseudo-control groups have included mental stimulation in the form of group discussions or mental tasks of some kind (e.g., Hassmén, Ceci, & Bäckman, 1992). Cognitive activity control groups have been criticised as they could be priming participants for the cognitive outcome measures (Miller et al., 2012). For example, cognitive training interventions have been effective at producing cognitive improvements (La Rue, 2010), and therefore suggests that mental activities are not an appropriate or true control group.

In a study which looked at the effects of mild aerobic training and cognitive training separately and together, the mild aerobic training group failed to demonstrate cognitive improvements after 4 months compared to mild aerobic training combined with cognitive training and compared to cognitive training alone (Shatil, 2013). It was concluded that the results indicated that the mild aerobic training was not driving the effect. However, there is evidence that the level of intensity could be a moderator of the effect. Reviews have indicated that mild levels of exercise intensity have failed to demonstrate an effect (Denkinger, Nikolaus, Denkinger, & Lukas, 2012) and that moderate levels of intensity are required to demonstrate a beneficial effect on cognitive performance. For resistance exercises, high intensity training does not appear to provide any additional effect over moderate intensity training (Cassilhas et al., 2007). While for aerobic exercise, moderate intensity training appears to provide larger effects compared to both high and low intensity training (Kramer & Erickson, 2007b).

The duration of exercise sessions and whole exercise program have been examined for their moderating effect in improving cognitive performance. It has been suggested that for most elderly it seems safe to recommend as much physical activity that is individually achievable, while 30 minutes five days per week represents the overall class A recommendation (Denkinger et al., 2012). Short durations of physical activity (<30 minutes) independent of weekly sessions seem to have little impact on cognitive abilities (Denkinger et al., 2012). Sessions which last between 31 and 45 minutes demonstrated the largest effects (Colcombe & Kramer, 2003; Miller et al., 2012). However, the data on the moderating effect of session duration is scarce and more studies utilising objective continuous measures of physical activity are needed (Denkinger et al., 2012). There have been indications that intensity may be more important than duration of physical activities. One study that found significant associations on numerous cognitive outcome measures with intensity of weekly physical activities did not find any associations for weekly duration of physical activities (Angevaren et al., 2007).

Reviews of the literature have indicated that long lasting exercise programs (> 6 months) and shorter programs (1-3 months) have demonstrated larger effect sizes (0.667 and 0.52 respectively) compared to medium length programs (3-6 months) (Clifford et al., 2010; Kramer & Erickson, 2007b). Positive effects have been demonstrated after only four weeks in older adults (Anderson-Hanley, Nimona, & Westena, 2010) and after six weeks in young adults, with little additional gains during the 6-12 weeks periods (Harada, Okagawa, & Kubota, 2004). Therefore, short as well as longer follow-up assessments in future RCTs would be useful to examine the trajectory of cognitive improvements. The rate of change in cognitive performance rather than the absolute gains from pre- to post-assessments has been cited as relevant to assessing the effect of aerobic fitness (Angevaren et al., 2008; Salthouse, 2006). Additionally, participants who are less physically fit and healthy may be more likely to drop out of the exercise program (particularly if it is of long duration and high intensity). This would result in a different composition of groups at the end of the study (Miller et al., 2012). Level of adherence by participants to the exercise programmes has also been suggested as a moderator of the effect on cognitive improvements. Low levels of adherence could contribute to a null effect (Hogervorst et al., 2012) as some individuals who were in exercise groups who had poor adherence could more appropriately fit into the control group (Clifford et al., 2009). For example, in one study attendance of exercise classes ranged from attending just three to 51 out of a total of 52 classes (Brown, Liu-Ambrose, Tate, & Lord, 2009). Additionally, another study reported an adherence rate of 69% for aerobic classes but participants reported completing the home practice on only 54% of all days (Oken et al., 2006). Level of adherence could result in different findings between studies. Level of adherence is important to consider and may indicate how feasible a specific exercise is in an older adult population and likelihood of participants continuing with the exercise after the intervention has ended. Psychological factors should be considered when designing an exercise intervention to improve adherence and feasibility, such as motivation and self-efficacy (Biddle & Mutrie, 2007).

Moderators: Cognitive Specificity

Another commonly explored explanation across reviews for the mixed results is the vast range of cognitive measures used (Angevaren et al., 2008; Clifford et al., 2009; Hogervorst et al., 2012; Kramer et al., 2003). A myriad of cognitive tests measuring different domains of cognitive performance have been used as outcome measures across studies. At least one hundred different tests have been used to look at the effect of physical activity on cognitive performance across all age groups and study designs (Etnier et al., 1997). Using a selection of cognitive tests can be useful for exploring the possible associations with physical activity across domains. However, it also increases the risk of finding an effect by chance (Type 1 errors). Cognitive ability is usually assessed either using a measure of global cognition, often the Mini Mental State Examination (MMSE; Folstein, Folstein, & McHugh, 1975) or with specific cognitive tests which assess different domains of cognitive performance. These have been categorised into the domains of i) memory, ii) cognitive speed, iii) executive function, and iv) response inhibition (Angevaren et al., 2008; Clifford et al., 2009). It has been suggested that the sensitivity of physical activity on cognitive performance is domain specific (Weingarten, 1973). However, consistent associations have not been found between physical activity and any of these domains. The evidence from meta-analyses in terms of which domains are the most sensitive is equivocal (Angevaren et al., 2008; Clifford et al., 2009; Hogervorst et al., 2012; Miller et al., 2012). The effect of exercise appears to be both broad and specific across cognitive domains (Kramer & Erickson, 2007b), in contrast to cognitive training which is reported to have a task-specific effect on cognitive performance and lacks generalizability to other related tasks (Kramer & Willis, 2002). All domains were found to demonstrate a positive association with physical activity in some studies, but not others. Even the association of specific cognitive tests was not consistent across studies and those showing the most consistent positive associations across studies were from a wide range of domains (Hogervorst et al., 2012).

A meta-analysis which included 18 RCTs which had an aerobic fitness component found robust but selective cognitive benefits with general positive effects on processing speed, controlled processing and visuospatial function. However, the strongest effect was shown on more complex tasks which required executive control processes (Colcombe & Kramer, 2003).

A more recent meta-analysis did not replicate these findings (Angevaren et al., 2008). This more recent meta-analysis included 11 RCTs, also of aerobic exercise in healthy older adults and concluded that the majority of comparisons yielded no significant results across the 33 cognitive outcome measures. However, they found that the largest positive effects were found for more simple cognitive tasks assessing motor function and auditory attention (with effect sizes of 1.17 and 0.50 respectively) with only moderate positive effects for cognitive speed (0.26) and visual attention (0.26). They also concluded that there was insufficient evidence to attribute the cognitive gains to improvements in cardiovascular fitness, as eight out of the 11 RCTs reported that cardiorespiratory fitness improved in the aerobic fitness group, but only 14% of this improvement coincided with improvements in cognitive performance. Although these two meta-analyses had similar selection criteria, Angevaren et al. (2008) used more strict exclusion criteria (using Cochrane criteria) compared to Colcombe and Kramer (2003). For example, they excluded studies which did not have a randomised controlled design. Only four of the same studies were included in both meta-analyses which could explain why that even though both assessed aerobic exercise specifically, they did not find comparable results.

A more recent systematic review corroborated the cognitive domain specific findings of Angevaren et al. (2008) as the strongest effects were also found in simple cognitive tasks, such as concentration and simple reaction time (Clifford et al., 2009). However, the results across the included studies were still mixed, with some cognitive tests showing an effect in some RCTs, but not others. Of the 20 RCTs included, six studies showed a clear positive effect of exercise on cognitive performance across tests, while 13 showed some positive effect on some cognitive tests, and seven studies showed no effect on any cognitive tests. It was suggested that the studies in this review reflected a 50% chance of finding an exercise effect on a simple concentration task, versus only a 32% chance on more complex cognitive tasks (Hogervorst et al., 2012). Thus, numerous reviews have concluded that a battery of cognitive tests should be agreed upon in order to be able to compare results between future studies more effectively (Angevaren et al., 2008; Clifford et al., 2009)

The variation across studies and between meta-analyses suggests that although the domain specific association between physical activity and cognitive ability cannot be ruled out, it cannot explain the wide variation across studies (Clifford et al., 2009).

Moderators: Participant Characteristics

It is likely that there is a complex relationship between physical activity and cognitive ability, with multiple mechanisms that interact and influence each other (Etnier & Labban, 2012). The variation in effect sizes across different samples of populations suggests that individual participant characteristics may also moderate the effect. There is evidence for gender as a moderating variable. Numerous reviews have highlighted that studies which included a higher proportion of females (> 50%) showed the largest effects, and that studies which included only men demonstrated little to no effects (Clifford et al., 2009; Kramer & Erickson, 2007a). This suggests that the potential cognitive gains may be larger for women.

Age has also been suggested as a moderator of the effect (Colcombe & Kramer, 2003; Etnier, 1997). A meta-analysis demonstrated that the effect size of physical activity on cognitive performance varied depending on participants' age, with the largest effect size of

0.69 for those aged 66 to 70 years old, followed by an effect size of 0.55 for those aged 71 to 80 years old, and the smallest effect size of 0.29 for those aged 55 to 65 years old (Colcombe & Kramer, 2003). However, another meta-analysis, which used different age groupings and also included younger participants found contrasting results. The largest effect was found for participants aged 40 to 60 years old and the effect found in participants aged 18 to 30 years old was larger than that for the association for participants aged 60 to 90 years old (Etnier et al., 1997). As this study assigned all older adults aged 60 to 90 years old into one broad group, it is difficult to assess at what age physical activity might be the most effective for improving cognitive ability in older adults. The moderating effect of age on this relationship is yet to be clearly established, and thus further research is needed (Miller et al., 2012).

Genetic status is another potentially moderating variable which has been discussed. The Apolipoprotein E epsilon 4 allele (APOE ε4) has been found to be a major risk factor for Alzheimer's disease. Physical activity has been shown prospectively to be protective against dementia in carriers but did not significantly affect non-carriers (Schuit, Feskens, Launer, & Kromhout, 2001). However, these findings have not been found consistently since (discussed in Clifford, Stock, Bandelow, Rahardjo, & Hogervorst, 2013; Podewils & Guallar, 2005) which further suggests that the relationship is complex with a number of moderating or mediating factors contributing to the effect.

Moderators: Baseline Cognitive Ability

The majority of RCTs have been carried out in cognitively healthy older adults. A smaller number have been carried out with older adults with subjective memory complaints (e.g., Lautenschlager, Cox, & Kurz, 2010), mild cognitive impairment (e.g., Baker et al., 2010), or evident dementia (e.g., Schwenk, Zieschang, Oster, & Hauer, 2010). A meta-analysis with strict inclusion criteria (using Cochrane criteria) - which included only two RCTs in the analysis – concluded there was insufficient evidence of a positive effect of exercise on cognitive performance in those with dementia (Forbes et al., 2008). A systematic review which included only four RCTs with participants with cognitive decline concluded that although some studies found positive effects there was insufficient evidence to establish a conclusion (Clifford et al., 2009). A larger meta-analysis was conducted which included a total of 2020 participants with cognitive impairment and dementia in the 30 included trials. They found an effect size of 0.57 for the effect of exercise on global cognition assessed by the MMSE (Heyn, Abreu, & Ottenbacher, 2004). An examination of this meta-analysis and another with cognitively healthy participants (Colcombe & Kramer, 2003) found similar effect sizes of exercise across various analyses (0.57 and 0.60 respectively). This suggests that older adults with or without early dementia may benefit similarly from exercise in this context (Kramer & Erickson, 2007a).

The Role of Psychosocial Factors

The majority of reviews of the literature neglect psychosocial factors which may play a role in the relationship of physical activity and cognitive outcomes. Psychosocial factors have occasionally been considered but usually only in terms of their influence on participation of physical activity (McAuley, Kramer, & Colcombe, 2004) and not as a mechanism through which physical activity could impact on cognitive outcomes. Exercise does not occur independently of the environment, and the biopsychosocial model of dementia (Clare, 2007; Kitwood, 1997) implicates the importance of considering the impact of the social context and environment for their role on cognitive outcomes. The consistent positive effects found in observational studies which have not been replicated in RCTs suggests potential scope for the contribution of psychosocial factors in the effect. Potential psychosocial mechanisms are neglected when this complex relationship is reduced to internal physiological mechanisms alone.

More recent reviews have considered the role of psychosocial factors in this relationship (Miller et al., 2012; Stock et al., 2012). A mediating relationship has been suggested due to the evidence for the psychological impact of the exercise intervention and the subsequent impact of this on cognitive performance (Stock et al., 2012). For example, exercise interventions have demonstrated positive effects on psychological outcomes including depression and self-efficacy (Callaghan, 2004; Callaghan, Khalil, Morres, & Carter, 2011; Katula, Sipe, Rejeski, & Focht, 2006; Stanton & Reaburn, 2013).

Additionally, in non-exercise related observation and intervention studies, psychosocial factors have been associated with improvements in cognitive performance, such as positive attitudes to ageing (e.g., Langer & Rodin, 1976), positive self-perceptions (e.g., Levy, Slade, Kunkel, & Kasl, 2002; Levy, 2003), better mood (e.g., Ganguli, Du, Dodge, Ratcliff, & Chang, 2006), social engagement (e.g., Saczynski et al., 2006) and mental stimulation (e.g., Salthouse, 2006).

The potential mechanisms through which psychosocial factors could mediate the positive effect of physical activity on cognitive outcomes has been discussed (Stock et al., 2012). The psychosocial factors discussed include self-efficacy, mood, attitudes towards ageing, and perceived control. It may be that the exercise intervention studies which facilitate psychosocial improvements result in larger cognitive gains through psychosocial mechanisms (Stock et al., 2012).

Pilot data has indicated that improvements in psychosocial factors, such as levels of depression are associated with improvements in cognitive performance (Stock, 2014). Additionally, the pilot data indicated that the association between psychosocial improvements and cognitive outcomes was independent to the association between increases in strength and cognitive outcomes. This suggests that there could be an additive effects of physiological and psychosocial mechanisms (Stock, 2014), which should be investigated in future RCTs with larger sample sizes.

The majority of reviews of exercise intervention studies have not taken into account the psychosocial factors of the relationship or have excluded studies in which participants were suffering from depression (Hertzog, Kramer, Wilson, & Lindenberger, 2009). Therefore, although, the impact of psychological factors on cognitive decline has been demonstrated in non-physical activity contexts (Hertzog et al., 2009), the potential psychosocial mechanisms on cognitive functioning in a physical activity context have not been widely investigated, and requires further research.

Conclusion

The extant literature of the protective effect of physical activity against cognitive decline is challenging to interpret due to the myriad of ways that the relationship has been investigated. The moderating effect of specific components of exercise interventions has been investigated and led to recommendations of type, duration and intensity of exercise that are more likely to lead to cognitive gains. However, it is not clear which domains of cognitive ability benefit the most from physical activity, due to the large variety of cognitive tests used. The effect is inconsistent across studies and appears to be both broad and specific across cognitive domains. Findings vary across reviews and meta-analyses, even between those with similar hypotheses. The effect also appears to be moderated by individual factors, such as gender, age, and genetic status. Despite the existing evidence, the relationship between physical activity and cognitive ability is still not fully understood. The role of psychosocial factors in this relationship has largely been neglected despite the evidence for their effect on cognitive outcomes in non-exercise contexts. Psychosocial mechanisms may offer an explanation for some of the inconsistent results between studies and pilot studies indicate that they may a role in the effect of exercise interventions on cognitive outcomes. Future RCTs should utilise the biopsychosocial model of dementia and cognitive decline to further assess the role of psychosocial factors in this relationship. A better understanding of their role would assist with exercise intervention design to maximise cognitive benefits. In relation to the preventative strategy against dementia, understanding the role of psychosocial factors in the relationship between physical activity and cognitive outcomes could contribute to physical activity recommendations for delaying the onset of dementia and prolonging independent living.

References

Abbott, R. D. R., White, L. L. R., Ross, G. W., Masaki, K. H., & Petrovitch, H. (2004). Walking and dementia in physically capable elderly men. *JAMA*, *292*(12), 1447–1453.

Age UK. (2012). *Later Life in the United Kingdom.* Retrieved October 3, 2013, from http://www.ageuk.org.uk/Documents/EN-GB/Factsheets/Later_Life_UK_factsheet.pdf?dtrk=true

Ahn Jo, S., Ahn, K., Kim, J. H., Kang, B. H., Kim, E., Jo, I., & Kim, D. K. (2006). ApoE-ε 4-dependent association of the choline acetyltransferase gene polymorphisms (2384G> A and 1882G> A) with Alzheimer's disease. *Clinica Chimica Acta*, *368*(1), 179–182.

Alzheimer's Society. (2007). Dementia UK: The full report. *Vasa*. Retrieved October 3, 2013, from http://medcontent.metapress.com/index/A65RM03P4874243N.pdf

American Psychiatric Association. (2013). *Highlights of Changes from DSM-IV-TR to DSM-5, Neurodevelopmental Disorders*. Retrieved from http://www.dsm5.org/Documents

Anderson-Hanley, C., Nimona, J. P., & Westena, S. C. (2010). Cognitive health benefits of strengthening exercise for community-dwelling older adults. *Journal of Clinical and Experimental Neuropsychology*, *32*(9), 996–1001.

Angevaren, M., Aufdemkampe, G., Verhaar, H., Aleman, A., & Vanhees, L. (2008). Physical activity and enhanced fitness to improve cognitive function in older people without known cognitive impairment (Review). *Cochrane Database of Systematic Reviews*, (3) CD005381.

Angevaren, M., Vanhees, L., Wendel-Vos, W., Verhaar, H. J. J., Aufdemkampe, G., Aleman, A., & Verschuren, W. M. (2007). Intensity, but not duration, of physical activities is related to cognitive function. *European Journal of Cardiovascular Prevention & Rehabilitation*, *14*(6), 825.

Baker, L. D., Frank, L. L., Foster-Schubert, K., Green, P. S., Wilkinson, C. W., McTiernan, A., Plymate, S. R., et al. (2010). Effects of aerobic exercise on mild cognitive impairment: a controlled trial. *Archives of Neurology*, *67*(1), 71–9. doi:10.1001/archneurol.2009.307

Barberger-Gateau, P, Fabrigoule, C., Helmer, C., Rouch, I., & Dartigues, J. F. (1999). Functional impairment in instrumental activities of daily living: an early clinical sign of dementia? *Journal of the American Geriatrics Society*, *47*(4), 456–62.

Barberger-Gateau, Pascale, Commenges, D., Gagnon, M., Letenneur, L., Sauvel, C., & Dartigues, J. F. (1992). Instrumental Activities of Daily Living as a screening tool for cognitive impairment and dementia in elderly community dwellers. *Journal of the American Geriatrics Society*, *40*(11), 1129–1134.

Barnes, D. E., Santos-Modesitt, W., Poelke, G., Kramer, A. F., Castro, C., Middleton, L. E., & Yaffe, K. (2013). The Mental Activity and eXercise (MAX) trial: a randomized controlled trial to enhance cognitive function in older adults. *JAMA Internal Medicine*, *173*(9), 797–804. doi:10.1001/jamainternmed.2013.189

Bherer, L., Erickson, K. I., & Liu-Ambrose, T. (2013). A Review of the Effects of Physical Activity and Exercise on Cognitive and Brain Functions in Older Adults. *Journal of Aging Research*, *2013*, 657508. doi:10.1155/2013/657508

Biddle, S., & Mutrie, N. (2007). *Psychology of physical activity: Determinants, well-being and interventions*. London: Routledge.

Bielak, A. (2010). How can we not “lose it” if we still don’t understand how to “use it”? Unanswered questions about the influence of activity participation on cognitive performance in older. *Gerontology*, *56*, 507–519. doi:10.1159/000264918

Blair, S., & Brodney, S. (1999). Effects of physical inactivity and obesity on morbidity and mortality: current evidence and research issues. *Medicine and Science in Sports and Exercise*, *31*, S646–62.

Bonner, A., & Cousins, S. (1996). Exercise and Alzheimer’s disease: benefits and barriers. *Activities, Adaptation & Aging*, *20*(4), 21–34.

Bothwell, M. (1995). Functional interactions of neurotrophins and neurotrophin receptors. *Annual Review of Neuroscience*, *132*(18), 223–253.

Bouchard, C., & Shephard, R. (1994). Physical activity fitness and health: the model and key concepts. In S. T. Bouchard C, Shephard RJ (Ed.), *Physical activity, fitness, and health: International proceedings and consensus statement.* (pp. 77–88). IL: Champaign: Human Kinetics.

Brookmeyer, R., Johnson, E., Ziegler-Graham, K., & Arrighi, H. M. (2007). Forecasting the global burden of Alzheimer’s disease. *Alzheimer’s & Dementia: the Journal of the Alzheimer’s Association*, *3*(3), 186–91. doi:10.1016/j.jalz.2007.04.381

Brown, A. D., McMorris, C. A., Longman, R. S., Leigh, R., Hill, M. D., Friedenreich, C. M., & Poulin, M. J. (2010). Effects of cardiorespiratory fitness and cerebral blood flow on cognitive outcomes in older women. *Neurobiology of Aging*, *31*(12), 2047–57. doi:10.1016/j.neurobiolaging.2008.11.002

Brown, A. K., Liu-Ambrose, T., Tate, R., & Lord, S. R. (2009). The effect of group-based exercise on cognitive performance and mood in seniors residing in intermediate care and self-care retirement facilities: a randomised controlled trial. *British Journal of Sports Medicine*, *43*(8), 608.

Bruscoli, M., & Lovestone, S. (2004). Is MCI really just early dementia? A systematic review of conversion studies. *International Psychogeriatrics*, *16*(2), 129–140.

Bull, F., & the Expert Working Groups. (2010). *Physical Activity Guidelines in the UK: Review and Recommendations. School of Sport, Exercise and Health Sciences, Loughborough University.*

Cabeza, R., Anderson, N. D., Locantore, J. K., & McIntosh, A. R. (2002). Aging Gracefully: Compensatory Brain Activity in High-Performing Older Adults. *NeuroImage*, *17*(3), 1394–1402. doi:10.1006/nimg.2002.1280

Callaghan, P. (2004). Exercise: a neglected intervention in mental health care? *Journal of Psychiatric and Mental Health Nursing*, *11*(4), 476–83. doi:10.1111/j.1365-2850.2004.00751.x

Callaghan, P, Khalil, E., Morres, I., & Carter, T. (2011). Pragmatic randomised controlled trial of preferred intensity exercise in women living with depression. *BMC Public Health*, *11*(1), 465. doi:10.1186/1471-2458-11-465

Carter, D. B. (2005). The interaction of amyloid-beta with ApoE. *Sub-cellular Biochemistry*, *38*, 255–72.

Caspersen, C. J., Powell, K. E., & Christenson, G. M. (1985). Physical activity, exercise, and physical fitness: definitions and distinctions for health-related research. *Public Health Reports*, *100*(2), 126.

Cassilhas, R. C., Viana, V. A. R., Grassmann, V., Santos, R. T., Santos, R. F., Tufik, S., & Mello, M. T. (2007). The impact of resistance exercise on the cognitive function of the elderly. *Medicine & Science in Sports & Exercise*, *39*(8), 1401–1407.

Clare, L. (2007). *Neuropsychological rehabilitation and people with dementia* (p. 192). East Sussex: Psychology Press.

Clifford, A., Bandelow, S., & Hogervorst, E. (2009). The Effects of Physical Exercise on Cognitive Function in the Elderly: A Review. In Q. Gariépy & R. Ménard (Eds.), *Handbook of Cognitive Aging: Causes, Processes and Effects* (pp. 109–150). New York: Nova Science Publishers, Inc.

Clifford, A., Stock, J., Bandelow, S., Rahardjo, T. B., & Hogervorst, E. (2013). Alzheimer's Disease and Dementia: A Midlife Approach to Treatment is Needed. In Atta-ur-Rahman (Ed.), *Frontiers in Clinical Drug Research – Alzheimer Disorders* (1st ed., Vol. 1, pp. 217–242). Bentham Science Publishers.

Colcombe, S. J., Kramer, A. F., Erickson, K. I., Scalf, P., McAuley, E., Cohen, N. J., Webb, A., et al. (2004). Cardiovascular fitness, cortical plasticity, and aging. *Proceedings of the National Academy of Sciences of the United States of America*, *101*(9), 3316.

Colcombe, S., & Kramer, A. F. (2003). Fitness effects on the cognitive function of older adults: A Meta-Analytic study. *Psychological Science*, *14*(2), 125–130. doi:10.1111/1467-9280.t01-1-01430

Crook, T., Bartus, R., & Ferris, S. (1986). Age associated memory impairment: Proposed diagnostic criteria and measures of clinical change—report of a national institute of mental health work group. *Developmental Neuropsychology*, *2*(4), 261–276.

Denkinger, M. D., Nikolaus, T., Denkinger, C., & Lukas, a. (2012). Physical activity for the prevention of cognitive decline: current evidence from observational and controlled studies. *Zeitschrift für Gerontologie und Geriatrie*, *45*(1), 11–6. doi:10.1007/s00391-011-0262-6

Department of Health. (2009). More help for dementia research. *Department of Health press release – 5 November 2009.* Retrieved October 3, 2013, from http://www.wired-gov.net/wg/wg-news-1.nsf/lfi/408275

Downs, M., Clare, L., & Anderson, E. (2008). Dementia as a Biopsychosocial Condition: Implications for Practice and Research. In B. Woods & L. Clare (Eds.), *Handbook of the Clinical Psychology of Ageing*. Chichester, UK: John Wiley & Sons, Ltd. doi:10.1002/9780470773185

Dubois, B., Feldman, H., & Jacova, C. (2007). Research criteria for the diagnosis of Alzheimer's disease: revising the NINCDS–ADRDA criteria. *The Lancet Neurology*, *6*, 734–746.

Etnier, J. L., Nowell, P. M., Landers, D. M., & Sibley, B. a. (2006). A meta-regression to examine the relationship between aerobic fitness and cognitive performance. *Brain Research Reviews*, *52*(1), 119–30. doi:10.1016/j.brainresrev.2006.01.002

Etnier, J. L., Salazar, W., Landers, D. M., Petruzzello, S. J., Han, M., & Nowell, P. (1997). The influence of physical fitness and exercise upon cognitive functioning: a meta-analysis. *Journal of Sport & Exercise Psychology*, *19*, 249–277.

Etnier, J., & Labban, J. (2012). Physical Activity and Cognitive Function: Theoretical Bases, Mechanisms, and Moderators. In E. O. Acevedo (Ed.), *The Oxford Handbook of Exercise Psychology*. New York: Oxford University Press.

Farrell, L., Hollingsworth, B., Propper, C., & Shields, M. A. (2013). The Socioeconomic Gradient in Physical Inactivity in England. *CMPO Working Paper Series*, *13/311*.

Fillit, H., Butler, R., O'Connell, A., Albert, M., Birren, J., Cotman, C., Greenough, W., et al. (2002). Achieving and maintaining cognitive vitality with aging. *Mayo Clinic Proceedings*, *77*(July), 681–696.

Folstein, M., Folstein, S., & McHugh, P. (1975). "Mini-mental state": a practical method for grading the cognitive state of patients for the clinician. *Journal of Psychiatric Research*, *23*(3), 189–198.

Forbes, D., Forbes, S., Dg, M., Wood, J., Culum, I., Morgan, D., & Markle-Reid, M. (2008). Physical activity programs for persons with dementia. *Cochrane Database of Systematic Reviews*, (3). doi:10.1002/14651858.CD006489.pub2.

Fratiglioni, L., Paillard-borg, S., & Winblad, B. (2004). An active and socially integrated lifestyle in late life might protect against dementia. *The Lancet Neurology*, *3*(6), 343–353.

Ganguli, M., Du, Y., Dodge, H. H., Ratcliff, G. G., & Chang, C.-C. H. (2006). Depressive Symptoms and Cognitive Decline in Late Life A Prospective Epidemiological Study. *Archives of General Psychiatry*, *63*(2), 153–160. doi:10.1001/archpsyc.63.2.153

Geda, Y. E., Roberts, R. O., Knopman, D. S., Christianson, T. J. H., Pankratz, V. S., Ivnik, R. J., Boeve, B. F., et al. (2010). Physical exercise, aging, and mild cognitive impairment: a population-based study. *Archives of Neurology*, *67*(1), 80–86.

Ghosh, A. (2010). Endocrine, metabolic, nutritional., and toxic disorders leading to dementia. *Annals of Indian Academy of Neurology*, *13*(Suppl 2), S63–8. doi:10.4103/0972-2327.74247

Gu, D., Dupre, M. E., Sautter, J., Zhu, H., Liu, Y., & Yi, Z. (2009). Frailty and mortality among Chinese at advanced ages. *The Journals of Gerontology. Series B, Psychological Sciences and Social Sciences*, *64*(2), 279–89. doi:10.1093/geronb/gbn009

Hamer, M., & Chida, Y. (2009). Physical activity and risk of neurodegenerative disease: a systematic review of prospective evidence. *Psychological Medicine*, *39*(1), 3–11. doi:10.1017/S0033291708003681

Harada, T., Okagawa, S., & Kubota, K. (2004). Jogging improved performance of a behavioral branching task: implications for prefrontal activation. *Neuroscience Research.*

Harridge, S., Magnusson, G., & Saltin, B. (1997). Life-long endurance-trained elderly men have high aerobic power, but have similar muscle strength to non-active elderly men. *Aging (Milan, Italy), 9(1-2), 80-87.*

Hassmén, P., Ceci, R., & Bäckman, L. (1992). Exercise for older women: a training method and its influences on physical and cognitive performance. *European Journal of Applied Physiology and Occupational Physiology*, *64*(5), 460–466.

Henderson, A. S., Jorm, A. F., Korten, A. E., Christensen, H., Jacomb, P. A., Easteal., S., Croft, L., et al. (1995). Apolipoprotein E allele∈ 4, dementia, and cognitive decline in a population sample. *The Lancet*, *346*(8987), 1387–1390.

Hertzog, C., Kramer, A. F., Wilson, R. S., & Lindenberger, U. (2009). Enrichment Effects on Adult Cognitive Development. *Journal of the Association for Psychological Science*, *9*(1), 1–65.

Heyn, P., Abreu, B. C., & Ottenbacher, K. J. (2004). The effects of exercise training on elderly persons with cognitive impairment and dementia: A meta-analysis. *Archives of Physical Medicine and Rehabilitation*, *85*(10), 1694–1704. doi:10.1016/j.apmr.2004.03.019

Hogervorst, E., Clifford, A., Stock, J., Xin, X., & Bandelow, S. (2012). Exercise to Prevent Cognitive Decline and Alzheimer's disease: For Whom, When, What, and (most importantly) How Much? *Journal of Alzheimer's Disease & Parkinsonism*, *02*(03). doi:10.4172/2161-0460.1000e117

Johnson & Johnson. (2012). Johnson & Johnson Announces Discontinuation Of Phase 3 Development of Bapineuzumab Intravenous (IV) In Mild-To-Moderate Alzheimer's Disease | Johnson & Johnson. Retrieved February 5, 2014, from http://www.jnj.com/news/product/johnson-and-johnson-announces-discontinuation-of-phase-3-development-of-bapineuzumab-intravenous-iv-in-mild-to-moderate-alzheimers-disease

Karp, A., Paillard-Borg, S., Wang, H.-X., Silverstein, M., Winblad, B., & Fratiglioni, L. (2006). Mental., physical and social components in Leisure Activities Equally Contribute to Decrease Dementia Risk. *Dementia and Geriatric and Cognitive Disorders*, *21*, 65–73.

Katula, J. a., Sipe, M., Rejeski, W. J., & Focht, B. C. (2006). Strength Training in Older Adults: An Empowering Intervention. *Medicine & Science in Sports & Exercise*, *38*(1), 106–111. doi:10.1249/01.mss.0000183373.95206.2f

Kiecolt-Glaser, J. K., Dura, J. R., Speicher, C. E., Trask, O. J., & Glaser, R. (1991). Spousal caregivers of dementia victims: longitudinal changes in immunity and health. *Psychosomatic medicine*, *53*(4), 345–62.

Kitwood, T. (1996). A dialectical framework for dementia. *Handbook of Clinical Psychology of Ageing*. Chichester: John Wiley & Sons Ltd.

Kitwood, T. (1997). *Dementia Reconsidered: The Person Comes First*. Buckingham: Open University Press.

Kivipelto, M., Ngandu, T., Fratiglioni, L., Viitanen, M., Kareholt, I., Winblad, B., Helkala, E. L., et al. (2005). Obesity and vascular risk factors at midlife and the risk of dementia and Alzheimer disease. *Archives of Neurology*, *62*(10), 1556–1560.

Kramer, A F, Hahn, S., McAuley, E., Cohen, N. J., Banich, M. T., Harrison, C., Chason, J., et al. (2001). Exercise, aging, and cognition: Healthy body, healthy mind. *Human factors interventions for the health care of older adults*, 91–120.

Kramer, Arthur F, Colcombe, S. J., Mcauley, E., Eriksen, K. I., Scalf, P., Jerome, G. J., Marquez, D. X., et al. (2003). Enhancing Brain and Cognitive Function of Older Adults Through Fitness Training. *Journal of Molecular Neuroscience, 20*, 213–221.

Kramer, Arthur F, & Erickson, K. I. (2007a). Capitalizing on cortical plasticity: influence of physical activity on cognition and brain function. *Trends in cognitive sciences*, *11*(8), 342–348. doi:10.1016/j.tics.2007.06.009

Kramer, Arthur F., & Erickson, K. I. (2007b). Effects of physical activity on cognition, well-being, and brain: human interventions. *Alzheimer's & Dementia*, *3*, S45–S51. doi:10.1016/j.jalz.2007.01.008

Kramer, Arthur F., & Willis, S. L. (2002). Enhancing the Cognitive Vitality of Older Adults. *Current Directions in Psychological Science*, *11*(5), 173–177. doi:10.1111/1467-8721.00194

La Rue, A. (2010). Healthy brain aging: Role of cognitive Reserve, cognitive stimulation, and cognitive exercises. *Clinics in Geriatric Medicine* (Vol. 26, pp. 99–111).

Langer, E. J., & Rodin, J. (1976). The effects of choice and enhanced personal responsibility for the aged: A field experiment in an institutional setting. *Journal of Personality and Social Psychology*, *34*(2), 191–198.

Launer, L. J., & Hofman, A. (1992). Studies on the incidence of dementia: the European perspective. *Neuroepidemiology*, *11*(3), 127–134.

Lautenschlager, N. T., Cox, K., Cyarto, E. V., Gold, B. T., & Keller, J. N. (2012). The influence of exercise on brain aging and dementia. *Biochimica et Biophysica Acta*, *1822*(3), 474–81. doi:10.1016/j.bbadis.2011.07.010

Lautenschlager, N. T., Cox, K., & Kurz, A. F. (2010). Physical activity and mild cognitive impairment and Alzheimer's disease. *Current Neurology and Neuroscience Reports*, *10*(5), 352–8. doi:10.1007/s11910-010-0121-7

Leon, A. S., & Sanchez, O. A. (2001). Response of blood lipids to exercise training alone or combined with dietary intervention. *Medicine & Science in Sports & Exercise*, *33*(6), S502–S515.

Levy, B. (2003). Mind matters: cognitive and physical effects of aging self-stereotypes. *The Journals of Gerontology. Series B, Psychological Sciences and Social Sciences*, *58*(4), 203–211.

Levy, B. R., Slade, M. D., Kunkel, S. R., & Kasl, S. V. (2002). Longevity increased by positive self-perceptions of aging. *Journal of Personality and Social Psychology*, *83*(2), 261–270. doi:10.1037//0022-3514.83.2.261

Lilly. (2010). Lilly Halts Development of Semagacestat for Alzheimer's Disease Based on Preliminary Results of Phase III Clinical Trials - Aug 17, 2010. Retrieved February 5, 2014, from http://lilly.mediaroom.com/index.php?s=9042&item=12812

Lindwall, M., Rennemark, M., & Berggren, T. (2008). Movement in mind: the relationship of exercise with cognitive status for older adults in the Swedish National Study on Aging and Care (SNAC). *Aging & Mental Health*, *12*(2), 212–20. doi:10.1080/13607860701797232

Liu-Ambrose, T, & Donaldson, M. G. (2009). Exercise and cognition in older adults: is there a role for resistance training programmes? *British Journal of Sports Medicine*, *43*(1), 25–7. doi:10.1136/bjsm.2008.055616

Liu-Ambrose, Teresa, Nagamatsu, L. S., Graf, P., Beattie, B. L., Ashe, M. C., & Handy, T. C. (2011). Resistance Training and Executive Functions. *Archives of Internal Medicine*, *170*(2), 170–178.

Luengo-Fernandez, R., Leal., J., & Gray, A. (2010). Dementia 2010 – The economic burden of dementia and associated research funding in the United Kingdom. *Cambridge: Alzheimer's Research Trust*. Retrieved October 13, 2014, from www.dementia2010.org/reports/Dementia2010Full.pdf

Madden, D. J., Blumenthal., J. A., Allen, P. A., & Emery, C. F. (1989). Improving aerobic capacity in healthy older adults does not necessarily lead to improved cognitive performance. *Psychology and aging*, *4*(3), 307–320.

McAuley, E., Kramer, A. F., & Colcombe, S. J. (2004). Cardiovascular fitness and neurocognitive function in older adults: a brief review. *Brain, behavior, and immunity*, *18*(3), 214–220. doi:10.1016/j.bbi.2003.12.007

Miller, D. I., Taler, V., Davidson, P. S. R. R., & Messier, C. (2012). Measuring the impact of exercise on cognitive aging: methodological issues. *Neurobiology of aging*, *33*(3), 622.e29–43. doi:10.1016/j.neurobiolaging.2011.02.020

Moul, J. L., Goldman, B., & Warren, B. (1995). Physical Activity and Cognitive Performance in the Older Population, 135–145.

Nagamatsu, L. S., Handy, T. C., Hsu, C. L., Voss, M., & Liu-Ambrose, T. (2012). Resistance training promotes cognitive and functional brain plasticity in seniors with probable mild cognitive impairment. *Archives of Internal Medicine*, *172*(8), 666–8. doi:10.1001/archinternmed.2012.379

Nakajima, S., Ohsawa, I., Ohta, S., Ohno, M., & Mikami, T. (2010). Regular voluntary exercise cures stress-induced impairment of cognitive function and cell proliferation accompanied by increases in cerebral IGF-1 and GST activity in mice. *Behavioural brain research*, *211*(2), 178–184.

Nelson, M. E., Rejeski, W. J., Blair, S. N., Duncan, P. W., Judge, J. O., King, A. C., Macera, C. a, et al. (2007). Physical activity and public health in older adults: recommendation from the American College of Sports Medicine and the American Heart Association. *Medicine and science in sports and exercise*, *39*(8), 1435–45. doi:10.1249/mss.0b013e3180616aa2

Office for National Statistics. (2009). *National population projections, 2008-based Statistical Bulletin*.

Office for National Statistics. (2013). *National Population Projections , 2012-based Statistical Bulletin*.

Oken, B. S., Zajdel, D., Kishiyama, S., Flegal., K., Dehen, C., Haas, M., Kraemer, D. F., et al. (2006). Randomized, controlled, six-month trial of yoga in healthy seniors: effects on cognition and quality of life. *Alternative Therapies in Health and Medicine*, *12*(1), 40–47.

Paillard-Borg, S., Fratiglioni, L., Xu, W., Winblad, B., & Wang, H.-X. (2012). An active lifestyle postpones dementia onset by more than one year in very old adults. *Journal of Alzheimer's disease: JAD*, *31*(4), 835–42. doi:10.3233/JAD-2012-120724

Petersen, R. C. (2004). Mild cognitive impairment as a diagnostic entity. *Journal of Internal Medicine*, *256*(3), 183–94. doi:10.1111/j.1365-2796.2004.01388.x

Petersen, Ronald C. (1999). Mild Cognitive Impairment: Clinical Characterization and Outcome. *Archives of Neurology*, *56*(3), 303. doi:10.1001/archneur.56.3.303

Petersen, Ronald C., Doody, R., Kurz, A., Mohs, R. C., Morris, J. C., Rabins, P. V., Ritchie, K., et al. (2001). Current Concepts in Mild Cognitive Impairment. *Archives of Neurology*, *58*(12), 1985. doi:10.1001/archneur.58.12.1985

Podewils, L., & Guallar, E. (2005). Physical activity, APOE genotype, and dementia risk: findings from the Cardiovascular Health Cognition Study. *American Journal of Epidemiology*, *161*(7), 639–651.

Rodin, J., & Langer, E. (1977). Long-term effects of a control-relevant intervention with the institutionalized aged. *Journal of Personality and Social Psychology*, *35*(12), 897–902.

Rogers, M., & Evans, W. (1993). Changes in skeletal muscle with aging: effects of exercise training. *Exercise & Sport Sciences Reviews*, *21*(1), 65–102.

Roth, D., & Goode, K. (2003). Association of physical activity and visual attention in older adults. *Journal of Aging and Health*, *15*(3), 534–547. Saczynski, J. S., Pfeifer, L. A., Masaki, K., Korf, E. S. C., Laurin, D., White, L., & Launer, L. J. (2006). The effect of social engagement on incident dementia: the Honolulu-Asia Aging Study. *American Journal of Epidemiology*, *163*(5), 433–40. doi:10.1093/ aje/kwj061

Salthouse, T. a. (2006). Mental Exercise and Mental Aging. Evaluating the Validity of the "Use It or Lose It" Hypothesis. *Perspectives on Psychological Science*, *1*(1), 68–87. doi:10.1111/j.1745-6916.2006.00005.x

Scarmeas, N., & Stern, Y. (2003). Cognitive reserve and lifestyle. *Journal of Clinical and Experimental Neuropsychology*, *25*(5), 625–633.

Schuit, A. J., Feskens, E. J., Launer, L. J., & Kromhout, D. (2001). Physical activity and cognitive decline, the role of the apolipoprotein e4 allele. *Medicine and Science in Sports and Exercise*, *33*(5), 772–7.

Schulz, R, O'Brien, a T., Bookwala, J., & Fleissner, K. (1995). Psychiatric and physical morbidity effects of dementia caregiving: prevalence, correlates, and causes. *The Gerontologist*, *35*(6), 771–91.

Schulz, Richard, & Martire, L. M. (2004). Family Caregiving of Persons With Dementia. *The American Journal of Geriatric Psychiatry*, *12*(3), 240–249.

Schwenk, M., Zieschang, T., Oster, P., & Hauer, K. (2010). Dual-task performances can be improved in patients with dementia A randomized controlled trial. *Neurology*, *74*(24), 1961–1968.

Shatil, E. (2013). Does combined cognitive training and physical activity training enhance cognitive abilities more than either alone? A four-condition randomized controlled trial among healthy older adults. *Frontiers in Aging Neuroscience*, *5*(March), 8. doi:10.3389/fnagi.2013.00008

Shephard, R. J. (2003). Limits to the measurement of habitual physical activity by questionnaires. *British Journal of Sports Medicine*, *37*(3), 197–206.

Singh-Manoux, A., Hillsdon, M., Brunner, E., & Marmot, M. (2005). Effects of physical activity on cognitive functioning in middle age: evidence from the Whitehall II prospective cohort study. *American Journal of Public Health*, *95*(12), 2252–8. doi:10.2105/AJPH.2004.055574

Sixsmith, A., Stilwell, J., & Copeland, J. (1993). "Rementia": Challenging the limits of dementia care. *International Journal of Geriatric Psychiatry*, *8*(12), 993–1000. doi:10.1002/gps.930081205

Smiley-Oyen, A. L., Lowry, K. A., Francois, S. J., Kohut, M. L., & Ekkekakis, P. (2008). Exercise, fitness, and neurocognitive function in older adults: the "selective improvement" and "cardiovascular fitness" hypotheses. *Annals of Behavioral Medicine*, *36*(3), 280–291. doi:10.1007/s12160-008-9064-5

Smith, G., Ivnik, R. J., Petersen, R. C., Malec, J. F., Kokmen, E., & Tangalos, E. (1991). Age-associated memory impairment diagnoses: Problems of reliability and concerns for terminology. *Psychology and Aging*, *6*(4), 551–558.

Snowdon, D. A. (2003). Healthy Aging and Dementia: Findings from the Nun Study. *Annals of Internal Medicine*, *139*(5), 450. doi:10.7326/0003-4819-139-5_Part_2-200309021-00014

Sofi, F., Valecchi, D., Bacci, D., Abbate, R., Gensini, G. F., Casini, A., & Macchi, C. (2010). Physical activity and risk of cognitive decline: a meta-analysis of prospective studies. *Journal of Internal Medicine*, *269*(1), 107–17. doi:10.1111/j.1365-2796.2010.02281.x

Solfrizzi, V., Panza, F., Colacicco, A. M., D'Introno, A., Capurso, C., Torres, F., Grigoletto, F., et al. (2004). Vascular risk factors, incidence of MCI, and rates of progression to dementia. *Neurology*, *63*(10), 1882–1891. doi:10.1212/01.WNL.0000144281.38555.E3

Stanton, R., & Reaburn, P. (2014). Exercise and the treatment of depression: A review of the exercise program variables. *Journal of Science and Medicine in Sport*, *17*(2), 177–182.

Stern, Y. (2002). What is cognitive reserve? Theory and research application of the reserve concept. *Journal of the International Neuropsychological Society*, *8*(03), 448–460. doi:10.1017/S1355617702813248

Stock, J. (2014). *Physical activity and cognitive ability in older adults: the role of psychosocial factors. A Doctoral Thesis*. Loughborough University.

Stock, J., Clifford, A., & Hogervorst, E. (2012). Exercise Interventions to Improve Cognitive Performance in Older Adults – Potential Psychological Mediators to Explain Variation in Findings Neurodegenerative Disorders Cognitive Ageing. *European Neurological Review*, *7*(2), 107–112.

Taaffe, D. R., Irie, F., Masaki, K. H., Abbott, R. D., Petrovitch, H., Ross, G. W., & White, L. R. (2008). Physical activity, physical function, and incident dementia in elderly men: the Honolulu-Asia Aging Study. *The Journals of Gerontology. Series A, Biological Sciences and Medical Sciences*, *63*(5), 529–535.

Taylor, A. H., Cable, N. T., Faulkner, G., Hillsdon, M., Narici, M., & Van Der Bij, A. K. (2004). Physical activity and older adults: a review of health benefits and the effectiveness of interventions. *Journal of Sports Sciences*, *22*(8), 703–25. doi:10.1080/02640410410001712421

Thies, W., Bleiler, L., & Alzheimer's Association. (2013). Alzheimer's disease facts and figures. *Alzheimer's & dementia: the Journal of the Alzheimer's Association*, *9*(2), 208–45. doi:10.1016/j.jalz.2013.02.003

Van Gelder, B., Tijhuis, M., & Kalmijn, S. (2004). Physical activity in relation to cognitive decline in elderly men The FINE Study. *Neurology*, *63*(12), 2316–2321.

Van Praag, H., Kempermann, G., & Gage, F. H. (1999). Running increases cell proliferation and neurogenesis in the adult mouse dentate gyrus. *Nature Neuroscience*, *2*(3), 266–270.

Voss, M. W., Prakash, R. S., Erickson, K. I., Basak, C., Chaddock, L., Kim, J. S., Alves, H., et al. (2010). Plasticity of brain networks in a randomized intervention trial of exercise training in older adults. *Frontiers in Aging Neuroscience*, *2*, 1–17. doi:10.3389/fnagi.2010.00032

Wang, H.-X., Karp, A., Winblad, B., & Fratiglioni, L. (2002). Late-life engagement in social and leisure activities is associated with a decreased risk of dementia: a longitudinal study from the Kungsholmen project. *American Journal of Epidemiology*, *155*(12), 1081–7.

Warburton, Darren E. R, Nicol, C. W., & Bredin, S. S. D. (2006). Health benefits of physical activity: the evidence. *Canadian Medical Association journal.*, *174*(6), 801–809. doi:10.1503/cmaj.051351

Warburton, Darren E. R., Gledhill, N., & Quinney, A. (2001a). Musculoskeletal fitness and health. *Canadian Journal of Applied Physiology*, *26*(2), 217–237. doi:10.1139/h01-013

Warburton, Darren E.R., Gledhill, N., & Quinney, A. (2001b). The effects of changes in musculoskeletal fitness on health. *Canadian Journal of Applied Physiology*, *26*(2), 161–216. doi:10.1139/h01-012

Weuve, J., Kang, J. H., Manson, J. E., Breteler, M. M. B., Ware, J. H., & Grodstein, F. (2004). Physical activity, including walking, and cognitive function in older women. *JAMA: the Journal of the American Medical Association*, *292*(12), 1454–61. doi:10.1001/jama.292.12.1454

Williams, P. T. (2001). Physical fitness and activity as separate heart disease risk factors: a meta-analysis. *Medicine and Science in Sports and Exercise*, *33*(5), 754–61.

Woods, B., Aguirre, E., Spector, A. E., & Orrell, M. (2012). Cognitive stimulation to improve cognitive functioning in people with dementia. *The Cochrane Database of Systematic Reviews*, *2*, CD005562. doi:10.1002/14651858.CD005562.pub2

World Health Organization. (2001). International Classification of Functioning , Disability and Health. Retrieved from http://www.sustainable-design.ie/arch/ICIDH-2Final.pdf

Yaffe, K., Barnes, D., Nevitt, M., Lui, L. Y., & Covinsky, K. (2001). A prospective study of physical activity and cognitive decline in elderly women: women who walk. *Archives of Internal Medicine*, *161*(14), 1703.

Zhao, C., Deng, W., & Gage, F. (2008). Mechanisms and functional implications of adult neurogenesis. *Cell*, *132*(4), 645–660.

In: Dementia
Editor: Pamela Tanner

ISBN: 978-1-63321-928-1

Chapter 6

Frontotemporal Lobar Degeneration

Marie-Therese Clerc[1]* and Armin von Gunten[1]
[1]Service Universitaire de Psychiatrie de l'Age Avancé, Département de Psychiatrie, Centre Hospitalier Universitaire Vaudois, Lausanne, Switzerland

Abstract

Frontotemporal lobar degeneration (FTLD) is an umbrella term covering a heterogeneous set of neurodegenerative disorders whose clinical presentation may be cognitive, behavioural., motor, or mixed. These syndromes frequently combine during the course of the disease. FTLD syndromes show considerable phenotypic overlap and variable histopathological and genetic correlations. Current neuropathological classification is based on specific types of protein deposits and their related genes.

Although infrequent in the general population, FTLD is nearly as common as Alzheimer's disease in patients below 65 years of age. Its scope extends from sporadic (60%) to familial forms (40%), some of the latter having an autosomal dominant inheritance pattern. Numerous mutations of several implicated genes have been described.

FTLD represents a diagnostic challenge owing to its mixed features. Implementation of various methods is required and consists of a clinical assessment, neuropsychological testing, structural or functional neuroimaging and, sometimes, genetic analysis looking for mutations. Additional CSF and blood biomarkers, some of them still under study, may provide information about FTLD genetic risk factors or exclude other diseases. To date, only an autopsy allows a definite diagnosis.

No therapies are currently available to cure or alter the evolution of FTLD disorders. Management strategies include pharmacological treatment of the signs and symptoms and non-pharmacological interventions for the patients, for instance skill-based compensation methods, environmental modifications or activity groups. Caregivers should be integrated in the process and offered support when needed (educational programmes, psychological follow-up, respite facilities, etc.). Genetic counselling may prove useful.

* Corresponding author: Marie-Therese.Clerc@chuv.ch.

Research aims at a better understanding of the biochemical pathways of the proteinopathies which will potentially lead to more efficient diagnosis tools and innovative drug strategies.

Introduction

More than a century ago, the Czech neuropsychiatrist Arnold Pick portrayed the clinical picture of several demented patients who presented with an atrophy of the frontal and temporal lobes. A few years later, Alois Alzheimer described the typical neuropathological lesions which he named Pick bodies. For several decades, both Pick's and Alzheimer's diseases have been the representatives of the degenerative dementias. The first international conference on frontotemporal dementia, in 1986, and the subsequent ones have promoted scientific exchange and generated important research activity [1]. This work has given birth to two distinct classifications, one clinical., the other one pathological., highlighting complementary aspects of the FTLD spectrum.

The term FTLD is based on the macroscopically predominant atrophy of the frontal and temporal lobes. It is also an umbrella term covering a heterogeneous group of neurodegenerative disorders. Indeed, clinical presentation may either be neuropsychiatric, i.e., behavioural variant frontotemporal dementia (bvFTD), progressive non fluent aphasia (PNFA) and semantic dementia (SD), or motor, i.e., corticobasal degeneration (CBD), progressive supranuclear palsy (PSP) and motor neuron disease (MND). Co-occurrence or a sequence of these syndromes is frequent during the course of the disease. In addition to this considerable clinical overlap, histopathological and genetic correlations prove to be inconstant. Each specific tissue pathology may cause several phenotypes and, conversely, each phenotype may be underpinned by various histopathological features. Current neuropathological classification is based on the various types of protein deposits grouped into three major categories: FTLD-tau, FTLD-TDP (transactive response DNA-binding protein 43) and FTLD-FUS (fused in sarcoma).

Research constantly redefines these issues. Novel diagnostic criteria attempt to better delineate the domain, additional genes are found to play a role. In short, recent classifications describe a growing complexity. This review chapter presents current knowledge and new insights in the FTLD spectrum (Figure 1).

Epidemiology

Estimation of FTLD prevalence and incidence is difficult to determine due to several factors. First, diagnosis is challenging, implying a risk of under- and over-diagnosis and misclassification [2]. Second, the rarity of FTLD in the population requires large-scale surveys which are seldom available. Third, the design of the studies (community-based, memory centre cohorts, autopsy series, etc.) inevitably induces biases and variable results.

FTLD prevalence estimates range from 2/100'000 to 35/100'000 persons in the general population [3, 4]. Overall incidence data are scarce and rates vary between 14/100'000 and 18/100'000 person-year [5, 6]. Age at presentation is around 50-60 years. This positions the disease among the young-onset dementias although its incipience can vary widely from the third to the ninth decade of life [7-10]. FTLD duration extends from one to fourteen years with a median survival estimated at 6-11 years from symptom onset and 3-4 years from diagnosis [10-16]. Age at onset, gender, education, family history and neuropsychiatric profile do not affect survival rates in FTLD [11, 13]. Most studies report a male preponderance in bvFTD and SD, and a female preponderance in PNFA [4, 8-10, 13].

Compared to Alzheimer's disease (AD), FTLD survival rate is lower, and cognitive and functional decline is more rapid [11, 12]. In living individuals over 65 years of age, FTLD ranks between the second or third most common causes of dementia [17, 18]. Its rank drops to the fourth or fifth in autopsy series [19, 20]. When considering early-onset dementia, most studies indicate AD as the main aetiology, followed by FTLD or vascular dementia [21]. In the age group 45- to 64-years, FTLD may be as frequent as AD [8].

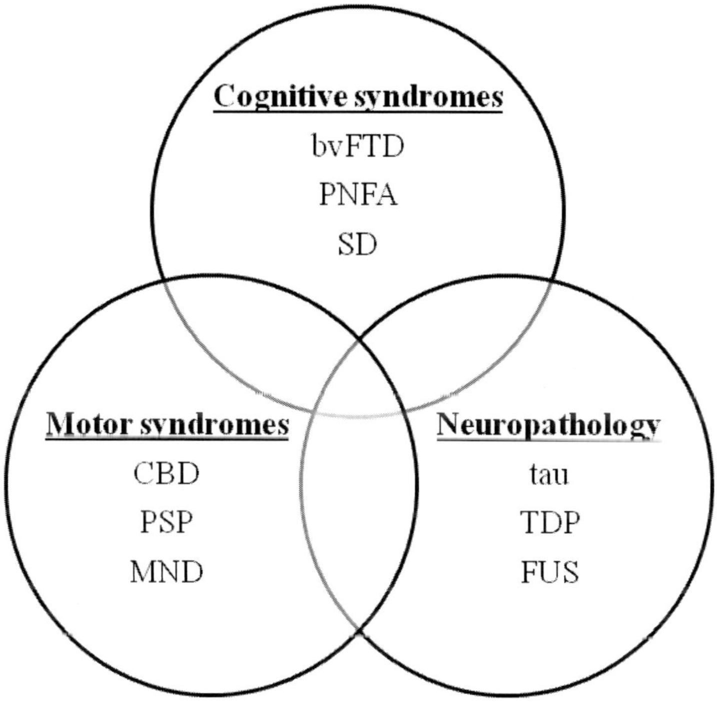

Figure 1. FTLD spectrum: bvFTD behavioural-variant frontotemporal dementia, PNFA progressive non-fluent aphasia, SD semantic dementia, CBD corticobasal degeneration, PSP progressive supranuclear palsy, MND motor neuron disease, TDP transactive response DNA-binding protein, FUS fused in sarcoma.

Clinical Aspects

From a clinical point of view, FTLD comprises various syndromes according to their presenting features. Ongoing debate prompted the revision of the former 1998 criteria [22]. New diagnostic criteria for FTLD cognitive and behavioural variants have been proposed in 2011 in order to improve diagnostic accuracy and sensitivity (Tables 1-4) [23, 24].

Table 1. Summary of bvFTD diagnostic criteria (adapted from Rascovsky, 2011)

Criteria	Rating
I. Progressive cognitive and/or behavioural deterioration	Compulsory
II. Possible bvFTD	≥ 3 symptoms (A-F) compulsory
A. early behavioural disinhibition	
B. early apathy	
C. early loss of empathy	
D. early repetitive, stereotyped or compulsive behaviour	
E. hyperorality and dietary changes	
F. specific neuropsychological profile	
III. Probable bvFTD	All symptoms (A-C) compulsory
A. meets criteria for II	
B. functional decline	
C. compatible imaging	
IV. bvFTD with definite FTLD pathology	≥ 2 symptoms compulsory
A. meets criteria for II or III	(A + either B or C)
B. histopathological evidence	
C. known genetic mutation	
V. Exclusionary criteria	A and/or B exclusionary
A. other non-degenerative nervous system or medical disorders	C admissible for II, exclusionary for III
B. psychiatric disorders	
C. incompatible biomarkers	

"Early" refers to symptom presentation within the first 3 years.

Table 2. Summary of PNFA diagnostic criteria (adapted from Gorno-Tempini, 2011)

Criteria	Rating
I. Clinically diagnosed PNFA	≥ 1 criterion (a-b)
a. agrammatism	AND
b. effortful speech with distorsions	≥ 2 criteria (c-e)
c. impaired comprehension of complex sentences	
d. spared comprehension of simple words	
e. spared object knowledge	
II. Imaging-supported PNFA	criteria (a) AND (b) compulsory
a. meets criteria for I	
b. supportive imaging	
III. PNFA with definite pathology	criterion (a) compulsory
a. meets criteria for I	AND
b. histopathological evidence	≥ 1 criterion (b-c)
c. known genetic mutation	

Table 3. Summary of SD diagnostic criteria (adapted from Gorno-Tempini, 2011)

Criteria	Rating
I. Clinically diagnosed SD	criteria (a) AND (b) compulsory
a. impaired confrontation naming	AND
b. impaired single-word comprehension	≥ 3 criteria (c-f)
c. impaired object knowledge	
d. surface dyslexia or dysgraphia	
e. spared repetition	
f. spared speech production	
II. Imaging-supported SD	criteria (a) AND (b) compulsory
a. meets criteria for I	
b. supportive imaging	
III. SD with definite pathology	criterion (a) compulsory
a. meets criteria for I	AND
b. histopathological evidence	≥ 1 criterion (b-c)
c. known genetic mutation	

A number of diagnostic issues, some of them addressed below, remain controversial and may indicate future perspectives:

- Whereas early episodic memory impairment has been reported in bvFTD cases, and therefore removed from the new definition, it remains an exclusion criterion for the primary progressive aphasias (PPA) [23, 25, 26]. The terminology itself ("aphasia") indicates overemphasis on language at the expense of other cognitive functions. Growing evidence questions the overly restrictive diagnostic criteria for PNFA and SD, such as the absence of early episodic memory impairment, or the preserved calculation and spatial orientation [27-31]. More flexible definitions and a reduced distinction between core and supportive features would better accommodate the variations of the clinical presentation.
- A second or benign form of bvFTD, called "phenocopy syndrome", has been described in patients who progress slowly or not at all, and do not show atrophy on MRI [32-34]. Although the aetiology of these phenocopies is unknown, some of them could reflect a mid-life decompensation of a psychiatric disorder. Personality disorders, autism spectrum disorders and chronic low-grade mood disorders are hypothetical candidates [34, 35]. Intriguingly, some unrelated patients display the same pathogenic mutation on chromosome 9 [36]. The precise nature of this entity still needs to be determined.
- A third type of PPA, the logopenic variant, has been coined by Gorno-Tempini in 2004 and added to her classification in 2011 [24]. Two recent studies, though, failed to support the reliability of its diagnostic criteria [37, 38]. Additionally, AD seems to be the most common underlying pathology [24]. This syndrome remains somewhat elusive.
- Current FTLD definitions leave little to no room to the overlapping syndromes. PSP, CBD and MND are not even mentioned in spite of a common neuropathological

classification and entangled clinical course [39-41]. While some patients reach enough criteria to deserve several diagnoses within the FTLD spectrum, in other cases, intermingled clinical features may alter the clinical and neuropsychological picture, making diagnosis difficult. This considerable overlap has given birth to the notion of a single nosographic category called "Pick complex" [42, 43].

Table 4. Additional criteria for the diagnosis of primary progressive aphasias (PNFA and SD), Gorno-Tempini et al. (2011)

Criteria	Rating
Inclusion criteria:	Criteria 1-3 compulsory
1. Most prominent clinical feature is difficulty with language.	
2. These deficits are the principal cause of impaired daily living activities.	
3. Aphasia should be the most prominent deficit at symptom onset and for the initial phases of the disease.	
Exclusion criteria:	Criteria 1-4 must be answered negatively
1. Pattern of deficits is better accounted for by other nondegenerative nervous system or medical disorders.	
2. Cognitive disturbance is better accounted for by a psychiatric diagnosis.	
3. Prominent initial episodic memory, visual memory, and visuoperceptual impairments	
4. Prominent initial behavioural disturbance	

FTLD motor syndromes are not devoid of cognitive and behavioural features of their own, which may present even in non-demented patients and before the onset of the motor symptoms.

PSP may be associated with bvFTD and PNFA [39, 41]. Its main cognitive features are due to fronto-subcortical dysfunction: apathy, slowness of information processing, impaired memory retrieval, decreased verbal fluency (letter greater than semantic), executive dysfunction (planning, attention shifting, abstraction, reasoning), utilization or imitation behaviour, frontal release signs (primitive reflexes), and other specific behavioural symptoms (disinhibition, irritability, stereotypy, rituals, gluttony, sweet tooth). Language disorders belong to the non-fluent type [44, 45].

CBD may also be associated with bvFTD and PNFA [39, 46]. Frontal lobe involvement predominates, especially in the early stage of the disease: decreased verbal fluency, concreteness in thinking, impaired reasoning, slowed information processing, lack of insight, poor information retrieval, impaired execution of sequential actions, frontal release signs. Personality changes may include apathy, lack of concern about personal behaviour or behaviour of others, disinhibition, perseveration, inattention. Other cognitive symptoms consist of motor speech disturbances (mainly non-fluent aphasia, apraxia of speech or global aphasia), variable episodic memory performance, acalculia, ideational (object use) apraxia, ideomotor (on command or imitation) apraxia, buccofacial apraxia, constructional (draw or copy) apraxia [45, 47, 48].

MND is a general term for a group of diseases whose most common form is amyotrophic lateral sclerosis (ALS). Up to 15% of FTLD patients and 30% of ALS patients present an overlap syndrome [49]. In the vast majority of cases, the mental symptoms precede the motor ones: they begin with changes in behaviour (apathy, stereotypies, greed, tendency to hoard things), cognition (impaired planning, memory deficits, mental rigidity, visuospatial dysfunction) and the emergence of psychiatric symptoms (depression, bipolar disorder, delusions, hallucinations, paranoid or catatonic psychosis). As the psychiatric symptoms tend to subside, the cognitive frontal-executive dysfunction becomes prominent. Patients show a behavioural syndrome (altered social conduct, emotional blunting, loss of insight, impaired emotional processing and recognition of facial emotions) and pronounced language disorders (reduced verbal fluency, verbal perseverations, echolalia, use of stereotypic expressions, impaired comprehension, selective semantic deficit in the knowledge of actions compared to objects, and in the production and comprehension of verbs, as opposed to nouns and adjectives) [50, 51].

Differential Diagnosis

Determination of the correct diagnosis is not only academically satisfying, but also of significant importance given its implications for management, prognosis and potential genetic counselling. The first step is to exclude any treatable or reversible condition which can mimic FTLD. This can be achieved by collecting the following information:

- past and present medical history: age at onset, course (acute, progressive, episodic), pace, cognitive domains involved and their chronology, behaviour, associated symptoms (neurological., psychiatric, others), degree of disability, assessment of co-morbidity.
- family history
- drugs: prescribed and over-the-counter, alcohol, other substances
- physical examination
- standard blood tests: complete blood cell count, C-reactive protein, renal and liver functions, folate, B12, TSH, electrolytes
- neuropsychological testing
- neuroimaging (preferably magnetic resonance imaging).

If these procedures prove non-diagnostic, further investigation is indicated according to the presumed diagnosis. A host of ancillary methods are available, such as lab tests (toxicology, infectiology, serum electrophoresis, autoantibodies, genetic analysis, urine analysis), lumbar puncture and CSF analysis, additional imaging (PET, SPECT, CT scan, DAT-scan, angiography, carotid duplex, cardiac echography, etc.), EEG, ENMG, specific tissue biopsy [52, 53]. The most frequent causes of dementia syndromes and their supportive tests are summarized in Table 5.

When any organic aetiology has been reasonably dismissed, a "functional" psychiatric diagnosis should be considered. Caution is warranted as a significant overlap blurs the distinction between FTLD and some other psychiatric disorders. Confounding biases include a similar clinical presentation, neuropsychology (e.g., executive dysfunction) and, to a certain extent, imaging (e.g., frontal hypoperfusion). Moreover, shared genetic vulnerabilities have been demonstrated, for instance, in reported families with genetic mutations causing FTLD in some members and schizophrenia in others who carry the same mutation [54-56]. Part of the difficulty is also due to the prolonged latency, up to 20 years, between the emergence of psychiatric symptoms and neurocognitive decline [57, 58]. Early-stage FTLD patients may present features of a major depressive disorder, bipolar disorder, schizophrenia, anxiety disorder, or adjustment disorder [59]. Less frequent diagnoses or behaviours that may eventually prove to be due to FTLD are conversion, attention deficit, attempted suicide, substance abuse, obsessive-compulsive disorder, pathological gambling, and antisocial behaviour [59-64].

Several indicators should arouse suspicion of FTLD in psychiatric patients: cognitive impairment, lack of emotional distress, progressive treatment-resistant illness, unusual psychiatric presentation, new onset of a psychiatric disorder in middle-aged and older patients, positive family history of dementia and/or neurological symptoms [65]. Conversely, late-onset psychiatric disorders may be supported by a positive personal or family history of affective or psychotic disorder, a long-term clinical observation over one or more years (by health professionals, family or caregivers), and the presence of specific symptoms rarely seen in FTLD (for instance feelings of worthlessness and poor self-esteem in depression, euphoria and insomnia in mania, obsessions in OCD, complex delusions in schizophrenia) [65, 66]. A thorough history and a consultation with a trained psychiatrist are highly advisable.

Complementary Investigations

Once a possible FTLD syndrome is suspected, the next challenge is to further characterize it. The various instruments available constitute a body of evidence which may support diagnosis if positive, but fail to exclude it if negative or inconclusive. They also lack specificity in accurately predicting the underlying pathology (i.e., definite FTLD diagnosis), but may prove useful to monitor disease progression and therapeutic responses.

Neuropsychological Profile

An interesting meta-analysis sought to identify the cognitive tests that best discriminate between AD and FTLD [67]. None of them was found contributory due to substantial overlap in the scores. The most significant differences between groups were measured in orientation, memory, visuomotor function and general cognitive ability tests (persons with AD performed more poorly than those with FTLD), and in language tests (persons with AD did better than those with FTLD). Another recent meta-analysis investigated the ability of 18 neurobehavioral scales to distinguish between AD and FTLD [68]. Four of them allowed an excellent discrimination, surpassing the cognitive tests, namely, the Schedules for Clinical Assessment in Neuropsychiatry, the Scale for Emotional Blunting, the Middleheim Frontality Score and the Frontal Behavior Inventory. Neuropsychologists are sometimes in the difficult position of attempting to determine whether poor performance in a cognitive domain is primary, or secondary to deficits in a different cognitive domain (e.g., executive dysfunction interfering with episodic memory), or due to behavioural abnormalities (e.g., reluctance to follow instructions) [69]. The cognitive tests and scores should therefore be used cautiously when considering differential diagnoses.

Table 5. Differential diagnosis of dementia

Type	Examples	Testing
Degenerative	AD, FTLD, Lewy bodies, Parkinson, Huntington, multiple system atrophy, prion disorders, CBD, PSP, MND	Medical history, physical examination, lab tests, imaging, EEG, ENMG, LP, neuropsychological testing
Inflammatory/Autoimmune/ Infectious	Systemic lupus erythematosus, Sjögren, Behçet, polyarteritis nodosa, sarcoidosis, celiac disease, Hashimoto's encephalitis, HSV, HIV, CMV, EBV, Lyme, syphilis, Whipple, tuberculosis, malaria, fungal meningitis	Lab tests, LP
Vascular	CNS vasculitis, macro/micro-infarcts, microangiopathic diseases, thrombotic thrombocytopenic purpura, hyperviscosity syndromes, chronic subdural hematoma	Lab tests, neuroimaging, carotid duplex, ECG, skin biopsy (CADASIL), muscle biopsy (vasculitis)
Neoplastic	Primary and secondary malignancies, paraneoplastic syndromes	Lab tests, LP, imaging
Toxic/ Metabolic	Uremia, hepatic encephalopathy, hypo/hyper-thyroidism, hyperPTH, hypo/hyper-corticism, porphyria, vitamin deficiencies, alcohol, drugs, heavy metal poisoning, Wilson	Lab tests, liver biopsy
Neurological	Hydrocephalus, epilepsy, multiple sclerosis	EEG, imaging
Psychiatric	Depression, schizophrenia, bipolar disorder, obsessive-compulsive disorder, conversion, etc.	Clinical assessment

AD Alzheimer's disease, CADASIL cerebral autosomal-dominant arteriopathy with subcortical infacts and leukoencephalopathy, CBD corticobasal degeneration, CMV cytomegalovirus, CNS central nervous system, EBV Epstein-Barr virus, ECG electrocardiogram, EEG electroencephalogram, ENMG electroneuromyogram, EBV Epstein-Barr virus, FTLD frontotemporal lobar degeneration, HIV human immunodeficiency virus, HSV herpes simplex virus, LP lumbar puncture, MND motor neuron disease, PSP progressive supranuclear palsy, PTH parathyroid hormone.

Screening tools are valuable in substantiating the clinical impression. They include the widely used Mini-Mental State Examination and the Montreal Cognitive Assessment, the latter being superior for bvFTD [70]. Frontal lobe functions can be assessed by bedside short scales, for instance the Frontal Assessment Battery [71]. Additional questionnaires are commonly used to check FTLD behavioural symptoms, e.g., the Neuropsychiatric Inventory or the Frontal Behavior Inventory [68, 72]. Finally, assessment of everyday functioning is part of the diagnostic work-up and measures basic and higher order skills, as in ADL (activities of daily living) and IADL (instrumental activities of daily living) scales [73].

Typical neuropsychological patterns which correspond to FTLD clinical phenotypes are based on formal neuropsychological testing [73]. They are described as an executive dysfunction with relative sparing of memory and visuospatial functions for bvFTD, a prominent nonfluent aphasia in the absence of initial episodic memory, visual memory, and visuoperceptual impairments for PNFA, and a profound semantic loss, preserved phonology, syntax, elementary perceptual processing, spatial skills, and day-to-day memorizing for SD [22-24]. As stated before, a great individual variability in the neuropsychological profile emphasizes the need to combine cognitive assessment with other tests and measures [73, 74].

Imaging Techniques

Based on the current diagnostic criteria, standard structural magnetic resonance imaging (MRI) has become a requisite. It should be noted that frontal and temporal atrophy are supportive features for FTLD, but their absence does not exclude the diagnosis [73]. As usual in FTLD, there is no one-to-one correspondence between neuroimaging and the clinical syndromes, genetic mutations or underlying pathology [75, 76]. MRI-based studies nonetheless disclose patterns of atrophy which may help identify the type of FTLD syndrome or distinguish it from other neurodegenerative disorders. bvFTD is characterized by an atrophy of the frontal lobes, involving medial., dorsolateral and orbitofrontal regions, as well as the thalamus and the anterior temporal lobes [75, 76, 77]. In PNFA, the atrophy is observed primarily in the posterior frontal premotor cortex, involving Broca's area and the superior premotor regions, but it has also been reported in the superior temporal gyrus and the striatum [76]. SD is associated with an atrophy of the left (sometimes right) anterior temporal lobe, especially in the inferior regions, the orbitofrontal lobe, insula, caudate nucleus, thalamus and contralateral temporal pole [76].

Recent imaging techniques help to sort through the various neurodegenerative disorders, provide a diagnosis at an earlier stage, and give insight into disease progression. Some of these techniques are recommended in the evaluation of FTLD, while others are used in research settings. It is beyond the scope of this chapter to develop all of them in detail, so only the main principles of each technique will be addressed.

Four additional MRI-based techniques are used in FTLD imaging [73, 75, 76]. *Voxel-based morphometry* converts structural MRI data in order to quantify changes of gray matter volume on a voxel-by-voxel basis. A voxel is a 3D pixel (*vo*lumetric pi*xel*). *Diffusion tensor imaging* (DTI) is part of an MRI protocol that measures the diffusion of water through brain tissue. Several parameters can be extracted such as mean and radial diffusivity and fractional anisotropy. DTI provides information on the integrity of white matter tracts. *Resting state functional MRI* (RS-fMRI) examines functional connectivity, namely the blood-oxygen-level dependent signals provided by the spontaneous neuronal activity in the brain at rest. It offers the advantage of not requiring active participation in specific tasks on the part of patients. RS-fMRI identifies increased or decreased activity in specific brain networks. *Arterial spin labelling perfusion MRI* (ASL) uses arterial blood as an endogenous tracer for perfusion. As perfusion and regional metabolism are coupled, ASL depicts functional deficiencies in a similar way as PET or SPECT (see below), but it is non-invasive and free of exposure to ionizing radiation and intravenous contrast agents.

Positron emission tomography (PET) is a functional imaging technique which uses radioactive isotopes [73, 75, 77]. The most common is 18-F-fluorodeoxyglucose (FDG-PET). The labelled glucose is taken up by the metabolically active cells, thus measuring brain activity. New amyloid PET imaging uses ligands such as Pittsburgh compound B (PiB) or 18-F-florbetapir, which bind to cerebral amyloid deposits and detect AD pathology in vivo.

Single-photon emission computed tomography (SPECT) is another functional imaging modality. The radio-labelled 99m-Tc-hexamethylpropylene amine oxime (HMPAO) crosses the blood-brain barrier and is taken up by brain tissue in proportion to blood flow, hence tracking cerebral perfusion [75]. A special type of SPECT, using 123-I-fluoropropyl-carbomethoxy-iodophenylnortropane (FP-CIT), is also called a DAT (dopamine transporter) scan [78]. DAT is responsible for the reuptake of dopamine in the synaptic cleft. The ligand, a cocaine analogue, allows in vivo assessment of nigrostriatal nerve integrity. It is a sensitive tool for the early diagnosis of Parkinson's disease and atypical parkinsonism, and for the differentiation of Lewy body dementia from AD.

Genetics

A positive family history is observed in 25-30% of FTLD cases, and an additional 10-15% of cases are hereditary with an autosomal dominant inheritance [79, 80]. Importantly, as new genes and mutations will likely be identified in the future, not finding a mutation does not exclude a genetic cause [73]. While sporadic cases are unlikely to display pathological mutations, seven genes have been involved so far in familial FTLD [79, 81].

MAPT (microtubule associated protein tau), located on chromosome 17, encodes a protein implicated in the cytoskeleton. 44 different mutations have been reported.

GRN (progranulin) was the second FTLD-related gene to be discovered on chromosome 17. It encodes progranulin, a cellular growth factor precursor. 69 different mutations have been reported.

C9orf72 (chromosome 9 open reading frame 72) mutation is characterized by a large expansion of a non-coding hexanucleotide (GGGGCC) repeat. C9orf72 gene encodes a ubiquitously expressed protein of unknown function.

Mutations in C9orf72, GRN and MAPT are the most common ones and together explain up to 40% of the familial cases [79].

Less frequently implicated genes are:

VCP (valosin-containing protein) on chromosome 9 encodes a member of the family of the ATPases. 17 different mutations have been described.

CHMP2B (charged multivesicular body protein 2B, sometimes also referred to as chromatin-modifying protein 2B) on chromosome 3 encodes a component of the endosomal-lysosomal complex. Only 4 different mutations have been described [81].

TARDBP (transactive response DNA-binding protein 43) on chromosome 1 encodes a nuclear protein called TPD or TPD-43, involved in RNA regulation. Abnormal TDP accumulation in neuronal and glial cytoplasm has been found in sporadic and genetic forms with mutations in TARDBP, GRN, VCP and C9orf72, suggesting a final common mechanism leading to cell death [82].

FUS (fused in sarcoma) on chromosome 16 encodes a multifunctional nuclear DNA/RNA binding protein [82].

As for diagnosis, genetic testing has a great value in neuropathological studies, when oriented by immunohistochemistry. The benefit of genetic screening in clinical practice proves much more difficult to assess. Identification of the genetic signature of FTLD subtypes is complicated by the clinical heterogeneity, variable expression, misdiagnoses, premature death due to other causes, missing or incomplete medical records and lost family histories [83]. Several algorithms guiding genetic screening have been proposed [81, 84-87]. Current recommendations, though, indicate that genetic testing should only be undertaken in specialist centres with expertise in genetic counselling, in patients with appropriate phenotype or a family history of an autosomal-dominant dementia, and with consent [73]. The topic of predictive genetic testing for at-risk family members will be addressed in the Management Strategies section.

Other Biomarkers

- Routine cerebrospinal fluid (CSF) analysis may help to rule out certain infectious causes (e.g., neurosyphilis, HIV, neuroborreliosis) [73]. Besides, CSF ratio tau/amyloid beta 1-42 is significantly lower in FTLD than AD [73, 88]. A wide range of novel CSF biomarkers, some of them promising (e.g., interleukine-17, fas), still require further validation [88-91]. Indeed, in 2010, an in-depth exploration of human CSF unmasked 745 previously undetected proteins [90]. The growing number of potential biomarkers highlights the need for rigorous evaluation of their diagnostic accuracy.
- No blood biomarker is currently recommended for the diagnosis of FTLD, except DNA analysis for genetic testing [73]. The challenge is obvious: peripheral blood has no direct connection with the brain; blood contains a mixture of thousands of proteins and peptides; its constituents are subject to a huge intra- as well as inter-individual variability [90]. In the particular case of known GRN mutations, the dosage of plasma progranulin might be considered as carriers display decreased levels, unlike non-carriers [85, 86]. It has also been reported that plasma TDP level, when detected by a highly sensitive assay, may rise along with the extension of TDP brain lesions [89, 90].

Neuropathology

A detailed neuropathological examination is mandatory for a definite diagnosis and subtyping of FTLD (Table 6) [92]. The neuropathological diagnostic procedure requires sampling of numerous brain regions, application of a panel of antibodies and staining methods, and identification of specific lesions [93, 94]. Categorization depends on the major component of the neuronal inclusions, reported as FTLD-tau, FTLD-TDP, and FTLD-FUS. As might be expected, atypical variants and mixed neurodegenerative aetiologies do exist. To date, Pick's disease is the sole FTLD cognitive syndrome with specific neuropathological hallmarks.

Table 6. Nomenclature for FTLD, adapted from Mackenzie et al., 2010

Molecular class	Neuropathological diagnosis	Associated genes
FTLD-tau	Pick's disease	MAPT
	Corticobasal degeneration	
	Progressive supranuclear palsy	
	Argyrophilic grain disease	
	Multiple system tauopathy with dementia	
	Neurofibrillary tangle predominant dementia	
	White matter tauopathy with globular glial inclusions	
	Unclassifiable	
FTLD-TDP	Type 1-4	GRN
	Unclassifiable	VCP
		C9orf72
		TARDBP
FTLD-FUS	Atypical FTLD with ubiquitinated inclusions	FUS
	Neuronal intermediate filament inclusion disease	
	Basophilic inclusion body disease	
FTLD-UPS	Frontotemporal dementia linked to chromosome 3	CHMP2B
FTLD-no inclusions		

CHMP2B charged multivesicular body protein 2B, C9orf72 chromosome 9 open reading frame 72, FUS fused in sarcoma, MAPT microtubule-associated protein tau, TARDBP transactive response DNA-binding protein, TDP transactive response DNA-binding protein 47, UPS ubiquitine-proteasome system, VCP valosin-containing protein.

Recent research activity indicates a trend to look for common traits and mechanisms which could unify these seemingly disparate disorders. Anatomically, the topographical distribution of the lesions seems to correlate better with clinical picture rather than the type of protein deposits [95]. At a molecular level, a theory develops the concept of a prion-like induction and spreading of the pathogenic proteins [96]. Other research demonstrates the role of the mammalian target of rapamycin (mTOR), a protein kinase which inhibits autophagy, in tau accumulation and aging [97]. Our understanding of neurodegenerative disorders is still limited and will require further research effort.

Risk Factors

Little is known about FTLD risk factors. Medical conditions include traumatic brain injury and, possibly, thyroid disease [98-100]. Exposure to environmental neurotoxins, e.g., manganese, could result in an increased risk for subsequent development of FTLD [4, 101]. Genetic risk factors, apart from known genetic mutations, are also involved. A positive family history of first- or second-degree relatives affected by Parkinson's disease, FTLD or another dementia, especially if age at onset is before 65, provides a reasonably effective means of detecting those at risk for an inherited form of FTLD [81]. Furthermore, some psychiatric disorders (e.g., schizophrenia, bipolar disorder) may represent the prodrome of a neurodegenerative disease as well as an independent risk factor for it, in the same way as depression may increase the risk for developing AD [54-59]. These hypotheses are difficult to differentiate due to considerable phenotypic variability, possible misdiagnoses and shared genetic features. Finally, a genome-wide association (GWA) study found that variant alleles of TMEM106B on chromosome 7, encoding an uncharacterized transmembrane protein, contribute to the risk for FTLD-TDP [79, 102]. Other FTLD-related genes and molecular pathways are currently being investigated [80, 82].

Management Strategies

Pharmacological Treatment

To date, no treatment or lifestyle intervention has proven successful in preventing or delaying the development of non-AD dementias [73].

Current recommendations and recent studies discourage the use of cholinesterase inhibitors and memantine in the treatment of FTLD cognitive deficits [69, 73, 103, 104]. FTLD is not a hypocholinergic dementia, hence no gain is expected from cholinesterase inhibition. Memantine, a NMDA glutamate receptor antagonist, might even hasten cognitive decline. No medication of any type has been shown to improve cognition [73, 105, 106].

As for FTLD behavioural and psychological symptoms of dementia (BPSD), some medications may be used in clinical practice in spite of insufficient evidence [73]. Indeed, symptomatic therapy can enhance quality of life and provide relief to the patients and their caregivers. Most studies show a decrease of serotoninergic receptors in the frontotemporal regions and raphe nuclei [69]. Selective serotonin reuptake inhibitors are considered safe and effective in treating mood and behavioural symptoms [69, 73, 105-107]. Sertraline, paroxetine, fluvoxamine, fluoxetine, and citalopram have all demonstrated some effect on depressive symptoms, disinhibition, carbohydrate craving, compulsions, verbal and motor stereotypies, sexually inappropriate behaviours, apathy and hyperorality. In one study, however, paroxetine seemed to worsen cognition [108]. Trazodone has a 5HT1a-agonist and 5HT2c-antagonist effect, and a modest selective serotonin reuptake inhibitor effect. It improves BPSD, including delusions, aggression, anxiety, irritability, depression, disinhibition, agitation, and eating disorders. Conventional and atypical antipsychotic agents may be prescribed for aggression, psychosis and agitation [73, 109]. Their efficacy must be carefully weighed against their significant side effects, especially extrapyramidal symptoms, higher mortality due to cardiac-related events and infections, weight gain, stroke, and accelerated cognitive decline [69, 73, 106].

Innovative approaches with existing drugs are being explored. There is some evidence for reduced dopamine transport in the putamen and caudate of FTLD patients [69]. Recent studies on dopaminergic agonists, such as amphetamines, tolcapone, and bromocriptine, suggested a decrease in risk-taking behaviours and an improvement of apathy, slowing and perseveration [69, 103, 105-107]. Monoamine oxidase inhibitors might be useful, given

FTLD serotoninergic and dopaminergic deficits. Indeed, selegiline may reduce BPSD [103, 107]. Mood stabilizers are potential neuroprotective therapies. Lithium reduces tau phosphorylation and aggregation, whereas valproate reduces amyloid plaques in animal models. Unfortunately, no efficacy has been conclusively demonstrated in clinical trials [106, 110]. Two neuropeptides, oxytocin and vasopressin, are involved in social cognition, i.e., recognition of facial expressions, empathy and cooperative behaviour, which are frequently affected in FTLD patients [69, 111]. Oxytocin has been shown to improve social behaviour, while vasopressin antagonists have raised theoretical interest.

New therapeutic targets could lead to the emergence of disease-modifying drugs. Protein-specific therapies include microtubule stabilizing agents and inhibition of enzymes which contribute to tau or TDP processing (phosphorylation, ubiquitination, expression, etc.) [103, 112, 113]. Many other molecules, e.g., neuroprotective peptides or antioxidants, are in pharmaceutical pipelines but have to face a number of limitations: compared with other therapeutic areas, CNS drugs have the lowest success rate in all phases of drug development; preclinical animal models have proven to be poor predictors when translated into clinical trials; in vivo diagnosis still awaits substantial improvement in the identification of the underlying proteinopathy, and in the measure of disease progression [103, 113, 114]. Finally, most neurodegenerative diseases are characterized by a long delay with neuropathological changes taking place before the presentation of clinical symptoms. Novel therapeutic strategies acknowledge the need for a better understanding and prevention of the degenerative cascades, for instance inflammation triggered by the pathogenic proteins [115, 116].

Non-pharmacological Treatment

Although a variety of interventions are used in different settings, there is insufficient evidence for recommending any of the non-pharmacological treatments addressing FTLD cognitive impairment and BPSD [73]. Since drug therapies for FTLD remain modestly effective and carry the risk of serious adverse effects, empirically-based strategies offer alternative options to relieve suffering and provide assistance to the patients and their families or caregivers. Each intervention should be individually tailored according to disease stage, symptoms pattern, needs, and available resources. Treatment is multidisciplinary and aims at improving daily functioning, managing symptoms and preserving quality of life.

Safety and Risk Management

Safety concerns are often associated with impaired cognitive functioning and impulsive behaviour. Environmental modifications may minimize risks and deleterious behaviour [117, 118]. They may include the removal of dangerous items (e.g., firearms), rearrangement of furniture to prevent falls or access to stairs, covering doorknobs to discourage elopement, installing door alarms to alert elopement attempts, locking the kitchen door to prevent binge-eating, etc. Evaluation by an occupational therapist may contribute to securing the patient's physical surroundings.

Financial problems may arise from neglected bills, impulsive or compulsive spending, or poor judgement (e.g., gifts to strangers) [65]. Limiting access to bank accounts and credit cards may prove necessary, as well as engaging in disability procedures. As FTLD frequently begins before 65, it may bring about a loss of income along with growing health care costs.

Families should be advised by a lawyer or social worker about financial planning. They should secure assets (e.g., life insurance) prior to genetic testing.

Assessment of driving ability should be made after diagnosis, with particular attention paid to visuospatial., visuoperceptual and executive abilities [73]. Referral to the local jurisdiction for a formal driving assessment helps to make the decision [65]. Cessation of driving will restrict the patient's autonomy, can undermine the patient-doctor relationship and cause conflicts between patient and family. The decision should therefore never be made lightly.

Behavioural Interventions

The objective of this approach is to target problematic behaviour identified by caregivers as most troublesome and to provide strategies to manage them effectively. BPSD may be conceptualized as a consequence of interacting factors which fall into three domains: patient (unmet needs, discomfort, incipient medical condition), caregiver (distress, communication style) and environment (clutter, hazards, general conditions) [119]. Potential triggers are identified and modified in order to improve well-being. For instance, adapting to the patient's abilities and simplifying daily tasks (e.g., clearing area of all items except those related to the present task) may alleviate excessive stress and concomitant agitation [117, 119, 120]. Improving caregiver communication skills reduces resistance to care among patients (e.g., informing patients about the upcoming task, or avoiding "elderspeak" such as "sweetie" or "good boy") [117]. Structuring the environment to facilitate participation may also prove useful (e.g., avoiding crowded or noisy places) [118].

Cognitive Interventions

Although no interventions can reverse the cognitive decline, it seems that a certain degree of improvement is possible in important skills such as memory or verbal communication, especially in progressive primary aphasia [117, 118]. For instance, structured oral reading of text enhances word production in PNFA [121]. Another study provides evidence that errorless learning ameliorates comprehension and naming deficits in SD [122]. Although maintenance of learning is variable, outcomes demonstrate that cognitive rehabilitation contributes to the treatment of neurodegenerative diseases.

Compensatory Devices and Interventions

Compensation means implementing new adaptive strategies when existing abilities are lost or insufficient for adequate functioning. The living environment should be simplified in order to promote self-reliance and a stable daily routine made of structured activities should be implemented [117, 118]. Physical interventions include exercise, assessment of swallowing and advice on dietary modifications, external aids for mobility and continence problems [117]. The learned dependency which occurs in the demented patients when the caregivers provide too much support is to be avoided. Whether by compassion or by irritation, caregivers may be tempted to do things for the patient instead of waiting for the patients to do them by themselves. These over-compensatory interactions lead to reduced activities of daily living [117, 118]. Caregiver's information and education promotes activity and preserves skills. Cognitive impairment may require external memory aids such as calendars, a diary, photo albums or electronic devices (e.g., tablets) [117, 118]. A wide array of communication strategies and tools may prove useful for language deficits, for instance written messages, drawing charts, photographs, etc.[118, 123].

Community Services

Home-based interventions and visits are usually available in high-income countries. They consist of multidisciplinary teams with occupational therapists, nurses, social workers and household maids, who provide support to FTLD patients and their families.

Specialized day hospitals and recreational centres benefit patients while giving families respite [124]. Unfortunately, finding a facility which will admit FTLD patients may prove difficult due to their younger age, disruptive behaviour, physical strength and preserved mobility [125].

Respite facilities, for instance short-duration nursing home placement, are another way to support families. Hospitalization is reserved for cases which cannot be handled otherwise (e.g., violent behaviour). Residential care must be considered when care needs exceed the capacity of the carer [65]. Families and patients often need time and active assistance to accept change and prepare emotionally for separation, so that early conversations about this topic are useful [65].

Caregiver Support

Caregiver burden in FTLD is higher than in AD [124, 126]. Several patient-dependent variables contribute to carer burden: young age, impaired anterograde memory and emotion recognition, diagnosis (FTLD), low impulse control and behavioural disturbances [126, 127]. However, the patient's gender, performance on general measure of cognition, disease duration, language skills, and the type of relationship (i.e., spouse vs other) between the patient and the carer do not influence carer burden [127]. Regarding carer variables, young age, depression, social isolation, neglected personal needs, and inadequate coping style to problem behaviours are predictive of carer burden [124, 126, 127].

Hence, support services have been developed to meet the needs of this population. Group or individual information and education programmes are modestly successful in reducing stress and burden [126, 127]. Support groups for families, which may be internet-based, prove beneficial by providing mutual self-help and allowing verbalization of feelings [124, 126]. Mental health care professional counselling and case management also have positive effects on burden and satisfaction of caregivers [73]. In some instances, psychosocial support proves insufficient owing to high levels of carer distress. Referral to a mental health professional for psychotherapy should then be considered [65]. Practical issues, such as access to care facilities, disability procedures, financial advice and evaluation of needs should be addressed systematically. Integration of the caregivers and family members into a team surrounding the patient ensures that everyone has a proper understanding of the situation.

Genetic Counselling

Regarding FTLD genetic counselling, no internationally shared guidelines are available. In their absence, the approach is similar to that used for Huntington's disease and consists of a three-step programme [73, 128]. The pre-test session comprises general information on the disease, on the test, on possible alternatives (e.g., DNA bank, research), and on their consequences. Additional investigation, such as neurological and psychological examinations, may be advisable, but should always be non-compulsory. A minimal interval of one month is necessary between the pre-test session and the decision to take the test in order to assimilate the information and make an informed decision. The result should be delivered as soon as possible after completion of the test. Follow-up sessions should be scheduled over two years in the post-disclosure period. These recommendations are intended to be individually tailored [128, 129].

Predictive testing is intended for at-risk family members of FTLD patients. Due to the complexity of FTLD genetics, it is highly recommended that the mutation be identified in an affected relative prior to pre-symptomatic testing of kindred [73, 84]. This requirement is sometimes extended to autosomal-dominant inheritance only, which may prove extremely difficult to establish and cause much frustration in families who fear that dementia in their family is genetic but have no way to prove it [83, 84]. As stated before, incomplete family history, misdiagnoses and psychiatric disorders may prevent exact determination of cases. Furthermore, mutations with incomplete or age-dependent penetrance contribute to the blurring of the picture [84].

If the index case cannot be tested or identified, the likelihood of a hereditary mutation is based primarily on a positive family history. A three-generation pedigree of family members with an FTLD disorder or another neurodegenerative disease must be collected [81]. Integration of several variables is required: family history, phenotype, age at onset, neuroimaging data and any other source of information (e.g., autopsy, progranulin plasma level, etc.). Should the family history be negative, the odds of finding a pathogenic mutation are less than 3% [84]. If the data point to a possible hereditary transmission of the disease, the next step is to decide which genes are the most likely candidates according to statistical probability. It is only at this point of the workup that adult family members are eligible for predictive testing [84-87].

Only a small proportion of those at risk requests testing [83, 129]. The most common reasons for testing are to further scientific research, to know if children are at risk, to plan for a medical and financial future, and to be relieved of anxiety [83]. The primary reasons of those who do not wish to pursue testing are to maintain hope, inability to cope with the stress of a positive result, and fear of knowing the future [83].

The impact of test results is difficult to predict and only slightly dependent on the outcome (positive or negative) [129]. Hence, support must be offered to carriers as well as non-carriers. Reactions depend on individual features such as baseline mood, ego strength, and coping strategies [129]. They range from relief, anxiety, depression or adjustment problems, to a decision not to procreate or divorce [83, 129].

End-of-life Issues

The scarcity of literature about end-of-life care in FTLD may translate the discomfort which many health professionals experience towards inevitable decline and death. Nevertheless, families and patients have to plan for their future and make decisions about the goals of care when there is still time and ability to discuss these matters [4]. The cognitive and physical progression of the signs and symptoms should be addressed pre-emptively during the follow-up sessions. The expressed will of the patients helps diminish the stress and guilt that some caregivers may feel about not doing enough or making the right decisions, for instance, about measures of comfort or referral to palliative care [65].

Anticipatory grief in dementia is equivalent in intensity and breadth to death-related grief [130]. However, the grief process is different for adult-child caregivers than for spouse caregivers, and depends upon the dementia stage [130]. Moreover, end-stage cognitive decline does not allow for patients and caregivers to grieve together. This experience of human condition may function as a starting point for clinical intervention [131, 132]. Support and guidance must therefore be adapted to fluctuating affective, intellectual and existential needs.

After the patient's death, contact with the family may address further issues, such as post-mortem brain examination, genetic implications of the disease and bereavement [65]. Anticipatory grief appears to alleviate post-death grief initially, but not in the long run, emphasizing the need for psychological follow-up to be offered upon request [130, 131].

Conclusion

Neurodegenerative disorders remain disconcerting and challenge our knowledge about their cause, their prevention and their treatment. The "airbag problem" theory may explain the lack of translational success despite the tremendous work and money invested in dementia research over the past thirty years. A recent and provocative paper describes it as an illustration of reverse causality [133].

The airbag theory questions beliefs about presumptive disease aetiology and suggests re-considering future research with an iconoclast state of mind. For instance, emerging evidence indicates that abnormal protein aggregation may not necessarily be the cause of neuronal toxicity and death [134]. This could partly explain why some individuals whose brain carries a heavy lesion burden remain cognitively healthy. Another part of the explanation could arise from the protective and adaptive mechanisms of the brain, such as neural genesis or neuroplasticity [135]. Obviously, a considerable amount of inter-individual variation exists.

Understanding why aging is the major risk factor for the development of neurodegenerative disorders may be a more promising approach than focusing on specific diseases, conditions or single aetiologies [136, 137]. Evolutionary theories provide valuable insight. Classical evolution theory predicts that genomes are inherently unstable because of the need for DNA variation as a substrate for evolution through natural selection [138]. Nonetheless, genetic control that drives aging is not optimized because evolutionary pressure decreases with age [138, 139]. Due to shorter life spans in the past, the antagonistic pleiotropy theory explains why some alleles, having a positive effect early in life and thus retained by selection, may accumulate in successive generations before uncovering their negative effects at an older age [139, 140]. These entangled concepts point to the need for interdisciplinary research in order to expand and nuance our knowledge of the aging processes, which might be the key to future treatments for those affected by these devastating diseases.

References

[1] Brun A, Gustafson L. The birth and early evolution of the frontotemporal dementia (FTD) concept. *J Mol Neurosci.* 2011 Nov; 45(3):324-9.

[2] Knopman DS, Robert RO. Estimating the number of persons with frontotemporal lobar degeneration in the US population. *J Mol Neurosci.* 2011 Nov; 45(3):330-5.

[3] Rosso SM, Donker Kaat L, Baks T, Joosse M, de Koning I, Pijnenburg Y, et al. Frontotemporal dementia in the Netherlands: patients characteristics and prevalence estimates from a population-based study. *Brain* 2003; 126:2016-22.

[4] Gilberti N, Turla M, Alberici A, Bertasi V, Civelli P, Archetti S, et al. Prevalence of frontotemporal lobar degeneration in an isolated population: the Vallecamonica study. *Neurol Sci.* 2012 Aug; 33(4):899-904.

[5] Knopman DS, Petersen RC, Edland SD, Cha RH, & Rocca WA. The incidence of frontotemporal lobar degeneration in Rochester, Minnesota, 1990 through 1994. *Neurology* 2004; 62:506-8.

[6] Garre-Olmo J, Genis Batlle D, del Mar Fernandez M, Marquez Daniel F, de Eugenio Huelamo R, Casadevall T, et al. Incidence and subtypes of early-onset dementia in a geographically defined general population. *Neurology* 2010; 75:1249-55.

[7] Rabinovici GD, & Miller BL. Frontotemporal lobar degeneration: epidemiology, pathophysiology, diagnosis and management. CNS Drugs 2010; 24(5):375-98.

[8] Ratnavalli E, Brayne C, Dawson K, & Hodges JR. The prevalence of frontotemporal dementia. *Neurology* 2002; 58:1615-21.

[9] Johnson JK, Diehl J, Mendez MF, Neuhaus J, Shapira JS, Forman M, et al. Frontotemporal lobar degeneration : Demographic characteristics of 353 patients. *Arch Neurol.* 2005; 62 :925-30.

[10] Hodges JR, Davies R, Xuereb J, Kril J, & Halliday G. Survival in frontotemporal dementia. *Neurology* 2003; 61:349-54.

[11] Roberson ED, Hesse JH, Rose KD, Slama BA, Johnson JK, Yaffe K, et al. Frontotemporal dementia progresses to death faster than Alzheimer disease. *Neurology* 2005; 65:719-25.

[12] Rascovsky K, Salmon DP, Lipton AM, Leverenz JB, DeCarli C, Jagust WJ, et al. Rate of progression differs in frontotemporal dementia and Alzheimer disease. *Neurology* 2005; 65:397-403.

[13] Kertesz A, Blair M, McMonagle P, & Munoz DG. The diagnosis and course of frontotemporal dementia. *Alzheimer Dis Assoc Disord* 2007; 21(2):155-163.

[14] Seelar H, Kamphorst W, Rosso SM, Azmani A, Masdjedi R, de Koning I, et al. Distinct genetic forms of frontotemporal dementia. *Neurology* 2008; 71:1220-6.

[15] Onyike CU. What is the life expectancy in frontotemporal lobar degeneration? *Neuroepidemiology* 2011; 37:166-7.

[16] Nunnemann S, Last D, Schuster T, Förstl H, Kurz A, & Diehl-Schmid J. Survival in a German population with frontotemporal lobar degeneration. *Neuroepidemiology* 2011; 37:160-5.

[17] McMurtray A, Clark DG, Christine D, & Mendez MF. Early-onset dementia: frequency and causes compared to late-onset dementia. *Dement Geriatr Cogn Disord* 2006; 21:59-64.

[18] Ikeda M, Ishikawa T, & Tanabe H. Epidemiology of frontotemporal lobar degeneration. *Dement Geriatr Cogn Disord* 2004; 17:265-8.

[19] Brunnström H, Gustafson L, Passant U, & Englund E. Prevalence of dementia subtypes: a 30-year retrospective survey of neuropathological reports. *Arch Gerontol Geritr* 2009; 49(1):146-9.

[20] Barker WW, Luis CA, Kashuba A, Luis M, Harwood DG, Loewenstein D, et al. Relative frequencies of Alzheimer disease, Lewy body, vascular and frontotemporal dementia, and hippocampal sclerosis in the State of Florida brain bank. *Alzheimer Dis Assoc Disord* 2002; 16(4):203-12.

[21] Vieira RT, Caixeta L, Machado S, Silva AC, Nardi AE, Arias-Carrion O et al. Epidemiology of early-onset dementia: a review of the literature. *Clin Pract Epidemiol Ment Health* 2013; 14(9):88-95.

[22] Neary D, Snowden JS, Gustafson L, Passant U, Stuss D, Black S, et al. Frontotemporal lobar degeneration: a consensus on clinical diagnostic criteria. *Neurology* 1998; 51:1546-54.

[23] Raskovsky K, Hodges JR, Knopman D, Mendez MF, Kramer JH, Neuhaus J, et al. Sensitivity of revised diagnostic criteria for the behavioural variant of frontotemporal dementia. *Brain* 2011; 134:2456-77.

[24] Gorno-Tempini ML, Hillis AE, Weintraub S, Kertesz A, Mendez M, Cappa SF, et al. Classification of primary progressive aphasia and its variants. *Neurology* 2011; 76:1006-14.

[25] Hornberg M, & Piguet O. Episodic memory in frontotemporal dementia: a critical review. *Brain* 2012; 135:678-92.

[26] Shinagawa S. Phenotypic variety in the presentation of fronto-temporal lobar degeneration. *Int Rev Psychiatry* 2013; 25(2):138-44.

[27] Pleizier CM, van der Vlies AE, Koedam E, Koene T, Barkhof F, van der Flier WM, et al. Episodic memory and the medial temporal lobe: not all it seems. Evidence from the temporal variants of frontotemporal dementia. *J Neurol Neurosurg Psychiatry* 2012; 83(12):1145-8.

[28] Grossman M, Xie SX, Libon DJ, Wang X, Massimo L, Moore P, et al. Longitudinal decline in autopsy-defined frontotemporal lobar degeneration. *Neurology* 2008 ; 70 :2036-45.

[29] Julien CL, Thompson JC, Neary D, & Snowden JS. Arithmetic knowledge in semantic dementia: is it invariably preserved? *Neuropsychologia* 2008; 46:2732-44.

[30] Clerc MT, Deprez M, Leuba G, Lhermitte B, Lopez U, & von Gunten A. Atypical association of semantic dementia, corticobasal syndrome, and 4R tauopathy. *Neurocase* 2013 (ahead of print) doi 10.1080/13554794.2013.841953

[31] Pengas G, Patterson K, Arnold RJ, Bird CM, Burgess N, & Nestor PJ. Lost and found: bespoke memory testing for Alzheimer's disease and semantic dementia. *J Alzheimer Dis.* 2010; 21(4):1347-65.

[32] Davies RR, Kipps CM, Mitchell J, Kril JJ, Halliday GM, & Hodges JR. Progression in frontotemporal dementia: identifying a benign behavioral variant by magnetic resonance imaging. *Arch neurol* 2006; 63(11):1627-31.

[33] Hornberger M, Shelley BP, Kipps CM, Piguet O, & Hodges JR. Can progressive and non-progressive behavioural variant frontotemporal dementia be distinguished at presentation? *J Neurol Neurosurg Psychiatry* 2009; 80:591-3.

[34] Kipps CM, Hodges JR, & Hornberger M. Nonprogressive behavioural variant frontotemporal dementia: recent developments and clinical implications of the "bvFTD phenocopy syndrome". *Curr Opin Neurol* 2010; 23(6):628-32.

[35] Piguet O, Hornberger M, Mioshi E, & Hodges JR. Behavioural-variant frontotemporal dementia: diagnosis, clinical staging, and management. *Lancet Neurol* 2011; 10(2):162-72.

[36] Khan BK, Yokoyama JS, Takada LT, Sha SJ, Rutherford NJ, Fong JC, et al. Atypical., slowly progressive behavioural frontotemporal dementia associated with C9ORF72 hexanucleotide expansion. *J Neurol Neurosurg Psychiatry* 2012; 83:358-64.

[37] Leyton CE, Villemagne VL, Savage S, Pike KE, Ballard KJ, Piguet O, et al. Subtypes of progressive aphasia: application of the International Consensus Criteria and validation using β-amyloid imaging. *Brain* 2011; 134:3030-43.

[38] Sajjadi SA, Patterson K, Arnold RJ, Watson PC, & Nestor PJ. Primary progressive aphasia. *Neurology* 2012; 78:1670-7.

[39] Kertesz A, McMonagle P, Blair M, Davidson W, & Munoz DG. The evolution and pathology of frontotemporal dementia. *Brain* 2005; 128:1996-2005.

[40] Boeve BF. Links between frontotemporal lobar degeneration, corticobasal degeneration, progressive supranuclear palsy, and amyotrophic lateral sclerosis. *Alzheimer Dis Assoc Disord* 2007; 21(4):S31-S38.

[41] Espay AJ, & Litvan I. Parkinsonism and frontotemporal dementia: the clinical overlap. *J Mol Neurosci* 2011; 45:343-9.

[42] Kertesz A. Pick complex: an integrative approach to frontotemporal dementia. *Neurologist* 2003; 9(6):311-7.

[43] Kertesz A, McMonagle P, & Jesso S. Extrapyramidal syndromes in frontotemporal degeneration. *J Mol Neurosci* 2011; 45(3): 336-42.

[44] Litvan I, Bhatia KP, Burn DJ, Goetz CG, Lang AE, McKeith I, et al. Movement Disorders Society Scientific Issues Committee report: SIC Task Force appraisal of clinical diagnostic criteria for parkinsonian disorders. *Mov Disord* 2003; 18(5):467-86.

[45] Kertesz A, & McMonagle P. Behavior and cognition in corticobasal degeneration and progressive supranuclear palsy. *J Neurol Sci* 2010; 289:138-43.

[46] Lee SE, Rabinovici GD, Mayo MC, Wilson SM, Seeley WW, DeArmond SJ, et al. Clinicopathological correlations in corticobasal degeneration. *Ann Neurol* 2011; 70:327-40.

[47] Mathew R, Bak TH, & Hodges JR. Diagnostic criteria for corticobasal syndrome: a comparative study. *J Neurol Neurosurg Psychiatry* 2012; 83:405-10.

[48] Graham NL, Bak TH, & Hodges JR. Corticobasal degeneration as a cognitive disorder. *Mov Disord* 2003; 18(11):1224-32.

[49] Lomen-Hoerth C. Clinical phenomenology and neuroimaging correlates in ALS-FTD. *J Mol Neurosci* 2011; 45:656-62.

[50] Bak TH. Motor neuron disease and frontotemporal dementia: one, two, or three diseases? *Ann Indian Acad Neurol* 2010; 13(2):S81-S88.

[51] Phukan J, Elamin M, Bede P, Jordan N, Gallagher L, Byrne S, et al. The syndrome of cognitive impairment in amyotrophic lateral sclerosis: a population-based study. *J Neurol Neurosurg Psychiatry* 2012; 83:102-8.

[52] Heinemann U, Gawinecka J, Schmidt C, & Zerr I. Differential diagnosis of rapid progressive dementia. *Eur Neurol Rev* 2010; 5(2):21-8.

[53] Geschwind MD, Shu H, Haman A, Sejvar JJ, & Miller BL. Rapidly progressive dementia. *Ann Neurol* 2008; 64(1):97-108.

[54] Schoder D, Hannequin D, Martinaud O, Opolczynski G, Guyant-Maréchal L, Le Ber I, et al. Morbid risk for schizophrenia in first-degree relatives of people with frontotemporal dementia. *Br J Psychiatry* 2010; 197(1):28-35.

[55] Momeni P, DeTucci K, Straub RE, Weinberger DR, Davies P, Grafman J, et al. Progranulin (GRN) in two siblings of a Latino family and in other patients with schizophrenia. *Neurocase* 2010; 16(3):273-9.

[56] Cooper JJ, & Ovsiew F. The relationship between schizophrenia and frontotemporal dementia. *J Geriatr Psychiatry Neurol* 2013; 26(3):131-7.

[57] Floris G, Borghero G, Cannas A, Di Stefano F, Murru MR, Corongiu D, et al. Bipolar affective disorder preceding frontotemporal dementia in a patient with C9orf72 mutation: is there a genetic link between these two disorders? *J Neurol* 2013; 160: 1155-7.

[58] Galimberti D, Fenoglio C, Serpente M, Villa C, Bonsi R, Arighi A, et al. Autosomal dominant frontotemporal lobar degeneration due to the C9ORF72 hexanucleotide repeat expansion: late-onset psychotic clinical presentation. *Biol Psychiatry* 2013; 74:384-91.

[59] Woolley JD, Khan BK, Murthy NK, Miller BL, & Rankin KP. The diagnostic challenge of psychiatric symptoms in neurodegenerative diseases: rates and risk factors for prior psychiatric diagnosis in patients with early neurodegenerative disease. *J Clin Psychiatry* 2011; 72(2):126-33.

[60] Mendez MF. The neurobiology of moral behaviour: review and neuropsychiatric implications. *CNS Spectr* 2009; 14(11):608-20.

[61] Synofzik M, Biskup S, Leyhe T, Reimold M, Fallgatter AJ, & Metger F. Suicide attempt as the presenting symptom of C9orf72 dementia. *Am J Psychiatry* 2012; 11:1211-3.

[62] Ibanez N. Atypical presentation of frontotemporal dementia masquerading as bipolar disorder and substance abuse: a case report. *W V Med J* 2012; 108(4):16-7.

[63] Pompanin S, Perini G, Toffanin T, Gnoato F, Cecchin D, Manara R, et al. Late-onset OCD as presenting manifestation of semantic dementia. *Gen Hosp Psychiatry* 2012; 34(1):102.e1-4.

[64] Manes FF, Torralva T, Roca M, Gleichgerrcht E, Bekinschtein TA, & Hodges JR. Frontotemporal dementia presenting as pathological gambling. *Nat Rev Neurol* 2010 ; 6(6) :347-52.

[65] Wylie MA, Shnall A, Onyike CU, & Huey ED. Management of frontotemporal dementia in mental health and multidisciplinary settings. *Int Rev Psychiatry* 2013; 25(2):230-6.

[66] Pose M, Cetkovich M, Gleichgerrcht E, Ibanez A, Torralva T, & Manes F. The overlap of symptomatic dimensions between frontotemporal dementia and several psychiatric disorders that appear in late adulthood. *Int Rev Psychiatry* 2013; 25(2):159-67.

[67] Hutchinson AD, & Mathias JL. Neuropsychological deficits in frontoemporal dementia and Alzheimer's disease: a meta-analytic review. *J Neurol Neurosurg Psychiatry* 2007; 78(9):917-28.

[68] Mathias JL, & Morphett K. Neurobehavioral differences between Alzheimer's disease and frontotemporal dementia: a meta-analysis. *J Clin Exp Neuropsychol* 2010; 32(7):682-98.

[69] Manoochehri M, & Huey ED. Diagnosis and management of behavioural issues in frontotemporal dementia. *Curr Neurol Neurosci Rep* 2012; 12(5):528-36.

[70] Freitas S, Simoes MR, Alves L, Duro D, & Santana I. Montreal Cognitive Assessment (MoCA): validation study for frontotemporal dementia. *J Geriatr Psychiatry Neurol* 2012; 25(3):146-54.

[71] Dubois B, Slachevsky A, Litvan I, & Pillon B. The FAB: a Frontal Assessment Battery at bedside. *Neurology* 2000; 55(11):1621-6.

[72] Valverde AH, Jimenez-Escrig A, Gobernado J, & Baron M. A short neuropsychologic and cognitive evaluation of frontotemporal dementia. *Clin Neurol Neurosurg* 2009; 111(3):251-5.

[73] Sorbi S, Hort J, Erkinjuntti T, Fladby T, Gainotti G, Gurvit H, et al. EFNS-ENS guidelines on the diagnosis and management of disorders associated with dementia. *Eur J Neurol* 2012; 19(9):1159-79.

[74] Mendez MF, Shapira JS, McMurtray A, Licht E, & Miller BL. Accuracy of the clinical evaluation for frontotemporal dementia. *Arch Neurol* 2007; 64:830-5.

[75] Rohrer JD, & Rosen HJ. Neuroimaging in frontotemporal dementia. Int Rev Psychiatry 2013; 25(2):221-9.

[76] Whitwell JL, & Josephs KA. Recent advances in the imaging of frontotemporal dementia. *Curr Neurol Neurosci Rep* 2012; 12(6):715-23.

[77] McGinnis SM. Neuroimaging in neurodegenerative dementias. *Semin Neurol* 2012; 32:347-360.

[78] Tatsch K, & Poepperl G. Nigrostriatal dopamine terminal imaging with dopamine transporter SPECT: an update. *J Nucl Med* 2013; 54:1331-8.

[79] Sieben A, van Langenhove T, Engelborghs S, Martin JJ, Boon P, Cras P, et al. The genetic and neuropathology of frontotemporal lobar degeneration. *Acta Neuropathol* 2012; 124:353-72.

[80] Cerami C, Scarpini E, Cappa SF, & Galimberti D. Frontotemporal lobar degeneration: current knowledge and future challenges. *J Neurol* 2012; 259:2278-86.

[81] Wood EM, Falcone D, Suh ER, Irwin JD, Chen-Plotkin AS, Lee EB, et al. Development and validation of pedigree classification criteria for frontotemporal lobar degeneration. *JAMA Neurol* 2013; 70(11):1411-7.

[82] Rademakers R, Neumann M, & Mackenzie IR. Recent advances in the molecular basis of frontotemporal dementia. *Nat Rev Neurol* 2012; 8(8):423-34.

[83] Quaid KA. Genetic counselling for frontotemporal dementias. *J Mol Neurosci* 2011; 45:706-9.

[84] Goldman JS, Rademakers R, Huey ED, Boxer AL., Mayeux R, Miller BL, et al. An algorithm for genetic testing of frontotemporal lobar degeneration. *Neurology* 2011; 76:475-83.

[85] Pelicano Paulos J, & Massano J. Clinical., genetic and neuropathological features of frontotemporal dementia: an update and guide. *Acta Med Port* 2013; 26(4):392-401.

[86] Borroni B, & Padovani A. Dementia: a new algorithm for molecular diagnostics in FTLD. *Nar Rev Neurol* 2013; 9(5):241-2.

[87] Van Langenhove T, van der Zee J, Gijselink I, Engelborghs S, Vanderberghe R, Vandenbulcke M, et al. Distinct clinical characteristics of C9orf72 expansion carriers compared with GRN, MAPT, and nonmutation carriers in a Flanders-Belgian FTLD cohort. *JAMA Neurol* 2013; 70(3):365-73.

[88] Grossman M. Biomakers to identify the pathological basis for frontotemporal lobar degeneration. *J Mol Neurosci* 2011; 45(3):366-71.

[89] Hales CM, & Hu WT. From frontotemporal lobar degeneration pathology to frontotemporal lobar degeneration biomarkers. *Int Rev Psychiatry* 2013; 25(2):210-20.

[90] Ghidoni R, Paterlini A, & Benussi L. Translational proteomics in Alzheimer's disease and related disorders. *Clin Biochem* 2013; 46(6):480-6.

[91] Hu WT, Trojanowski JQ, & Shaw LM. Biomarkers in frontotemporal lobar degenerations – Progress and challenges. *Prog Neurobiol* 2011; 95(4):636-48.

[92] Mackenzie IR, Neumann M, Bigio EH, Cairns NJ, Alafuzoff I, Kril J, et al. Nomenclature and nosology for neuropathologic subtypes of frontotemporal lobar degeneration: an update. *Acta Neuropathol* 2010; 119:1-4.

[93] Toledo JB, Brettschneider J, Grossman M, Arnold SE, Hu WT, Xie SX, et al. CSF biomarkers cutoffs: the importance of coincident neuropathological diseases. *Acta Neuropathol* 2012; 124:23-35.

[94] Mackenzie IR, Neumann M, Cairns NJ, Munoz DG, & Isaacs AM. Novel types of frontotemporal lobar degeneration: beyond tau and TDP-43. *J Mol Neurosci* 2011; 45(3):402-8.

[95] Arnold SE, Toledo JB, Appleby DH, Xie SX, Wang LS, Baek Y, et al. Comparative survey of the topographical distribution of signature molecular lesions in major neurodegenerative diseases. *J Comp Neurol* 2013; 521:4339-55.

[96] Jucker M, & Walker LC. Pathogenic protein seeding in Alzheimer's disease and other neurodegenerative disorders. *Ann Neurol* 2011; 70(4):532-40.

[97] Caccamo A, Magri A, Medina DX, Wisely EV, Lopez-Aranda MF, Silva AJ, et al. mTOR regulates tau phosphorylation and degradation: implications for Alzheimer's disease and other tauopathies. *Aging Cell* 2013; 12:370-80.

[98] Rosso SM, Landweer EJ, Houtermann M, Donker Kaat L, van Duijn CM, & van Swieten JC. Medical and environmental risk factors for sporadic frontotemporal dementia: a retrospective case-control study. *J Neurol Neurosurg Psychiatry* 2003; 74:1574-6.

[99] Kiraly MA, & Kiraly SJ. Traumatic brain injury and delayed sequelae: a review – Traumatic brain injury and mild traumatic brain injury (concussion) are precursors to later-onset brain disorders, including early-onset dementia. *ScientificWorldJournal* 2007; 7:1768-76.

[100] Jawaid A, Rademakers R, Kass JS, Kalkonde Y, & Schulz PE. Traumatic brain injury may increase the risk for frontotemporal dementia through reduced progranulin. *Neurodegenerative Dis* 2009; 6:219-20.

[101] Squitti R, Gorgone G, Panetta V, Lucchini R, Bucossi S, Albini E, et al. Implications of metal exposure and liver function in Parkinsonian patients resident in the vicinity of ferroalloy plants. *J Neural Transm* 2009; 116:1281-7.

[102] Van Deerlin VM, Sleiman PM, Martinez-Lage M, Chen-Plotkin A, Wang LS, Graff-Radford NR, et al. Common variants at 7p21 are associated with frontotemporal lobar degeneration with TDP-43 inclusions. *Nat Genet* 2010; 42(3):234-9.

[103] Kerchner GA, Tartaglia MC, & Boxer AL. Abhorring the vacuum: use of Alzheimer's disease medications in frontotemporal dementia. *Expert Rev Neurother* 2011; 11(5):709-17.

[104] Hodges JR. Hope abandoned: memantine therapy in frontotemporal dementia. *Lancet Neurol* 2013; 12:121-3

[105] Nardell M, & Tampi RR. Pharmacological treatments for frontotemporal dementias: a systematic review of randomized controlled trials. *Am J Alzheimers Dis Other Demen* 2014; 29(2):123-32.

[106] Weder ND, Aziz R, Wilkins K, & Tampi RR. Frontotemporal dementia: a review. *Ann Gen Psychiatry* 2007; 6:15

[107] Portugal MdaG, Marinho V, & Laks J. Pharmacological treatment of frontotemporal lobar degeneration: systematic review. *Rev Bras Psiquiatr* 2011; 33(1):81-90.

[108] Deakin JB, Rahman S, Nestor PJ, Hodges JR, & Sahakian BJ. Paroxetine does not improve symptoms and impairs cognition in frontotemporal dementia: a double-blind randomized controlled trial. *Psychopharmacology* 2004; 172:400-8.

[109] Gareri P, De Fazio P, Manfredi VGL, & De Sarro G. Use and safety of antipsychotics in behavioural disorders in elderly people with dementia. *J Clin Psychopharmacol* 2014; 34:109-23.

[110] Lauterbach EC, & Mendez MF. Psychopharmacological neuroprotection in neurodegenerative diseases, part III: criteria-based assessment: a report of the ANPA committee on research. *J Neuropsychiatry Clin Neurosci* 2011; 23:242-60.

[111] Finger EC. New potential therapeutic approaches in frontotemporal dementia: oxytocin, vasopressin, and social cognition. *J Mol Neurosci* 2011; 45:696-701.

[112] Brunden KR, Trojanowski JQ, Smith III AB, Lee V, & Ballatore C. Microtubule-stabilizing agents as potential therapeutics for neurodegenerative disease. *Bioorg Med Chem* 2013 (ahead of print, doi: 10.1016/j.bmc.2013.12.046).

[113] Boxer AL., Gold M, Huey E, Hu WT, Rosen H, Kramer J, et al. The advantages of FTD drug development (part 2 of FTD: the next therapeutic frontier). *Alzheimers Dement* 2013; 9(2):189-98.

[114] Boxer AL., Gold M, Huey E, Gao FB, Burton EA, Chow T, et al. Frontotemporal degeneration, the next therapeutic frontier: molecules and animal models for frontotemporal degeneration drug development. *Alzheimers Dement* 2013; 9(2):176-188.

[115] Golde TE, Borchelt DR, Giasson BI, & Lewis J. Thinking laterally about neurodegenerative proteinopathies. *J lin Invest* 2013; 123(5):1847-55.

[116] Piguet O. Frontotemporal dementia – time to target inflammation? *Nat Rev Neurol* 2013; 9(6):304-5.

[117] Buchanan JA, Christenson A, Houlihan D, & Ostrom C. The role of behaviour analysis in the rehabilitation of persons with dementia. *Behav Ther* 2011; 42(1):9-21.

[118] Kortte KB, & Rogalski EJ. Behavioural intervention for enhancing life participation in behavioural variant frontotemporal dementia and primary progressive aphasia. *Int Rev Psychiatry* 2013; 25(2):237-45.

[119] Gitlin LN, Winter L, Dennis MP, Hodgson N, & Hauck WW. Targeting and managing behavioral symptoms in individuals with dementia: a randomized trial of a nonpharmacological intervention. *J Am Geriatr Soc* 2010; 58:1465-74.

[120] Gitlin LN, Winter L, Dennis MP, Hodgson N, & Hauck WW. A biobehavioral home-based intervention and the well-being of patients with dementia and their caregivers. *JAMA* 2010; 304(9):983-91.

[121] Henry ML, Meese MV, Truong S, Babiak MC, Miller BL, & Gorno-Tempini ML. Treatment for apraxia of speech in nonfluent variant primary progressive aphasia. *Behav Neurol* 2013; 26:77-88.

[122] Jokel R, & Anderson ND. Quest for the best: effects of errorless and active encoding on word re-learning in semantic dementia. *Neuropsychol Rehabil* 2012; 22(2):187-214.

[123] Fried-Oken M, Beukelmann DR, & Hux K. Current and future AAC research considerations for adults with acquired cognitive and communication impairments. *Assist Technol* 2011; 24(1):56-66.

[124] Shnall A, Agate A, Grinberg A, Huijbregts M, Nguyen MQ, & Chow TW. Development of supportive services for frontotemporal dementias through community engagement. *Int Rev Psychiatry* 2013; 25(3):246-52.

[125] Chemali Z, Withall A, & Daffner KR. The plight of caring for young patients with frontotemporal dementia. *Am J Alzheimers Dis Other Demen* 2010; 25(2):109-15.

[126] Nunnemann S, Kurz A, Leucht S, & Diehl-Schmid J. Caregivers of patients with frontotemporal lobar degeneration: a review of burden, problems, needs, and interventions. *Int Psychogeriatr* 2012; 24(9):1368-86.

[127] Miller LA, Mioshi E, Savage S, Lah S, Hodges JR, & Piguet O. Identifying cognitive and demographic variables that contribute to carer burden in dementia. *Dement Geriatr Cogn Disord* 2013; 36:43-49.

[128] IHA/WFN. International Huntington Association and the World Federation of Neurology Research Group on Huntington's Chorea. Guidelines for the molecular genetics predictive test in Huntington's disease. *J Med Genet* 1994; 31:555-9.

[129] Tibben A. Predictive testing for Huntington's disease. *Brain Res Bull* 2007; 72(2-3):165-71.

[130] Meuser TM, & Marwit SJ. A comprehensive, stage-sensitive model of grief in dementia caregiving. *Gerontologist* 2001; 41(5):658-70.

[131] Ettema EJ, Derksen LD, & van Leeuwen E. Existential loneliness and end-of-life care: a systematic review. *Theor Med Bioeth* 2010; 31:141-69.

[132] McLennon SM, Habermann B, & Rice M. Finding meaning as a mediator of burden on the health of caregivers of spouses with dementia. *Aging Ment Health* 2011; 15(4):522-30.

[133] Krstic D, & Knuesel I. The airbag problem – a potential culprit for bench-to-bedside translational efforts: relevance for Alzheimer's disease. *Acta Neuropathol Commun* 2013; 1:62.

[134] Liu R, Yang G, Nonaka T, Tetsuaki A, Jia W, & Cynader MS. Reducing TDP-43 aggregation does not prevent its cytotoxicity. *Acta Neuropathol Commun* 2013; 1:49.

[135] Holman C, & de Villers-Sidani E. Indestructible plastic: the neuroscience of the new aging brain. *Front Hum Neurosci* 2014; 8:219.

[136] Walhovd KB, Fjell AM, & Espeseth T. Cognitive decline and brain pathology in aging – need for a dimensional., lifespan and systems vulnerability view. *Scand J Psychol* 2014; 55(3):244-54.

[137] Hu F, & Liu F. Targeting tissue-specific metabolic signalling pathways in aging: the promises and limitations. *Protein Cell* 2014; 5(1):21-35.

[138] Vijg J. Aging genomes: A necessary evil in the logic of life. *Bioessays 2014*; 36:282-92.

[139] Nussey DH, Froy H, Lemaitre JF, Gaillard JM, & Austad SN. Senescence in natural populations of animals: Widespread evidence and its implications for bio-gerontology. *Ageing Res Rev* 2013; 12(1):214-25.

[140] Blagosklonny MV. Why the disposable soma theory cannot explain why women live longer and why we age. *Aging* 2010; 2(12):884-7.

In: Dementia
Editor: Pamela Tanner

ISBN: 978-1-63321-928-1

Chapter 7

Risk Factors for Alzheimer's Disease

R. A. Armstrong*
Vision Sciences, Aston University, Birmingham, UK

Abstract

A large number of possible risk factors have been associated with Alzheimer's disease (AD).

This chapter discusses the validity of the major risk factors that have been identified including age, genetics, exposure to aluminum, head injury, malnutrition and diet, mitochondrial dysfunction, vascular disease, immune system dysfunction, and infection and proposes a hypothesis to explain how these various risk factors may cause AD pathology.

Rare forms of early-onset familial AD (FAD) are strongly linked to the presence of specific gene mutations, viz. mutations in *amyloid precursor protein (APP)* and *presenilin (PSEN1/2)* genes. By contrast, late-onset sporadic AD (SAD) is a multifactorial disorder in which age-related changes, genetic risk factors, such as allelic variation in *apolipoprotein E (Apo E)* gene, vascular disease, head injury and risk factors associated with diet, immune system, mitochondrial function, and infection may all be involved.

These risk factors interact to increase the rate of normal aging ('allostatic load') which over a lifetime results in degeneration of neurons and blood vessels and as a consequence, the formation of abnormally aggregated 'reactive' proteins such as β-amyloid (Aβ) and tau leading to the development of senile plaques (SP) and neurofibrillary tangles (NFT) respectively. Life-style changes that may reduce the allostatic load and therefore, the risk of dementia are discussed.

Keywords: Alzheimer's disease (AD), Risk factors, Aging, Genetics, Environmental factors, Allostatic load

* Corresponding author: Dr R.A.Armstrong, Vision Sciences, Aston University, Birmingham B4 7ET, UK (Tel 0121-204-4102, Fax 0121-204-4048, Email R.A.Armstrong@aston.ac.uk)

Introduction

Cognitive impairment together with the formation of a characteristic pathology, viz., extracellular senile plaques (SP) and intracellular neurofibrillary tangles (NFT) are regarded as the defining features of Alzheimer's disease (AD) (Khatchaturian, 1985; Mirra et al., 1991). The term AD was first used in 1910 by Kraepelin based on the clinical and pathological description of Alzheimer's original cases (Alzheimer, 1907). Of the two cases originally described by Alzheimer, however, both had numerous SP, but only one had significant numbers of NFT (Graeber et al., 1997), thus identifying the pathological heterogeneity characteristic of AD (Armstrong et al., 2000), and creating difficulties in establishing a single theory as to its cause.

As a result, many theories have been proposed as possible causes of AD (Armstrong, 2013), including exacerbation of aging, genetic factors, exposure to aluminum, head injury, malnutrition and diet, mitochondrial dysfunction, vascular disease, immune system dysfunction, and infectious agents. However, no single theory has gained universal acceptance and it has become increasingly recognized that AD is a multifactorial disorder, especially the common late-onset sporadic form of the disease (SAD). As a consequence, a large number of risk factors have been implicated in AD (Table 1). The objective of this chapter is to review the validity of the major risk factors that have been identified including: (1) age, (2) genetic factors, (3) exposure to aluminum, (4) head injury, (5) diet and malnutrition, (6) mitochondrial dysfunction, (7) vascular factors, (8) immune system factors, and (9) infection. A hypothetical model is proposed to explain how these various risk factors could result in the pathology characteristic of AD. In addition, life-style changes which could reduce the risk of developing dementia are discussed.

Age As a Risk Factor

Age is often regarded as the most important risk factor for AD. With advancing age, the prevalence of the disease increases to an estimated 19% in individuals 75-84 years of age (Knopman, 2001) and to 30-35% (Ferri et al., 2005), possibly up to 50% for those older than 85 years. That AD may be an accelerated form of aging is largely based on the observation that the many of the pathological changes in AD are similar to those present in normal aging apart from their severity (Reisberg, 1983; Rossor and Mountjoy, 1986). Hence, in cognitively normal brain, there is an age-related reduction in brain volume and weight, enlargement of ventricles, and loss of synapses and dendrites in selected areas (Imhof et al., 2007). Accompanying these changes are the characteristic pathological features of AD, including SP and NFT (Fig 1). Hence, in 60 normal elderly cases (Mann et al., 1987), 32/60 had no SP, although 30/60 were younger than 65 years, 13/60 had SP in the hippocampus, and 12/60 had SP in temporal cortex. It was concluded that it was not possible to distinguish early-stage AD from normal aging at post-mortem (Mann et al., 1987). In addition, the density of neuritic plaques (NP), which incorporate dystrophic neurites (DN), and SP with a distinct 'core' ('classic' plaques), may not be significantly different in AD and aging (Bell and Ball, 1990). In the study of Bergeron et al. (1987), SP have been observed in 60% of normal elderly cases, albeit at lower density than in AD. Similarly, Arrigada et al. (1992) reported SP in most normal individuals older than 55 years of age and concluded that there could be a 'continuum' of pathological change from elderly non-demented brains, early stage AD, to advanced AD (Armstrong, 2012a).

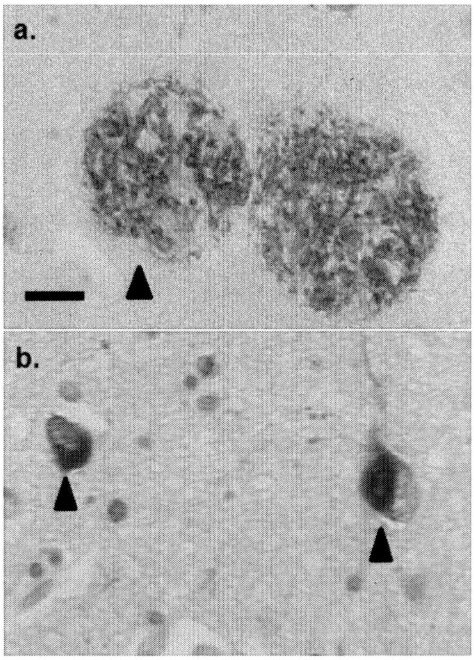

Figure 1. The 'signature' pathological lesions of Alzheimer's disease (AD): (a) senile plaques (SP) (arrow) (Aβ immunohistochemistry), (b) neurofibrillary tangles (NFT) (arrows) (tau immunohistochemistry), Magnification bar = 10 μm).

Whether NFT also occur as a result of normal aging is more controversial. Some studies suggest that the majority of cognitively normal individuals have minimal NFT (Knopman et al., 2003) and also less astrocytosis and microglial reaction (Coria et al. 1993). By contrast, Bouras et al. (1993) found that all non-demented cases had NFT in lamina II of the entorhinal cortex and in sector CA1 of the hippocampus. Moreover, in non-demented individuals, NFT were more numerous in medial temporal lobe and cortical association areas when a memory deficit was present suggesting NFT could be related to memory loss in non-demented as well as demented cases (Guillozet et al., 2003). In medial temporal lobe, the perforant path, which connects the entorhinal cortex to the dentate gyrus, appears to be sensitive to the development of NFT in AD and these changes may be distinct from those seen in normal aging even in the oldest individuals (Garcia-Sierra et al., 2003).

Two further aging processes may be involved in AD. First, an age-related breakdown of myelin (Bartzokis, 2011), although other studies suggest that myelin loss occurs late in AD and is secondary to neuronal degeneration (Brun, 1983). Second, there is loss of cells in the locus caeruleus (LC), which provides an input of noradrenaline to the cortex via terminal varicosities, and stimulates microglia to suppress production of Aβ (Heneka et al., 2010). NFT appear early in the LC in aging, mild cognitive impairment (MCI), and in AD (Grudzien et al., 2007). Loss of cells in the LC may therefore induce an age-related impairment of the blood brain barrier, thus implicating factors associated with the vascular system (Mann, 1985).

Table 1. Risk factors associated with Alzheimer's disease

Grouping	Risk factor
Demographic	Age
	Gender
Genetics	*Amyloid precursor protein (APP)*
	Presenilin 1 and 2 (PSEN1/2)
	Apolipoprotein E (Apo E)
	Triggering receptor expressed on myeloid cells 2 (TREM 2)
	Estrogen receptor gene (ESR)
	Hemochromatosis gene (HFE)
	Clusterin gene (CLU)
	Histocompatibility locus antigen (HLA Class III)
	Transferrin gene (Tf)
Lifestyle	Lack of exercise
	Lack of social engagement
	Lack of cognitive activity
	Smoking
	Alcohol
	Poor diet
	Increasing stress
	Education level
Co-morbidity	High blood pressure
	Poorly controlled type-2 diabetes
	High blood cholesterol
	Head trauma
	Congestive heart failure
	Oral infections
	Stroke
	Obesity
	Micro-infarcts
	Hypertension
	Depression
	Cancer
Environmental	Aluminum
	Viruses, e.g., Epstein-Barr virus (EBV), Human herpes virus 6 (HHV-6)
	Surgery/anesthesia
	Vitamin deficiency
	Military service
	Pesticides
	Organic solvents

These studies suggest that the differences between AD and the normal elderly are largely quantitative rather than qualitative and that there may be a 'continuum' of pathological change connecting these cases (Armstrong, 2012b). An important question, therefore, is whether AD is an exacerbation of normal aging resulting from enhanced spread of pathology along anatomical pathways (Armstrong, 2013).

Genetic Risk Factors

In the 1990s, strong evidence emerged of the connection between some forms of early-onset familial AD (FAD) and specific genetic factors. Hence, small numbers of cases were linked to mutations of *amyloid precursor protein (APP)* gene (Chartier-Harlin et al., 199, Goate et al., 1991) and a larger subgroup to mutations of *presenilin* genes *(PSEN1/2)* (Levy-Lahad et al., 1995; Sherrington et al., 1993). Moreover, allelic variation in the *apolipoprotein E (Apo E)* gene on chromosome 19 was identified as a significant risk factor, especially in late-onset sporadic AD (SAD) (Saunders et al., 1993; Strittmatter et al., 1993).

APP

Cleavage of *APP* results in the formation of a variety of Aβ peptides (Greenberg, 1995), the most common being $A\beta_{42,}$ found largely in SP, whereas the more soluble $A\beta_{40}$ is also found in association with cerebral microvessels (Miller et al., 1993) and may develop later in the disease (Delacourte et al., 2002). In addition, mutations of *APP* within the Aβ coding region may result in the deposition of $A\beta_{38}$ in vessel walls, especially in cases with extensive cerebral amyloid angiopathy (CAA) (Moro et al., 2012). Causation of AD could also be attributable to early soluble peptide oligomers (Gessel et al., 2012), which vary with the type of mutant, thus providing a genetic basis for variation in pathogenesis among FAD cases. The discovery of Aβ led to the formulation of the 'Amyloid Cascade Hypothesis' (ACH), the most influential model of the molecular pathology of AD developed over the last 25 years (Hardy and Higgins, 1992) (Fig 2). Essentially, the ACH proposes that the deposition of Aβ peptides is the initial pathological event in AD leading to the formation of SP and NFT, and then to cell death and clinical dementia (Hyman and Tanzi, 1992). Hence, risk factors which result in the formation of Aβ have been given considerable prominence in AD.

PSEN1/2

FAD is also linked to mutations of *PSEN1/2* genes (Levy-Lahad et al., 1995; Sherrington et al., 1993), and is the most common form of early-onset FAD. Full length PSEN is composed of nine trans-membrane domains located on the endoplasmic reticulum membrane. Endoproteolytic cleavage of PSEN and assembly into γ-secretase complex is followed by transport to the cell surface, thus potentially influencing APP processing (Honarnejad and Hermis, 2012). Hence, mutant *PSEN1* could enhance 42-specific-γ-secretase cleavage of normal APP resulting in increased deposition of amyloid-forming species (Sudoh et al., 1998). Nevertheless, PSEN may have a variety of other functions. First, PSEN may also act via loss of function by a reduction in γ-secretase activity (Wolfe, 2012). Second, the *PSEN1* gene may be involved in notch signaling (Steiner et al., 1999) and therefore important in cell differentiation. Third, *PSEN1/2* genes may also be involved via the perturbation of cellular calcium homeostasis (Zatti et al., 2006) or in interactions with the transcriptional coactivator cAMP-response element binding (CREB-binding) protein which plays a key role in regulating gene expression (Francis et al., 2006). Fourth, *PSEN1* may also mediate neuroprotective functions by ephrin-B (Barthet et al., 2013) and a decline in such protection could also be involved in AD.

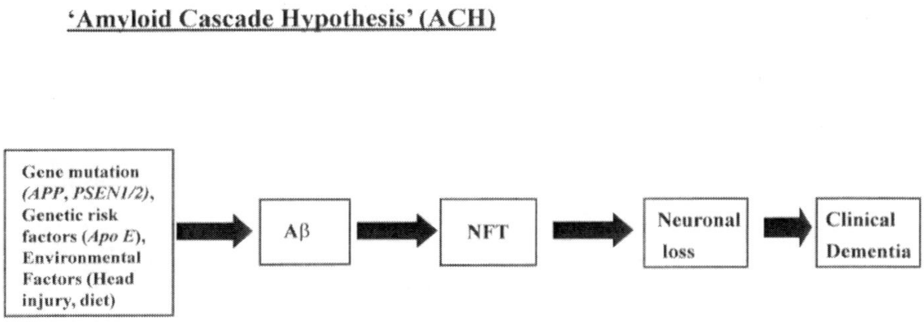

Figure 2. The Amyloid Cascade Hypothesis (ACH). The ACH proposes that the deposition of β-amyloid (Aβ) peptides is the initial pathological event in AD leading to the formation of senile plaques (SP) and neurofibrillary tangles (NFT), and then to cell death and clinical dementia. Other abbreviations: *Amyloid precursor protein* mutations (*APP*), *Presenilin genes 1 and 2* mutations (*PSEN1/2*, *Apolipoprotein E* (Apo E).

Apo E

Allelic variation in the *Apo E* gene is a major risk factor in SAD, individuals with AD having 2-3 times the frequency of allele ε4 compared with normal control cases (Saunders et al., 1993; Strittmatter et al., 1993). In addition, allele ε4 may accelerate the development of AD pathology within the aging brain (Oyama et al., 1995) and hence, may be associated with an earlier disease onset (Gomez-Isla et al., 1996). The majority of studies also report increased amyloid deposition and therefore SP, in individuals expressing allele ε4 (Beffort and Poirier, 1996; Berr et al., 1994; Polvikoski et al., 1995).

Other Genes

APP and *PSEN1/2* genes together account for less than 5% of all AD cases (Grazini et al., 2006; Hoenicka, 2006). Hence, SAD is more likely to be multifactorial with the potential involvement of many genetic and other types of risk factors. Hence, genome-wide studies have revealed genes associated with AD on chromosomes 6, 9, 10, 11, 12, 14, 18, 19 (Sillen et al., 2006; Burns et al., 2011) with the most compelling case for a gene on chromosome 12 (Panja et al., 2006). Further studies have mapped this gene to 12q13, a region which encompasses the vitamin D receptor (VDR) gene (Wang et al., 2011). This gene is a major mediator of the activity of vitamin D and insufficiency of this vitamin could therefore be a risk factor for AD. Additional genes which have recently been reported as possible risk factors include *glyceraldehyde-3-phosphate dehydrogenase* (*GAPDH*) (Allen et al., 2010), a rare variant of *the triggering receptor expressed on myeloid cells 2 (TREM2)* gene (Ruiz et al., 2014), genetic variation in the *estrogen receptor (ESR)* gene (Ryan et al., 2014), polymorphisms of the *clusterin (CLU)* gene (Ponomareva et al., 2013), and the *transferrin (Tf)* gene (Wang et al., 2013).

Aluminum

Much of the evidence that aluminum is a risk factor for AD is controversial (Armstrong et al., 1996). First, epidemiological studies (Graves et al., 1990; Neri and Hewitt, 1991; Martyn, 1992) have found little correlation between aluminum in the environment and AD. Second, out of 13 studies, in which gross brain tissue has been analyzed for aluminum, 9/13 found increased levels in AD brain, while 4/13 found no significant differences compared with control brains (Basun et al., 1991). The significance of an enhanced level of aluminum in brain is also controversial since damaged brains could accumulate aluminum (Armstrong et al., 1996). Third, the presence of aluminum may be linked to the formation of SP and NFT. Aluminum has been reported to be associated with the cores of classic Aβ deposits (Edwardson et al., 1986) but not in all studies (Landsberg et al., 1992) and it is unclear whether this type of SP is especially frequent in AD. Aluminum has also been detected in pyramidal neurons containing NFT (Perl and Brody, 1980; Perl and Pendlebury, 1986). Aluminum may bind to DNA and affect processing of cytoskeletal proteins resulting in the formation of NFT, although there is little evidence that aluminum can bind significantly to DNA (Dobson et al., 1993; Martyn, 1992). Fourth, patients with renal failure and exposed to high concentrations of aluminum do not develop cellular NFT (Perl and Brody, 1980). Fifth, whether or not exposure of experimental animals (Crapper et al., 1978) or cell cultures (Seil et al., 1969) to aluminum results in NFT formation is controversial. Experimentally induced cytoskeletal change usually results in the formation of straight 10 nm filaments, unlike the majority of NFT, which are composed of 20 – 24 nm twisted filaments (Terry and Pena, 1965), and which have different molecular composition to those of AD (Grunde-Iqbal et al., 1985). Sixth, neuropsychological conditions, which arise from acute exposure to aluminum, such as dialysis dementia (Arieff, 1985) or bladder irrigation (Murphy et al., 1992) in which a 1% alum solution is used to treat hemorrhagic cystitis, probably have little significance apart from demonstrating that aluminum in acute doses can be neurotoxic. Hence, the evidence does not suggest that aluminum is a significant risk factor for AD. However, a recent study in Australia reported significantly increased mortality from AD among miners exposed to aluminum dust (Peters et al., 2013) suggesting that some aspects of the aluminum hypothesis could be worth revisiting.

Head Injury

A number of studies suggest that previous head injury could be a risk factor for AD. Hence, in survivors of head injury, APP is observed in neuronal perikarya and in dystrophic neurites surrounding Aβ deposits, as observed in AD (Gentleman et al., 1993). Subsequently, it was shown that specific neurons in the medial temporal lobe secreted large quantities of APP and that there were more APP-immunoreactive neurons in these areas in head injury patients (McKenzie et al., 1994). Hence, increased expression of APP in head trauma cases may be an acute phase response to neuronal injury (Roberts et al., 1994), the overexpression of APP leading to the deposition of Aβ. Several acute phase proteins are localized within Aβ deposits in AD including amyloid-P, complement factors, and α-antichymotrypsin (Kalaria et al., 1993). Furthermore, Regland and Gottfries (1992) proposed that APP maintains cell function by supporting neuronal growth and survival. The possible neurotrophic action of APP is supported by the observation that it shares structural features with the precursor for epidermal growth factor. In addition, NFT may be part of the neurons response to injury (Wisniewski et al., 1994). These studies suggest that the formation of Aβ and tau as a result of brain injury could lead to AD pathology.

Diet and Malnutrition

Abalan (1984) was one of the first investigators to propose that malnutrition could be a risk factor for AD. This hypothesis was based on clinical observation of AD patients who often exhibited emaciation and cachexia, urinary tract infections, terminal bronchopneumonia, and low triceps skinfold. Low serum albumin, iron, folate, tryptophan, vitamin B12, and cerebral metabolism of glucose and oxygen were also present. These symptoms suggest a protein calorie malnutrition syndrome in AD which could result in the development of NFT due to a chronic nutritional deficiency of calcium/magnesium. A problem with this type of hypothesis, however, is in determining cause and effect, as malnutrition could be a consequence of mental state of the patient (Abalan, 1984). A more direct demonstration of a link between diet and AD was reported by Sparks et al. (1994) in which deposition of Aβ was induced in rabbits fed with high levels of dietary cholesterol. Moreover, although dietary cholesterol does not normally cross the blood brain barrier; in cholesterol-fed rabbits both enlarged ventricles and a reduction in cerebral vessels were observed (Schreurs et al., 2013). In addition, McCaddon and Kelly (1994) found in a human family carrying an APP_{717} mutation, that individuals with AD had a greater vitamin B12 deficiency compared with unaffected members. It was concluded that this link was unlikely to be a consequence of impaired dietary intake; further evidence that vitamin B12 deficiency could be a risk factor for AD.

Mitochondrial Dysfunction

Theories suggesting that mitochondrial dysfunction may be involved in AD have a long history (Blass and Zemcov, 1984) and rely on several lines of evidence. First, an early change in AD is the presence of swollen and distorted mitochondria accompanied by a decline in cerebral metabolic rate (Blass and Zemcov, 1984). Second, there is a deficiency of enzymes involved in carbohydrate utilization in AD including such mitochondrial markers as phosphofructokinase (PFK) and pyruvate dehydrogenase (Blass and Zemcov, 1984). Third, part of the familial aggregation of AD may be accounted for by excess maternal versus paternal inheritance consistent with mitochondrial inheritance. Hence, a genomic analysis of 1007 individuals suggested that possession of specific haplotypes could reduce AD risk, and therefore, there may be haplotypes, the possession of which would be risk factors for AD

(Ridge et al., 2012). The possibility of a genetic origin of mitochondrial dysfunction in AD has also led to the formulation of the 'mitochondrial cascade hypothesis' (MCH) in which it is mitochondrial dysfunction that is the root cause of the events leading to AD pathology (Swerdlow, 2012). Fourth, 'adaptor protein evolutionarily conserved signaling intermediate in Toll pathway' (ECSIT) is a protein which may act as a molecular sensor, ascertaining cell homeostasis in response to oxidative damage by Aβ (Soler-Lopez et al., 2012). Protective molecules could then be specifically activated in response and this failure could result in severe mitochondrial damage, promote apoptosis, and result in synaptic dysfunction and neuronal death (Soler-Lopez et al., 2012).

Vascular Disease

Several studies suggest that cardiovascular disease (CVD) could be a risk factor for AD (Liu et al., 2014). First, CVD may induce amyloid deposits and affect the age of onset of AD while deposition of Aβ can trigger cardiovascular degeneration (Lee et al., 2014). Second, individuals with congestive heart failure have a higher risk of dementia, especially vascular dementia (VD) (Hjelm et al., 2014). Third, obesity has been consistently associated with the presence of dementia, higher midlife body mass index (BMI) proportionally increasing AD risk (Tolppanen et al., 2014). Fourth, small infarcts and micro-bleeds are often associated with increasing Aβ burden in the brain (Benedictus et al., 2013). Fifth, an overall correlation has been established between various vascular risk factors and the neuropsychological symptoms of AD, but no individual vascular risk factor could predict change in any single neuropsychological feature (Steinberg et al., 2014).

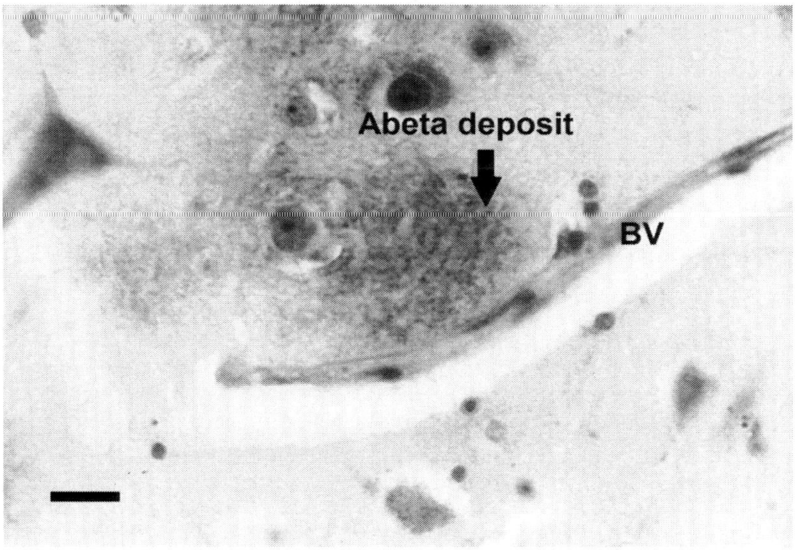

Figure 3. β-amyloid (Aβ) deposit (arrow) adjacent to a cerebral microvessel (BV) in the parahippocampal gyrus in a case of Alzheimer's disease (AD) (Aβ immuno-histochemistry Magnification bar = 10 μm).

A greater vascular involvement in the formation of SP has been observed in aging than in AD (Bell and Ball, 1990). Hence, SP have been observed in frontal and temporal cortex in 15/20 patients with critical stenosis, most often in the depths of the gyri (Sparks et al., 1990). Vascular factors may therefore be involved in SP formation and SP may not always be causally related to dementia. A further study of non-demented patients with critical coronary artery disease suggested that some patients had similar densities of SP to AD, numbers of SP being directly proportional to the duration of arterial disease (Sparks et al., 1990). In addition, there may a close link between ischaemic brain episodes and sporadic AD (SAD) suggesting that vascular factors could aggravate the progression of the disease (Pluta et al., 2012a,b).

Several studies have found evidence of pathology affecting the cerebral micro-vessels in AD. First, blood vessels with collapsed or degenerated endothelia are evident in more than 90% of AD cases (Kalaria and Hedera, 1995) and occur concurrently with Aβ deposition. Second, Tian et al. (2006) found that blood vessels underwent degenerative changes in AD accompanied by Aβ deposition and loss of smooth muscle cells. Third, Attems et al. (2004) found that $A\beta_{42}$ was deposited within the glia limitans rather than capillary walls. Fourth, some studies have found spatial correlations between Aβ deposits and blood vessels (Fig 3) suggesting that degeneration of blood vessels or diffusion of substances from vessels could be involved in the formation of Aβ deposits, therefore, supporting the hypothesis that vascular factors could be risk factors for AD (Perlmutter and Chui, 1990; Perlmutter et al., 1990; Miyakawa et al., 1992) By contrast, other studies conclude that the spatial correlations observed between Aβ deposits and blood vessels are fortuitous and arise because of the presence of high densities of capillary profiles and Aβ (Kawai et al., 1990; Luthert and Williams, 1991).

Vascular factors may also interact with genetics as risk factors for AD. Hence, plasma Aβ may be increased in FAD as well as in SAD (Su et al., 1999). In addition, a proportion of FAD cases exhibit CAA similar to that observed in SAD, viz., the deposition of Aβ in and around major blood vessels. Mutations of the *APP* gene within the Aβ region are often associated with familial CAA (Shin et al., 2003) while *APP* mutations outside the Aβ region result in a pathology deficient in $A\beta_{40,}$ and with lower levels of CAA (Kumar-Singh, 2008). In addition, possession of one or more *Apo E* ε4 alleles could also be linked to vascular pathology and significantly increase the risk of AD. In transgenic mice, for example, *Apo E* markedly promotes CAA associated vessel damage (Fryer et al., 2003).

Risk Factors Involving the Immune System

Several lines of evidence support the presence of immune system dysfunction in AD (Nandy, 1983, Rogers and Luber-Narod 1988; McGeer et al., 1991). First, complement proteins associated with the 'classical' pathway (Nandy, 1983), brain reactive antibodies (McGeer et al., 1991, immunoglobulins (Eikelenboom and Stam, 1982; Ishii and Haga, 1976), circulating immune complexes (CIC) in peripheral tissue and cerebral blood vessels (Heinonen et al., 1993), helper/inducer and cytotoxic/suppressor T-cells (McGeer et al., 1991), and abundant reactive microglia (McGeer et al., 1991) have all been observed in AD. Complement system proteins may act as pattern recognition molecules mediating the uptake of Aβ by glial cells which express complement receptors (Veerhuis, 2011). Second, alterations in the major histocompatibility locus (MHC) antigens have also been demonstrated (Walford and Fortoul, 1983) suggesting either increased resistance or susceptibility to a specific antigen in AD (Cohen et al., 1982; Henschke et al., 1978). Hence, several genes encoding the inflammatory mediators have been implicated in AD susceptibility, especially those of HLA class III region (Maggioli et al., 2013). Some of these immune reactions could be a response to the pathological processes of AD and especially to the deposition of Aβ. However, immune reactions could also be a response to an environmental factor, which would then be a significant risk factor for AD.

Infectious Agents As a Risk Factor

One of the first studies to suggest that infection could be a risk factor for AD was reported by Wisniewski et al. (1981) who suggested that invasion by a virus could cause activation of microglia and pericytes and ultimately, Aβ deposition. In addition, Libikova et al. (1975) suggested that the virus *herpes simplex* (HSV), to which antibodies may be observed in cerebral spinal fluid (CSF) in AD, could induce abnormal protein formation resulting in NFT. This type of theory has been given further credibility by observations of marked structural and biochemical alterations in regions of the AD brain associated with olfaction, most notably the olfactory bulb and entorhinal cortex (Doty et al., 1987); the olfactory system being a possible point of entry into the brain for an infectious agent or protein (Mann et al., 1987). Hence, viruses introduced into body cavities and organs often result in high titers of the virus in olfactory epithelium, olfactory bulb, and other brain regions. Nevertheless, HSV does not typically enter the brain via the olfactory system (Salazar et al., 1983) which argues against this common virus as a risk factor for AD. More recently, however, DNA from peripheral blood leucocytes and brain of AD patients has been analyzed for cytomegalovirus (CMV), Epstein-Barr virus (EBS), and human herpes virus 6 (HHV-6), the data suggesting that EPV and HHV-6 could be risk factors for the cognitive decline and progression to AD (Carbone et al., 2014). In addition, recent research suggests that dental infections could be a possible risk factor for AD (Rolim et al., 2014), a higher prevalence of the disease being observed in those patients with orofacial pain and periodontal infection.

Discussion and Conclusion

What are the Major Risk Factors for AD?

There is a clear association between AD and the processes of normal aging (Richardz-Saltburger et al., 2010), all features of AD being observed to some extent in aging cognitively normal brain (Reisberg, 1983). In addition, in rodent models of AD, the most important factors influencing the onset of 'AD' are often age-specific including: (1) perturbation of ribosomal and oxidative phosphorylation pathways, (b) changes in genes associated with the hypothalamic-pituitary-adrenal function, and (3) changes in insulin signaling (Jackson et al., 2013).

The theory which has had the most longevity and impact in AD research is the ACH (Hardy and Higgins, 1992) and hence, genetic risk factors related to Aβ deposition have often been given the greatest prominence. Genes directly linked to AD however, account for only a small proportion of cases; the *APP* and *PSEN1/2* genes together accounting for less than 5% of AD (Hoenicka, 2006). Genome-wide studies suggest that genes associated with AD may exert only very small risk effects over the disease as a whole. However, allelic variation in *Apo E* is likely to be an exception and is regarded as a significant risk factor in AD, especially in late-onset forms of the disease (O'Bryant et al., 2013). In addition, there are likely to be synergistic interactions between genes and other risk factors such as the presence of stroke, vascular disease, and diabetes that will increase the risk of AD (Percy et al., 2014).

Of the remaining risk factors that have been discussed, exposure to aluminum and other metals has been largely discounted, although there is some evidence that aluminum could accumulate in the brain and interact with processes that result in Aβ deposition and tau formation (Armstrong et al., 1995). However, study of diet, malnutrition, and head injury suggest that these could be additional risk factors for AD. In addition, there is evidence that of an association between AD and CVD (Lee et al., 2014), and that risk factors associated with CVD are also likely to be relevant to AD.

Immune system and mitochondrial dysfunction could also be implicated in AD and there may be several genes linked to these processes which may be identified as risk factors. In addition to the risk factors discussed in this review, a variety of further non-genetic factors have been associated with AD including exposure to pesticides, organic solvents, volatile anesthetics, various aspects of lifestyle, smoking, alcohol, coffee, degree of physical activity and cognitive activity (Jiang et al., 2013) (Table 1). It is likely that future research will identify many more such risk factors.

How Do Risk Factors Result in AD Pathology?

The study of the various risk factors associated with AD suggests that, with the exception of some forms of early-onset FAD, it is not primarily a disease linked to defective genes but a complex syndrome dependent on the rate of aging and indirectly influenced by genetic risk factors and the environment. A hypothesis which describes how these various risk factors may result in AD pathology is shown in Figure 4.

The primary factor in this scheme is age-dependent breakdown of anatomical systems and pathways within the brain and the consequent loss of synapses (Carroll 2002). The extent of this aging effect, which begins early in life, is mediated by the degree of lifetime stress (the 'allostatic load'). The brain is the ultimate mediator of stress-related mortality through hormonal changes resulting in hypertension, glucose intolerance, CVD, and immunological problems (Carroll, 2002). The consequence is gradual synaptic disconnection, neuronal degeneration, and the upregulation of genes which determine the production of reactive and breakdown products (Armstrong et al., 2002; Regland and Gottfries, 1992; Wallace et al., 1993). Second, in a small number of families, specific *APP* or *PSEN* mutations directly influence the outcome of this age-related degeneration by determining the solubility and/or toxicity of the molecular product. Cells have mechanisms to protect against the accumulation of misfolded and aggregated proteins including the ubiquitin system and the phagosome-lysosome system. Neuronal degeneration in individuals with specific mutations results in the accelerated formation of Aβ and tau, and then a further phase of 'secondary' neurodegeneration, which overwhelms these protection systems; early-onset FAD is the result of this process.

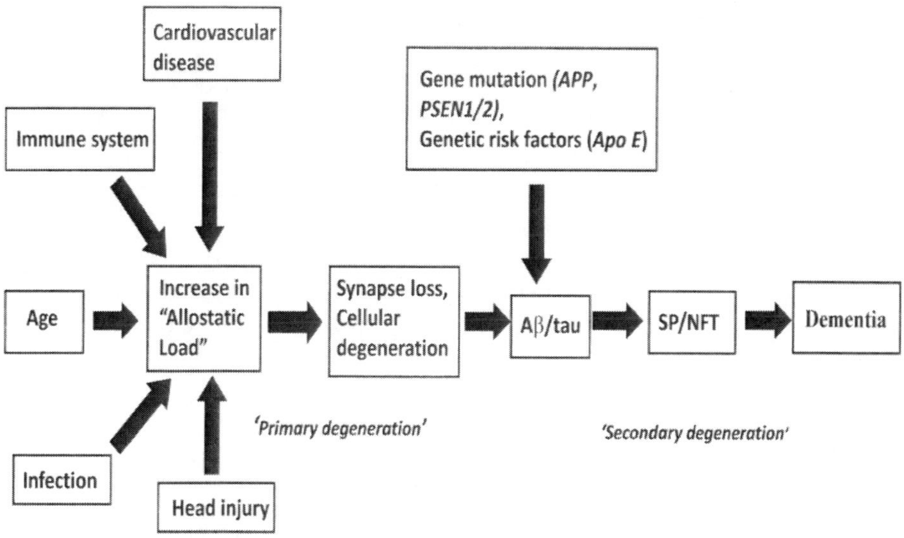

Figure 4. A scheme of how the various risk factors associated with Alzheimer's disease (AD) may cause the pathology associated with the disease. The various risk factors act in combination to increase the rate of normal aging ('allostatic load'), leading to degeneration of neural pathways and blood vessels and resulting in the formation of β-amyloid (Aβ) and tau and then senile plaques (SP) and neurofibrillary tangles (NFT). Other abbreviations: Apolipoprotein E gene (Apo E), Amyloid precursor protein gene (APP), Presenilin genes 1 and 2 (PSEN1/2).

By contrast, in individuals without specific genetic mutations, but where more complex genetic and environmental risk factors are present, the outcome of age-related loss of synapses is mainly soluble and smaller quantities of insoluble proteins which are degraded by the cellular protection systems and do not significantly accumulate to form SP and NFT. With advancing age, however, the protective systems become less effective resulting in slowly accumulating quantities of Aβ and tau. The result of these insidious processes is that the cellular protection systems do not become overwhelmed until much later in life, the consequence being late-onset SAD.

How could the Risk of AD be Reduced?

The implication of the proposed scheme is that it suggests life-style changes implemented over a life time could contribute to significantly reducing the risk of AD, especially SAD. This could be a potentially valuable insight given an increasingly aging population in many countries with enhanced levels of dementia and cognitive impairment. Hence, strategies are needed that will reduce the degree of 'allostatic load' over a life time and consequently, slow age-related decline. For example, healthy fit middle-age adults tend to have fewer chronic conditions later in life and therefore, a lesser burden of chronic disease before death (Rantanen, 2013). It has been suggested that physical exercise can modify metabolism, brain processes, and preserve cognition if suitable structured exercise programs can be developed which are specific to the individual., of sufficient intensity and duration, and which comprise several different components (Kirk-Sanchez and McGough, 2014).

In addition, there is growing evidence that increased cognitive activity later in life could reduce the risk of AD (Jonaitis et al., 2013; Solas et al., 2013). Three aspects may influence cognitive performance in later life: (1) the level of education, (2) occupational complexity, and (3) the degree of cognitive leisure activity (Jonaitis et al., 2013). In a study of the effect of these variables on cognitive performance of middle-aged adults at risk of AD, it was shown that some of the variance attributed to education was more closely related to the degree of cognitive activity.

There is also evidence that dietary changes could reduce the risk of AD. In Japan, for example, the rate of AD has risen markedly in the last decade associated with increased consumption of alcohol and animal products and a reduction in 'traditional' diets (Grant, 2014). There is no current evidence that cessation of smoking reduces the risk of AD. Nevertheless, smoking is regarded as a risk factor for many chronic diseases, although its specific effects on the brain are unclear (Chang et al., 2014). It is possible that smoking may damage endothelial cells of cerebral micro-vessels, increasing the chance of CVD and therefore, Aβ deposition in the brain and ultimately AD.

In conclusion, many risk factors have been associated with AD including those related to on aging, genetics, aluminum, head trauma, diet and nutrition, vascular and immunological factors, and exposure to infectious agents. With the exception of early-onset FAD, it is proposed that AD is a multifactorial disorder in which external and internal risk factors act together and non-specifically to increase the rate of normal aging ('allostatic load'). The consequent enhanced degeneration of neural pathways and blood vessels results in the formation of abnormally aggregated proteins such as β-amyloid and tau which then spread through the brain. Life-style changes which act to reduce the allostatic load could potentially slow the rate of aging and therefore the risk of AD.

References

Abalan F. Alzheimer's disease and malnutrition: a new aetiological hypothesis. *Med. Hypoth.* 1984; 15: 385-393.

Allen M, Cox C, Belbin O, Ma L, Bisceglio GD, Wilcox SL, Howell CC, Hunter TA, Culley O, Walker LP, Carrasquillo MM, Dickson DW, Petersen RC, Graff-Radford NR, Younkin SG, Ertekin-Taner N. Association and heterogeneity at the GAPDH locus in Alzheimer's disease. Neurobiol Aging 2012; 33: DOI: 10.1016/j.neurobiolaging. 2010.08.002.

Alzheimer A. On a peculiar disease of the cerebral cortex. Allgemeine Zeitschrift fur Psychiatrie und Psychish-Gerichtlich Medicin 1907; 64: 146-148.

Arieff AI. Aluminum and the pathogenesis of dialysis encephalopathy. *Am. J. Kidney Dis* 1985; 6: 317-321.

Armstrong RA. β-amyloid (Aβ) deposition in cognitively normal brain, dementia with Lewy bodies, and Alzheimer's disease: a study using principal components analysis (PCA). *Folia Neuropathol.* 2012a; 50: 130-139.

Armstrong RA. On the classification of neurodegenerative disorders: discrete entities, overlap or continuum? *Folia Neuropathol.* 2012b; 50: 201-218.

Armstrong RA. What causes Alzheimer's disease? *Folia Neuropathol* 2013; 51: 169-188.

Armstrong RA, Winsper SJ, Blair JA. Hypothesis: is Alzheimer's disease a metal-induced immune disorder? *Neurodegeneration* 1995; 4: 107-111.

Armstrong RA, Winsper SJ, Blair JA. Aluminum and Alzheimer's disease: Review of possible pathogenic mechanisms. *Dementia* 1996; 7: 1-9.

Armstrong RA, Nochlin D, Bird TD (2000) Neuropathological heterogeneity in Alzheimer's disease: A study of 80 cases using principal components analysis. *Neuropathology* 2000; 20: 31-37.

Armstrong RA, Cairns NJ, Lantos PL. Are pathological lesions in neurodegenerative disorders the cause or the effect of the degeneration? *Neuropathology* 2002; 22: 114-127.

Arriagada PV, Marzloff K, Hyman BT. Distribution of Alzheimer-type pathologic changes in non-demented elderly individuals matches the pattern in Alzheimer's disease. *Neurology* 1992; 42: 1681-1688.

Attems J, Lintner F, Jellinger K. Amyloid beta peptide 1-42 highly correlates with capillary cerebral amyloid angiopathy and Alzheimer disease pathology. *Acta. Neuropathol* 2004; 107: 283-291.

Barthet G, Dunys J, Shao ZP, Xuan Z, Ren YM, Xu JD, Arbez N, Mauger G, Bruban J, Georgakopoulos A, Shioi J, Robakis NK. Presenilin mediates neuroprotective functions of ephrin-B and brain-derived neurotrophic factor and regulates ligand-induced internalization and metabolism of EphB2 and TrkB receptors. *Neurobiol. Aging* 2013; 34: 499-510.

Bartzokis G. Alzheimer's disease as homeostatic response to age-related myelin breakdown. *Neurobiol Aging* 2011; 32: 1341-1371.

Basun H, Forssell LG, Wellerberg L, Winblad B. Metals and trace elements in plasma and cerebrospinal fluid in normal ageing and Alzheimer's disease. *J. Neural. Transm.* 1991; 4; 231-258.

Beffert U, Poirier J. Apolipoprotein E, plaques, tangles and cholinergic dysfunction in Alzheimer's disease. *Ann. NY Acad. Sci.* 1996; 777: 166-174.

Bell MA, Ball MJ. Neuritic plaques and vessels of visual cortex in aging and Alzheimer's dementia. *Neurobiol. Aging* 1990; 11: 359-370.

Benedictus, MR, Goos JDC, Binnewwijzend MAA, Muller M, Barkhof F, Scheltens P, Prins ND, van der Flier WM. Specific risk factors for microbleeds and white matter hyperintensities for Alzheimer's disease. *Neurobiol. Aging*. 2013; 34: 2488-2494.

Bergeron C, Ranalli PJ, Miceli PN. Amyloid angiopathy in Alzheimer's disease. *Can. J. Neurol. Sci.* 1987; 14: 564-569.

Berr C, Hauw JJ, Delaere P, Duyckaerts C, Amouyel P. Apolipoprotein E allele □4 is linked to increased deposition of the amyloid-β-peptide (Aβ) in cases with or without Alzheimer's disease. *Neurosci. Lett.* 1994; 178: 221-224.

Blass JP, Zemcov A. Alzheimer's disease- a metabolic systems degeneration. *Neurochem. Pathol.* 1984; 2: 103-114.

Bouras C, Hof PR, Morrison JH. Neurofibrillary tangle densities in the hippocampal formation in a non-demented population define subgroups of patients with differential early pathologic changes. *Neurosci. Lett.* 1993; 153: 131-135.

Brun A. An overview of light and electron microscopic changes. In: Reisberg B (ed.) Alzheimer's disease. The Standard Reference. Macmillan, London and New York, pp 37-45, 1983.

Burns LC, Minster RL, Demirci FY, Barmada MM, Ganguli M, Lopez OL, deKosky ST, Kamboh MI. Replication study of genome-wide associated SNPs with late-onset Alzheimer's disease. *Am. J. Med. Genet: B. Neuropsych. Genet.* 2011; 156B: 507-512.

Carbone I, Lazzarotto T, Ianni M, Porcellini E, Forti P, Masliah E, Gabrielli L, Licastro F. Herpes virus in Alzheimer's disease: related to progression of the disease. *Neurobiol. Aging* 2014, 35: 122-129.

Carroll BJ. Ageing, stress and the brain. Endocrine Facets of Ageing, *Novartis Foundation Symposium* 2002; 242: 26-36.

Chang RCC, Ho YS, Wong S, Gentleman SM, Ng HK. Neuropathology of cigarette smoking. *Acta. Neuropathol.* 2014; 127: 53-69.

Chartier-Harlin MC, Crawford F, Houlden H, Warren A, Hughes D, Fidani, L, Goate A, Rossor M, Rocques P, Hardy J, Mullan M. Early onset Alzheimer's disease caused by mutations at codon 717 of the □-amyloid precursor protein gene. *Nature* 1991: 353: 844-846.

Cohen D, Eisdorfer C, Walford R. Histocompatibility antigens (HLA) and patterns of cognitive loss in dementia of the Alzheimer type. *Neurobiol. Aging* 1982; 2: 277-280.

Coria F, Moreno A, Rubio I, Garcia MA, Morato E, Major F. The cellular pathology associated with Alzheimer α-amyloid deposits in non-demented aged individuals. *Neuropath Appl Neurobiol* 1993; 19: 261-268.

Crapper DR, Karlik S, de Boni U. Aluminum and other metals in senile (Alzheimer) dementia. *Aging* (NY) 1978; 7: 471-489.

Delacourte A, Sergeant N, Champain D Wattez A, Maurage CA, Lebert F, Pasquier F and David JP. Nonoverlapping but synergetic tau and amyloid precursor protein pathologies in sporadic Alzheimer's disease. *Neurology* 2002; 59: 398-407.

Dobson CB, Templer J, Day JP, Itzhaki RF. Aluminum and Alzheimer's disease: Sites of aluminum-binding in human neuroblastoma cells. *Biochem. Soc. Trans.* 1993; 21: P32.

Doty RL, Reyes PF, Gregor T. Presence of both odor identification and detection deficits in Alzheimer's disease. *Brain Res. Bull* 1987; 18: 597-600.

Edwardson JA, Klinowski J, Oakley AE, Perry RH, Candy JM. Aluminosilicates and the ageing brain: Implications for the pathogenesis of Alzheimer's disease. *Ciba Found Symp.* 1986; 121: 160-179.

Eikelenboom P, Stam FC. Immunoglobulins and complement factors in senile plaques. Acta Neuropathol 1982; 57: 239-242.

Ferri CP, Prince M, Brayne C, Brodaty H, Fratiglioni L, Ganguly M et al. Global prevalence of dementia: a Delphi consensus study. *Lancet* 2005; 366: 2112-2117.

Francis YI, Stephanou A, Latchman DS. CREB-binding protein activation by presenilin 1 but not by its M146L mutant. *Neuroreport* 2006; 17: 917-921.

Fryer JD, Taylor JW, DeMattos RB, Bates KR, Paul SM, Parsadamian M, Holtzman DM. Apolipoprotein E markedly facilitates age-dependent cerebral amyloid angiopathy and spontaneous hemorrhage in amyloid precursor protein transgenic mice. *J. Neurosci.* 2003; 23: 7889-7896.

Garcia-Sierra F, Hauw JJ, Duyckaerts C, Wischik CM, Luna-Munoz J, Mena R. The extent of neurofibrillary pathology in perforant pathway neurons is the key determinant of dementia in the very old. *Acta. Neuropathol.* 2000; 100: 29-35.

Gentleman SM, Nash MJ, Sweeting CJ, Graham DI, Roberts GW. β-amyloid precusor protein (βAPP) as a marker for axonal injury after head injury. *Neurosci. Lett.* 1993; 160: 139-144.

Gessel MM, Bernstein S, Kemper M, Teplow DB, Bowers MT. Familial Alzheimer's disease mutations differentially alter amyloid beta protein oligomerization. *ACS Chem. Neurosci.* 2012; 3: 909-918.

Goate R, Chartier-Harlin MC, Mullan M, Brown J, Crawford F, Fidani L, Giuffra L, Haynes A, Irving N, James L, Mant R, Newton P, Rooke K, Roques P, Talbot C, Pericak-Vance M, Roses A, Williamson R, Rossor M, Owen M and Hardy J. Segregation of a missense mutation in the amyloid precursor protein gene with familial Alzheimer's disease. *Nature* 1991; 349: 704-706.

Gomez-Isla T, West HL, Rebeck GW, Harr SD, Growdon JH, Locascio JJ, Perls TT, Lipsitz LA, Hyman BT. Clinical and pathological correlates of apolipoprotein E □4 in Alzheimer's disease. *Anns. Neurol.* 1996; 39: 62-70.

Graeber MB, Kosel S, Egensperger R, Banati RB, Muller U, Bise K, Hoff P, Moller HJ, Fujisawa K and Mehraein P. Rediscovery of the case described by Alois Alzheimer in 1911: historical., histological and molecular genetic analysis. *Neurogenetics* 1997; 1: 73-80.

Grant WB. Trends in diet and Alzheimer disease during the nutrition transition in Japan and developing countries. *J. Alz. Dis.* 2014; 38: 611-620.

Graves AB, White E, Koepsell TD, Reifler BV, van Belle G, Larson EB. The association between aluminum containing products and Alzheimer's disease. *J. Clin. Epidemiol.* 1990; 43: 35-44.

Grazini M, Prabas J, Silva F, Oliveira S, Santana I, Oliveira C. Genetic basis of Alzheimer's dementia: role of mitochondrial DNA mutations. *Genes, Brain, and Behaviour* 2006; 5 (supp 2): 92-107.

Greenberg BD. The COOH-terminus of the Alzheimer amyloid Aβ peptide: Differences in length influence the process of amyloid deposition in Alzheimer brain, and tell us something about relationships among parenchymal and vessel-asssociated amyloid deposits. *Amyloid* 1995; 21: 195-203.

Grudzien A, Shaw P, Wientraub S, Bigio E, Mash DC, Mesulam MM. The locus caeruleus neurofibrillary degeneration in aging, mild cognitive impairment and early Alzheimer's disease. *Neurobiol. Aging* 2007; 28: 327-335.

Grunde-Iqbal I, Wang GP, Iqbal K, Wisniewski HM. Alzheimer's paired helical filaments: identification of polypeptides with monoclonal antibodies. *Acta. Neuropathol.* 1985; 68: 279-283.

Guillozet AL., Weintraub S, Mash DC, Mesulam MM. Neurofibrillary tangles, amyloid, and memory in aging and mild cognitive impairment. *Arch. Neurol.* 2003; 60: 729-736.

Hardy JA, Higgins GA. Alzheimer's disease: the amyloid cascade hypothesis. *Science* 1992; 256: 184-185.

Heinonen O, Syrjanen S, Soininen H, Talasmenii S, Kaski M, Mantyjarvi R, Syrjanen K, Riekkinen P. Circulating immune complexes in sera from patients with Alzheimer's disease, multi-infarct dementia, and Down's syndrome. *Neurosci. Lett.* 1993; 149: 67-70.

Heneka MT, Nadrigny F, Regen T, Martinez-Hernandez A, Dumitrescu-Oziniek L, Terivel D, Jardanhazi-Kurutz D, Walter J, Kirchoff F, Hanisch UK, Kummer MP. Locus caeruleus controls Alzheimer's disease pathology by modulating microglial function through norepinephrine. *Proc. Natl. Acad. Sci. USA* 2010; 107: 6058-6063.

Henschke PJ, Bell DA, Cape RDT. Alzheimer's disease and HLA. *Tissue Antigens* 1978; 12: 132-135.

Hjelm C, Brostrom A, Dahl A, Johansson B, Fredrikson M, Stromberg A. factors associated with increased risk for dementia in individuals age 80 years or older with congestive heart failure. *J. Cardiovasc Nurs.* 2014; 29: 82-90.

Hoenicka J. Genes in Alzheimer's disease. *Revista de Neurolgia* 2006; 42: 302-305.

Honarnejad K, Herms J. Presenilins: Role in calcium homeostasis. *Int. J. Biochem. Cell. Biol.* 2012; 44: 1983-1986.

Hyman BT, Tanzi RE. Amyloid, dementia and Alzheimer's disease. *Curr. Opin. Neurol. Neurosurg.* 1992; 5: 88-93.

Imhof A, Kovari E, von Gunten A, Gold G, Rivara CB, Herrmann FR, Hof PR, Bouras C, Glannakopoulos P. Morphological substrates of cognitive decline in nonagenarians and centenarians: A new paradigm? *J. Neurol. Sci.* 2007; 257: 72-79.

Ishii T, Haga S. Immuno-electron microscopic localisation of immunoglobulins in amyloid fibrils of senile plaques. *Acta. Neuropathol.* 1976; 20: 372-378.

Jackson HM, Soto I, Graham LC, Carter GW, Howell GR. Clustering of transcriptional profiles identifies changes to insulin signalling as an early event in a mouse model of Alzheimer's disease. *BMC Genomics* 2013; 14: Article No 831.

Jiang T, Yu JT, Tian Y, Tan L. Epidemiology and aetiology of Alzheimer's disease: From genetic to non-genetic factors. *Curr. Alz. Res.* 2013; 10: 852-867.

Jonaitis E, La Rue A, Mueller KD, Koscik RL, Hermann B, Sager MA. Cognitive activities and cognitive performance in middle-aged adults at risk for Alzheimer's disease. *Pyschol. Aging* 2013; 28: 1004-1014.

Kalaria RN, Bhatt SU, Perry G, Lust WD. The amyloid precursor protein in ischaemic brain injury and chronic hypoperfusion. Proc 7th Inter Study Group on Pharm Mem Dis Assoc with *Aging* 1993; 291-294.

Kalaria R, Hedera P. Differential degeneration of the cerebral microvasculature in Alzheimer's disease. *Neuroreport* 1995; 6: 477-480.

Kawai M, Kalaria R, Harik S, Perry G. The relationship of amyloid plaques to cerebral capillaries in Alzheimer's disease. *Am. J. Pathol.* 1990; 137: 1435-1446.

Khatchaturian ZS. Diagnosis of Alzheimer's disease. Arch Neurol 1985; 42: 1097-1005.

Kirk-Sanchez NJ, McGough EL. Physical exercises and cognitive performance in the elderly: Current perspectives. *Clin Interven Aging* 2014; 9. DOI: 10.2147/CIA.S39506

Knopman DS. An overview of common non-Alzheimer dementias. *Clinics in Ger Med* 2001; 17: 281.

Knopman DS, Parisi JE, Salviati A, Floriach-Robert M, Boeve BF, Ivnik RJ, Smith GE, Dickson DW, Johnson KA, Petersen LE, McDonald WC, Braak H, Petersen RC. Neuropathology of cognitively normal elderly. *J. Neuropathol. Exp. Neurol.* 2003; 62: 1087-1095.

Kumar-Singh S. Cerebral amyloid angiopathy: pathogenic mechanism and link to dense amyloid plaques. *Genes, Brain & Behaviour* 2008; 7: 67-82.

Landsberg JP, McDonald B, Watt F. Absence of aluminum in neuritic plaque cores in Alzheimer's disease. *Nature* 1992; 360: 65-68.

Lee CW, Shih YH, Kuo YM. Cerebrovascular pathology and amyloid plaque formation in Alzheimer's disease. *Curr. Alz. Res.* 2014; 11: 4-10.

Levy-Lahad E, Wasco W, Poorkaj P, Romano DM, Oshima J, Pettingell WH, Yu C, Paul D, Jondro PD, Schmidt SD, Wang K, Crowley AC, Fu Y, Guenette SY, Galas D, Nemens E, Wijsman EM, Bird TD, Schellenberg GD and Tanzi RE. Candidate gene for chromosome 1 familial Alzheimer's disease locus. *Science* 1995; 269: 973-977.

Libikova H, Pogady J, Weidermann V. Search for herpetic antibodies in CSF in senile dementia and mental retardation. Acta. Virol. 1975; 19: 493-495.

Liu GY, Yao LF, Liu JF, Jiang YS, Ma GD, Chen ZG, Zhao B, Li KS. Cardiovascular disease contributes to Alzheimer's disease: evidence from large-scale genome-wide association studies. *Neurobiol. Aging.* 2014; 35: 786-792.

Luthert P, Williams J. A quantitative study of the coincidence of blood vessels and A4 protein deposits in Alzheimer's disease. *Neurosci. Lett.* 1991; 126: 110-112.

Maggioli E, Boicchi C, Zorzetto M, sinforiani E, Cereda C, Ricevuti G, Cuccia M. The human leucocyte antigen class III haplotype approach: New insights in Alzheimer's disease inflammation hypothesis. *Curr. Alz. Res.* 2013; 10: 1047-1058.

Mann DMA. The neuropathology of Alzheimer's disease: a review with pathogenetic, aetiological., and therapeutic considerations. *Mech. Ageing Dev.* 1985; 31: 213-255.

Mann DMA, Tucker CM, Yates PO. Topographic distribution of senile plaques, neurofibrillary tangles in the brains of non demented persons of different age. *Neuropath App Neurobiol* 1987; 13: 123-139.

Martyn CN. The epidemiology of Alzheimer's disease in relation to aluminum. *Ciba Found Symp* 1992; 169: 69-79.

McCaddon A, Kelly CL. Familial Alzheimer's disease and vitamin B12 deficiency. *Age and Ageing* 1994; 23: 334-337.

McGeer PL, McGeer EG, Kawamata T, Yamada T, Akiyama H. Reactions of the immune system in chronic degenerative neurological diseases. *Can. J. Neurol. Sci.* 1991; 18: 376-379.

McKenzie JE, Gentleman SM, Roberts GW, Graham DI, Royston MC. Increased numbers of βAPP-immunoreactive neurons in the entorhinal cortex after head injury. *Neuroreport* 1994; 6: 161-164.

Miller DL, Papayannopoulos IA, Styles J, Bobin SA, Lin YY, Biemann K, Igbal K. Peptide compositions of the cerebrovascular and senile plaque core amyloid deposits of Alzheimer's disease. *Arch. Biochem. Biophys.* 1993; 301: 41-52.

Mirra SS, Heyman A, McKeel, D, Sumi SM, Crain BJ, Brownlee LM, Vogel FS, Hughes JP, van Belle G, Berg L. The consortium to establish a registry for Alzheimer's disease (CERAD). Part II Standardization of the neuropathologic assessment of Alzheimer's disease. *Neurology* 1991; 41: 479-486.

Miyakawa T, Katsuragi S, Yamashita K, Ohuchi K. Morphological study of amyloid fibrils and preamyloid deposits in the brain with Alzheimer's disease. *Acta. Neuropathol.* 1992; 83: 340-346.

Moro ML, Giaccone G, Lombardi R, Indaco A, Uggetti A, Morbin M, Saccucci S, Di Fede G, Catania M, Walsh DM, Denmarchi A, Rozemuller A, Bogdanovic N, Bugiani F, Ghetti B, Tagliavini F. APP mutations in the A beta coding region are associated with abundant cerebral deposition of A beta 38. *Acta. Neuropathol.* 2012; 124: 809-821.

Murphy CP, Cox RI, Harden EA, Stevens DA, Heize MM, Herzig RH. Encephalopathy and seizures induced by intravesical alum irrigations. *Bone Marrow Transpl.* 1992; 10: 383-385.

Nandy K. Immunological factors. In: Reisberg B (ed.) Alzheimer's disease. The Standard Reference. Macmillan, London and New York, pp 135-138, 1983.

Neri LC, Hewitt D. Aluminum, Alzheimer's disease and drinking water. *Lancet* 1991; 338: 390.

O'Bryant SE, Johnson L, Reisch J, Edwards M, Hall J, Barber R, Devous MD, Royall D, Singh M. Risk factors for mild cognitive impairment among Mexican Americans. *Alz Dement* 2013; 9: 622-631.

Oyama F, Shimada H, Oyama R, Ihara Y. Apolipoprotein E genotype, Alzheimer pathologies and related gene expression in the ageing population. *Mol. Brain Res.* 1995; 29: 92-98.

Panja F, Colacicco A, D'Introno A, Capurso C, Liaci M, Capurso S, Capurso A, Solfrizzi V. Candidate genes for late-onset Alzheimer's disease: Focus on chromosome 12. *Mech. Age Dev. 2006*; 127: 36-47.

Percy M, Somerville MJ, Hicks M, Garcia A, Colelli T, Wright E, Kitaygorodsky J, Jiang A, Ho V, Parpia A. Risk factors for development of dementia in a unique six-year cohort study. 1. An exploratory, pilot study of involvement of the E4 allele of apolipoprotein E, mutations of the hemochromatosis-HFE gene, Type 2 diabetes, and stroke. *J. Alz. Dis.* 2014; 38: 907-922.

Perl DP, Brody AR. Alzheimer's disease: X-ray spectrometric evidence of aluminum accumulation in neurofibrillary tangle-bearing neurons. *Science* 1980; 208: 297-299.

Perl DP, Pendlebury WW. Aluminum neurotoxicity: Potential role in the pathogenesis of neurofibrillary tangle formation. *Can. J. Neurol. Sci.* 1986; 13: 441-445.

Perlmutter L, Chui C. Microangiopathy, the vascular basement membrane and Alzheimer's disease: A review. *Brain Res. Bull* 1990; 24: 677-686.

Perlmutter L, Chui C, Saperia D, Athanikar J. Microangiopathy and the colocalisation of heparan sulfate proteoglycan with amyloid in senile plaques of Alzheimer's disease. *Brain Res.* 1990; 508: 9-11.

Peters S, Reid A, Fritschi L, de Klerk N, Musk AW. Long-term effects of aluminum dust inhalation. *Occup. Env. Med.* 2013; 70: 864-868.

Pluta R, Jabłoński M, Czuczwar SJ. Postischemic dementia with Alzheimer phenotype: selectively vulnerable versus resistant areas of the brain and neurodegeneration versus β-amyloid peptide. *Folia Neuropathol.* 2012a; 50: 101-109.

Pluta R, Kocki J, Maciejewski R, Ulamek-Koziol M, Jabłoński M, Bogucka-Kocka A, Czuczwar SJ. Ischemia signalling to Alzheimer-related genes. *Folia Neuropathol.* 2012b, 50: 322-329.

Polvikoski T, Sulkava R, Haltia M, Kainulainen K, Vuorio A, Verkkoniemi A, Niinisto L, Halonen P, Kontula K. Apolipoprotein E, dementia and cortical deposition of β-amyloid protein. *New Engl. J. Med.* 1995; 333: 1242-1247.

Ponomareva N, Anfreeva T, Protasova M, Shagam L, Malina D, Goltsov A, Fokin V, Mitrofanov A, Rogaev E. Age-dependent effect of Alzheimer's risk variant of CLU on EEG alpha rhythm in non-demented adults. *Front Aging Neurosci* 2013; 5: Article No UNSP 86.

Rantanen T. Midlife fitness predicts less burden of chronic disease in later life. *Clin. J. Sports Med.* 2013; 23: 499-500.

Regland B, Gottfries CG. The role of amyloid β-protein in Alzheimer's disease. *Lancet* 1992; 340: 467-469.

Reisberg B. Alzheimer's disease. The Standard Reference. Macmillan, London and New York, 1983.

Richartz-Salzburger E, Stransky E, Laske C, Kohler N. Premature immunosenescence: a pathogenic factor in Alzheimer's disease. Nervenarzt 2010; 81: 837-843.

Ridge PG, Maxwell TJ, Corcoran CD, Norton MC, Tschanz JT, O'Brien E, Kerber RA, Cawthorn RM, Munger RG, Kauwe JSK. Mitochondrial genomic analysis of late-onset Alzheimer's disease reveals protective haplogroups H6A1A/H6A1B: The Cache County study on memory and aging. *Plos One* 2012; 7: article e45134.

Roberts GW, Gentleman SM, Lynch A, Murray L, Landon M, Graham DI. β-amyloid protein deposition in the brain after severe head injury: implications for the pathogenesis of Alzheimer's disease. *J. Neurol. Neurosurg. Psychiatr.* 1994; 57: 419-425.

Rogers J, Luber-Narod J. Immunoactions in nervous system: brief review with special emphasis on Alzheimer's disease. *Drugs Dev. Res.* 1988; 15: 227-235.

Rolim TD, Fabri GMC, Nitrini R, Anghinah R, Teixeira MJ, de Sequeira JTT, Cestari JAF, de Sequera SRDT. Oral infections and orofacial pain in Alzheimer's disease: A case-control study. *J. Alz. Dis.* 2014; 38: 823-829.

Rossor M, Mountjoy CQ. Post-mortem neurochemical changes in Alzheimer's disease compared with normal ageing. *Can. J. Neurol. Sci.* 1986; 13: 499-502.

Ruiz A, Dois-Tcardo O, Bullido MJ, Pastor P, Reodriguez-Rodriguez E, de Munain AL., de Pancorbo MM, Perez-Tur J, Alvarez V, Antonelli A et al. Assessing the role of the TREM2 p.R47H variant as a risk factor for Alzheimer's disease and frontotemporal dementia. *Neurobiol Aging* 2014; 35: Article number 444.e1.

Ryan J, Carriere I, Carcaillion L, Dartigues JF, Auriacombe S, Rouand O, Berr C, Ritchie K, Scarabin PY, Ancelin ML. Estrogen receptor polymorphisms and incident dementia: The prospective 3C study. *Alz. and Dement.* 2014; 10: 27-35.

Salazar AM, Brown P, Gajdusek DC, Gibbs CJ. Relation to Creutzfeldt-Jakob disease and other unconventional virus diseases. In: Reisberg B (ed.) Alzheimer's disease. The Standard Reference. Macmillan, London and New York, pp 311-318, 1983.

Saunders A, Strittmater W, Schmechel D, St. George-Hyslop P, Pericak-Vance M, Joo S, Rose B, Gasella J, Crapper-MacLachan D, Albersts M, Hulette C, Crain B, Goldgaber D, Roses A. Association of apolipoprotein E allele e4 with late-onset familial and sporadic Alzheimer's disease. *Neurology* 1993; 43: 1467-1472.

Schreurs BG, Smith-Bell CA, Lemieux SK. Dietary cholesterol increases ventricular volume and narrows cerebrovascular diameter in a rabbit model of Alzheimer's disease. *Neuroscience* 2013; 254: 61-69.

Seil FJ, Lampert PW, Katzo I. Neurofibrillary spheroids induced by aluminum phosphate in dorsal root ganglia neurons in vitro. *J. Neuropathol. Exp Neurol,* 1969; 28: 74.

Sherrington R, Rogaev EI, Liang Y, Rogaeva EA, Levesque G, Ikeda M, Chi H, Lin C, Li G, Holman K, Tsuda T, Mar L, Foncin JF, Bruni AC, Moulese MP, Sorbi S, Rainero I, Pinessi L, Nee L, Chumakov I, Pollen D, Brookes A, Sauseau P, Polinski RJ, Wasco RJ, Dasilva HAR, Haines JL, Pericak-Vance MA, Tanzi RE, Roses AD, Fraser PE, Rommens JM and St George-Hyslop PH. Cloning of a gene bearing missense mutations in early onset familial Alzheimer's disease. *Nature* 1993; 375: 754-760.

Shin Y, Cho HS, Fukumoto H, Shimizu T, Shirasawa T, Greenberg SM, Rebeck GW A beta species, including IsoAsp23 Abeta, in Iowa-type familial cerebral amyloid angiopathy. *Acta. Neuropathol.* 2003; 105: 252-258.

Sillen A, Forsell C, Lilius L, Axwlman K, Bjork B, Onkamo P, Kere J, Winblad B, Graff C. Genome scan on Swedish Alzheimer disease families. *Mole Psy* 2006; 11: 182-186.

Solas M, Aisa B, Tordera RM, Mugueta MC, Ramirez MJ. Stress contributes to the development of central insulin resistance during aging: Implication for Alzheimer's disease. *Biochem. Biophys. Acta: Mole basis Dis.* 2013; 1832: 2332-2339.

Soler-Lopez M, Badiola N, Zanzoni A, Aloy P. Towards Alzheimer's root cause: ECSIT as an integrating hub between oxidative stress, inflammation and mitochondrial dysfunction. *Bioessays* 2012; 34: 532-541.

Sparks DL, Hunsaker JC, Scheff SW, Kryscio RJ, Henson JL, Markesbery WR. Cortical senile plaques in coronary artery disease, aging and Alzheimer's disease. *Neurobiol. of Aging* 1990; 11: 601-607.

Sparks DL, Scheff SW, Hunsaker JC, Liu H, Landers T, Gross DR. Induction of Alzheimer-like β-amyloid immunoreactivity in the brains of rabbits with dietary cholesterol. *Exp. Neurol.* 1994; 126: 88-94.

Steinberg M, Hess K, Corcoran C, Mielke MM, Norton M, Breitner J, Green R, Leoutsakos J, Welsh-Bohmer K, Lyketsos C. Vascular risk factors and neuropsychiatric symptoms in Alzheimer's disease: the Cache County Study. *Int. J. Ger. Psych.* 2014; 29: 153-159.

Steiner H, Capell A, Leimer U, Haass C. Genes and mechanisms involved in beta-amyloid generation and Alzheimer's disease. *Eur. Arch. Psych. and Clin. Neurol.* 1999; 249: 266-270.

Strittmatter WJ, Wiesgraber KH, Huang DY, Dong LM, Salvesen GS, Pericak-Vance M, Schmechel D, Saunders AM, Goldgaber D, Roses D. Binding of human apolipoprotein E to synthetic amyloid-β-peptide: isoform specific effects and implications for late-onset Alzheimer's disease. *Proc. Natl. Acad. Sci.* 1993; 90: 8098-8102.

Su GC, Arendash GW, Kalaria RN, Bjugstad KB, Mullan M Intravascular infusions of soluble beta-amyloid compromise the blood brain barrier, activate central nervous system glial cells and induce peripheral hemorrhage. *Brain Research* 1999; 818: 105-117.

Sudoh S, Kawamura Y, Sato K. Wang R, Saido TC, Oyama F, Sakaki Y, Komano H, Yanagisawa K. Presenilin-1 mutations linked to FAD increase the intracellular levels of amyloid beta protein 1-42 and its n-terminally truncated variant(s) which are generated at distinct sites. *J. Neurochem.* 1998; 71: 1535-1543.

Swerdlow RH. Mitochondria and cell bioenergetics: increasingly recognised components and a possible etiologic cause of Alzheimer's disease. *Antiox Redux. Sign.* 2012; 16: 1434-1463.

Terry RD, Pena C. Experimental production of neurofibrillary degeneration. *J. Neuropathol Exp. Neurol.* 1965; 24: 200-210.

Tian J, Shi J, Smallman R, Iwatsubo T, Mann D. Relationships in Alzheimer's disease between the extent of A beta deposition in cerebral blood vessel walls, as cerebral amyloid angiopathy, and the amount of cerebrovascular smooth muscle cells and collagen. *Neuropathol. Appl. Neurobiol.* 2006; 32: 332-340.

Tolppanen AM, Ngandu T, Kareholt I, Laatikainen T, Rusanen M, Soininen H, Kivipelto M. Midlife and late-life body mass index and late-life dementia: Results from a prospective population-based cohort. *J. Alz. Dis.* 2014; 38: 201-209.

Veerhuis R. Histological and direct evidence for the role of complement in the neuroinflammation of Alzheimer's disease. *Curr. Alz. Res.* 2011; 8: 34-58.

Walford RL, Fortoul T. Histocompatibility locus antigens in Alzheimer's disease. In: Reisberg B (ed.) Alzheimer's disease. The Standard Reference. Macmillan, London and New York, pp 166-169, 1983.

Wallace WC, Bragin V, Robakis NK, Sambamurti K, Vanderputten D, Merril CR, Davis KL, Santucci AC Haroutunian V. Increased biosynthesis of Alzheimer amyloid precursor protein in the cerebral cortex of rats with lesions of the nucleus basalis of Meynert. *Mole Brain Res.* 1991; 10: 173-178.

Wang LY, Hara K, Van Baaren JM, Price JC, Beecham GW, Gallins PJ, Whitehead PL, Wang GF, Lu CR, Slifer MA, Zuchner S, Martin ER, Mash D, Haines JL, Pericak-Vance MA, Gilbert JR. Vitamin D receptor and Alzheimer's disease: a genetic and functional study. *Neurobiol. Aging* 2012; 33: DOI: 10.1016/j.neurobiolaging.2011.12.038.

Wang Y, Xu SL, Liu Z, Lai C, Xie ZH, Zhao CP, Wei Y, Bi JZ. Meta-analysis on the association between the Tf gene rs1049296 and Alzheimer's disease. *Can. J. Neurokl. Sci.* 2013; 40: 691-697.

Wisniewski HM, Moretz RC, Lossinsky AS. Evidence for the induction of localised amyloid deposits and neuritic plaques by an infectious agent. Ann Neurol 1981; 10: 517-522.

Wisniewski T, Ghiso J, Frangione B. Alzheimer's disease and soluble Aβ. *Neurobiol. Aging* 1994; 15: 143-152.

Wolfe MS. Processive proteolysis by gamma-secretase and the mechanism of Alzheimer's disease. *Biol. Chem.* 2012; 393: 899-905.

Zatti G, Burgo A, Giacomello M, Barbiero L, Ghidoni R, Sinigaglia C, Florean C, Bagnoli S, Binetti G, Sorbi S, Pizzo P, Fasolata C. Presenilin mutations linked to familial Alzheimer's disease reduce endoplasmic reticulum and Golgi apparatus calcium levels. *Cell. Calcium* 2006; 39: 539-550.

In: Dementia
Editor: Pamela Tanner
ISBN: 978-1-63321-928-1

Chapter 8

Dementia: Prevalence, Mortality Rates, Risk Factors and Management Strategies

Andrew Linton[1], Emma Louise Cunningham[2], Peter Passmore[3] and Stephen Todd[4]

[1]Geriatric and General Internal Medicine,
Queens University Belfast, Belfast, Northern Ireland
[2]Centre for Public Health, Queen's University Belfast, Belfast, Northern Ireland
[3]Memory Clinic, Belfast City Hospital., Queens Univeristy Belfast,
Belfast Northern Ireland
[4]Queen's University of Belfast, Belfast, Northern Ireland

Abstract

Dementia is a progressive global cognitive dysfunction resulting in cognitive and functional impairment. An accurate prognosis is helpful for the patient, family, healthcare professionals and also for planning of future health and social care resources. The incidence and prevalence of dementia is rising. Alzheimer's disease (AD) accounts for 60-80% of dementia cases, with vascular dementia (VaD) the next most common. There is also an increased mortality in patients with dementia with Lewy bodies and frontotemporal dementia.

Median survival from time of onset of dementia is 3.3-11.7 years and from diagnosis is 3.2-6.6 years. There is an increased risk of death with dementia (hazard ratio (HR) 2-4) which can result from the disease itself, and comorbidities which may be associated with the disease process. Typical risk factors predicting outcomes in dementia, such as age of onset, gender and education, are often not supported by studies with varying outcomes. Increased mortality is associated with older age, but more life years will be lost in younger sufferers. Male gender is associated with a higher mortality (HR 1.2-1.9). Ethnicity and education do not have strong associations with mortality. People who carry the APOE ε4 allele have an increased risk of developing AD (RR 3.2) and mortality doubles when AD is present. Reviewing the often heterogeneous study data on dementia makes comparisons difficult.

Excess mortality in AD patients may be associated with the disease itself (adjusted HR 1.55 in AD versus non AD dementia). The common causes of death in dementia are cardiovascular, cerebrovascular and pneumonia. VaD patients have higher mortality from cardiovascular disease than AD.

Current management is based around early diagnosis, support, education and the use of cholinesterase inhibitors and a NMDA receptor antagonist.

Introduction

Dementia has many definitions and translates from the Latin-"without mind". Diagnosing dementia itself is not always straightforward. Clinicians and researchers often use the Diagnostic and Statistical Manual of Mental Disorders (DSM) 4 to diagnose dementia. The DSM-3 preceded this and, when comparing data from previous decades which used the DSM-3, it is important to realise the limitations of this data. Previous cognitive tests such as the Mini-Mental State Examination (MMSE) lacked specificity for early and less common dementias, such as frontotemporal. Newer cognitive tests, such as the Addenbrookes Cognitive Examination 3 Revised (2005) is more comprehensive and includes testing of executive functioning, which is lacking in the MMSE. [1]

The fifth edition of DSM (DSM-5) has been released by the American Psychiatric Association and classifies the dementia under Major and Mild Neurocognitive disorder. The new classification requires cognitive difficulty (memory, language, and learning) and the major disorder also requires the cognitive difficulty to interfere with everyday activities. These can be further sub-divided into their aetiological subtypes. The mild Neurocognitive disorder classification allows less disabling symptoms and reflects that, in some cases, this is a "pre-dementia state". It is also possible to specify if there is "behavioural disturbance", or not. In addition DSM-5 has also expanded to include HIV and traumatic brain related dementias. [2]

Other widely used criteria are the NINCDS/ADRDA (National Institute of Neurological Communication Disorders and Stroke and Alzheimer's disease and Related Disorder Association) for AD and International Classification of Diseases and Related Health Problems, 10th Revision (ICD-10). [3]

More recent diagnostic criteria are suggested by the European and American Consensus Criteria on AD. This recognises a preclinical dementia state, mild cognitive impairment (MCI) and full AD. This is important as 50% of patients with MCI will go on to develop a dementia. [4]

Prevalence

The incidence and prevalence of dementia is rising. It is more common with increasing age and within an aging global population, this will place demands on healthcare systems, families, and general society. Accurate data is of interest to affected individuals, families and also for healthcare planning. There are almost a million people in the UK with dementia and this figure is expected to double by 2050. [5] Providing an accurate prognosis to a patient and or family is difficult. General trends from studies can be utilised, however the data can often be heterogeneous and needs treated with caution. One problem is the date of onset of symptoms will likely precede the date of diagnosis and studies often use different variables when considering morbidity, mortality, and prognosis. Studies that come from memory outpatient clinics will have different characteristics than population based studies. [6]

Dementia Subtypes

Alzheimer's disease (AD) accounts for 60-80% of dementia cases. Neuronal synaptic function is disrupted by extracellular beta-amyloid plaques and neurone dysfunction and death results from intracellular tau protein tangles. The onset of AD brain disease occurs well before clinical symptoms become apparent. The only absolute method of confirming definite AD is by brain tissue biopsy or post-mortem examination. This is rarely performed and so most diagnoses are clinical and classified as possible or probable.

Vascular dementia (VaD) is the next most common subtype accounting for about 10% of cases. It is acknowledged that there is an overlap in pathology of AD and VaD, i.e., there may well be degenerative cerebrovascular disease in AD patients and vice versa. Mixed dementia, in which there is more than one causative aetiology, probably accounts for more cases than previously thought.

Dementia with Lewy bodies occurs as a result of Lewy body deposition in the brain cortex, but again Alzheimer pathology can coexist. Visual hallucinations and Parksinsonian features tend to predominate and there is less memory impairment in the early stages of the dementia. Fronto-temporal dementia includes progressive non-fluent aphasia, behavioural variant and semantic dementia. It tends to occur in those aged under 65yrs and has a more aggressive course. There are stronger genetic links compared to AD, and it tends to cluster in families.

Table 1. Prevalence of main Dementia subtypes [5]

Dementia subtype	Prevalence of Subtype	Key Features
Alzheimer's Dementia	60-80%	Insidious progressive global impairment of cognition and activities of daily living(ADLs)
Vascular Dementia	10%	Stepwise decline in cognition. Ischaemic cerebrovascular disease (CVD)
Mixed Dementia	10%	Features of both AD and CVD
Fronto-temporal Dementia	5%	Younger onset 45-65yrs Speech, language and behavioural problems
Parkinson's Dementia	1%	Preceding Parkinson's Disease. Hallucinations
Dementia with Lewy Bodies	2%	Hallucinations, fluctuant nature.
HIV related Dementia	Rare	Known HIV
Creutzfeldt–Jakob disease (CJD) Dementia	Rare	Young age, myoclonic jerks, rapid progression

There is an increased prevalence of Parkinson's dementia as Parkinson's disease progresses. The pathology results from Lewy bodies, but Tau protein and amyloid are often also present. [5]

When reviewing the data and population statistics, it is important to recognise that many dementias may be mixed, but that most will be AD.

Prevalence

Statistics from the United States (US) estimate that in 2014, 5.2 million Americans have dementia, of which 5 million are over 65yrs. It is estimated that half of these persons are undiagnosed. The estimated prevalence of dementia in the US population is 15% aged 65-74yrs, 44% aged 75-84yrs and 38% persons aged over 85yrs. [7] There is estimated to be an increase in the prevalence of AD in the US from 4.7million in 2010 to 13.8million in 2050. The largest increase will be in those aged over 85yrs, due to increasing survival in an aging population. [8] This will put a strain on increasingly under pressure healthcare systems.

The Aging, Demographics And Memory Study (ADAMS) in the US estimates that the prevalence of dementia in woman aged over 65yrs is 16% and for men 11%. The proportion of dementia patients who are female is estimated at 2/3. Age matched studies have not demonstrated that there is an increased incidence of dementia in females at a particular age and so these statistics are explained by the longer life expectancy of females. This results in a rising prevalence in an aging population. The lifetime risk for a person aged 65yrs who does not have dementia of developing AD is estimated at 20% for a woman and 17% for a man. The higher risk in females again reflects the longer life expectancy. [9]

Mortality

Survival time in dementia is increasing. There are several reasons for this. The time from onset of symptoms is now more often specified than time from actual diagnosis. The public and medical services are more aware of the disease and more likely to diagnose it rather than simply pacifying patients and families with a notion of benign old age "forgetfulness". A diagnosis is also more likely to be sought as there are pharmacological treatments available, which were not previously. Better care for dementia and other disease processes is also increasing life expectancy.

Several studies have compared the mortality of patients with dementia compared to cognitively normal individuals. This has demonstrated that dementia increases mortality, with hazard ratios (HR) of between 1.4 to 5.2. [6] Median survival from time of onset of dementia is 3.3-11.7 years and from diagnosis is 3.2-6.6 years. This may be partly as a result from the disease itself, but is largely influenced by comorbidities and complications of the disease process.

Mortality is highest in the first year of diagnosis. This may be as a result of diagnosis made during hospitalisation for other pathology, or other times of "crisis". [10]

Dementia Subtypes

Mortality varies across the dementias. Patients over 65yrs with dementia are 2-4 times more likely to die. [11] AD has a more favourable outcome in terms of loss of life years, compared to the other dementia subtypes, particularly in older persons, as the disease and its consequences takes time to manifest. AD is associated with a 1.5-3 relative risk (RR) of death. A younger age of diagnosis is associated with increased relative loss of life years in VaD, perhaps reflecting other vascular related disease in the patient. AD does not have as strong an association with age of onset.

Fronto-temporal dementia tends to occur in those aged less than 65yrs, in contrast with AD. Survival is shorter with the median survival being 4.2 years, compared to 6 years for AD. Since the disease affects younger people, the loss of life years is much greater than in AD. There is also a more rapid deterioration in cognition and function. [12]

While considering mortality you need to consider the disease itself, consequences of impaired cognition and functionality, and association with relevant comorbidities. AD tends to be an insidious progressive disease and mortality is usually related to complications of loss of function, such as pneumonia and dehydration, rather than due to AD itself. [13] The presence of psychotic symptoms has also been shown to reduce survival in AD patients. [14]

Cause of Death and Co-Morbidities

Comorbidities which accumulate as individuals age are associated with increased mortality. In dementia, hypertension, stroke and diabetes mellitus increase mortality. Rates of co-morbidity in AD compared to non-AD patients admitted to hospital show that the most prevalent were pneumonia 9.8% (RR 2.8), eating disorder 6.4% (RR 6.4), urinary tract infections (RR 4.1) and epilepsy (RR 4.6). Pneumonia was the most common cause of death in both groups in hospital. Cardiovascular disease, hypertension and type 2 diabetes mellitus were noted to be less common in AD patients. [15]

There are higher rates of cardiovascular and cerebrovascular disease in VaD compared to AD. Pneumonia was the most common cause of death (57%) in a post mortem study of dementia patients in the UK. The second most common cause of death was cardiovascular disease (16%), followed by pulmonary embolism (14%). There was no difference between the VaD and AD groups. [16]

Dementia is often stated as a contributory cause of death on certification and rarely the primary cause. [13] A review of death certification in the US showed that AD appeared on the death certificate in any form in only 12.3% of patients who had AD. This may be because of lack of awareness of the diagnosis, the idea that AD was not a cause of death, or there may be sensitivities to stating AD on the death certificate. [17]

Conversely a study in Northern Ireland (Todd S et al. Cause of death in Alzheimer's disease: a cohort study. Q J Med May 2013:1-7) observed a higher rate of AD recorded on death certificates of AD patients. 25.5% stated the underlying cause of death, while 63.5% had AD recorded somewhere in the certificate. [18] This may be related to local variation in practice and a higher awareness of AD. However, mortality over the 5.7 year follow up period was less in the AD group of patients. 48.9% survived, compared to only 26.2% of the non-AD dementia patients. The cause of death in two thirds of patients was cardiovascular disease or stroke. There was a lower prevalence of hypertension among the AD patients 28.9%, compared to 51.5% in the other dementia patients. The cardiovascular mortality was only 39% in AD patients who died. [18] This is in keeping with the higher mortality rates for VaD and reflects their vascular risk factors. [19]

Another study has observed that the death rate from strokes was 42% in VaD, compared to 8.8% in AD. Dementia free patients were more likely to die from cancer (40%) or cardiovascular disease (25%). [13]

In 2010 in the US 83,494 deaths were directly attributed to AD, after a review of death certificates. However, many patients will die of complications from dementia, such as dehydration and aspiration pneumonia. In the same year, 600,000 people who died in the US had a diagnosis of AD. Medi-Care estimates that in the US 1 in 3 deaths at any particular time are in patients with a diagnosis of AD. [5]

There was a higher requirement for oral nutritional support in the AD patients-24%, compared to 9.2% in other dementia patients and 9.9% overall. [19] This reflects the longer survival times in AD and the loss of function that develops, such as impaired swallow mechanism and loss of thirst reflex. Rather than dying from the AD itself, dehydration is a common complication and cause of mortality.

Age

Increased mortality is associated with older age, with each additional year of life resulting in a mortality risk HR of 1.04-1.07. Average future life expectancy from onset of symptoms of dementia is 8.6 years aged 65 years, and only 1.8 years aged 85years. One study showed that the additional mortality from dementia in the ‘oldest old’, greater then 85yrs, is less than in younger subjects 65-74 years, mortality RR 7.24 fell to 2.2. This reflects the burden of multisystem disease in the older person. [6] A diagnosis of AD aged 65yrs leads to a reduction of approximately 67% in remaining life span, whilst at 90yrs leads to a reduction of 39%. [20]

A study comparing mortality in community dwelling patients with AD versus cognitively normal persons observed a mortality rate of 45.5% in the AD group, compared to 27% in the control group. Comparing age at diagnosis of AD groups demonstrates that patients aged over 80 years had an adjusted HR of 4.57 compared to persons younger than 65 years. [21]

More life years will be lost in younger sufferers, although they may live longer with their dementia than older patients, as they may lack comorbid diseases associated with older age.

Gender

Whilst females have a higher risk of dementia, resulting from a longer life expectancy and possible genetic influences, their mortality is less than males. The adjusted HR for male mortality in dementia is 1.74, compared to females in AD. This may be because their diagnosis presents at an earlier stage than males, as impaired functioning from loss of ADLs may become more easily apparent with household tasks. Male mortality in general is higher in the general population aged over 65 years. [21]

The exaggerated risk of death in females is higher in VaD than AD. The adjusted HR for death in VaD in females is 6.5 and 3.3 for men in one study. [13]

Disease Severity

Perhaps unsurprisingly, disease severity has shown a strong association with mortality in dementia. Those with a baseline MMSE of 0-15/30 had an adjusted HR of 3.57, compared to adjusted HR of 1.75 with an MMSE 16-23/30.

This study also observed that those with functionally poor status had increased mortality. A baseline Barthel score <17 had an adjusted HR of 2.23, compared to an adjusted HR 1.26 for those scoring 18-19. [6]

Ethnicity

Ethnicity does not have strong associations with mortality. Most population studies have tended to involve Caucasian populations. There is limited evidence that mortality with dementia is higher in Caucasian and Black populations and lower in Hispanic populations. [22]

Genetics

Dementia patients who carry the ApoE ε4 allele have an increased mortality with an adjusted HR 1.31 in one study. Those with one ε4 allele and AD have been observed to have a 77% chance of increased all-cause mortality, compared to non-carriers. It was also noticed that dementia patients who carry this gene have a lower mean BMI than cognitively normal participants. Carriers were also observed to have an increased risk of death from cardiovascular disease. Observational data suggests that there is an additional positive association between ApoE ε4 status and mortality in females compared to men, however this may be as a result of their longer life expectancy. [23]

In summary, age and functional ability tend to be the strongest predictors of death in dementia patients. [13]

Risk Factors

This section looks risk factors for dementia. Typical risk factors predicting outcomes in dementia, such as age of onset, gender, education, are often not supported by studies with varying outcomes.

Age

Age is the most common risk factor for AD, but the disease itself results in more neuro-degeneration than is explained by simply aging physiology. A prognostic study found the mean age of diagnosis of dementia was 85 years. [20] This reflects the insidious nature of the disease and often later presentation at diagnosis.

Shortening of chromosomal telomeres with time reflects the aging process. Analysis also shows an association with shortening telomeres and mortality and dementia. It is unknown if this association reflects the increased incidence of dementia with aging, or whether shorting telomeres and the increased risk of mutations could cause dementia. [24]

MCI

About 10% of patients over 65 years have mild cognitive impairment (MCI). There is an increased risk of dementia with MCI, but this does not inevitably lead to dementia. It may represent an early stage in the diagnosis in some cases, but in others it does not progress. Further investigation is needed to identify risk factors for MCI patients who will develop AD.

Genetics

Family history is a risk factor for AD. Having one or more first degree relatives affected by AD increases the risk of disease development.

ApoE ε4 is associated with AD and is thought to interfere with amyloid production. The ApoE ε4 allele is carried by about a quarter of the population and has an increased risk of developing AD (RR 3.2). The risk is higher in patients who are homozygous, which increases the risk of developing AD by ten times. There is no difference in gender distribution. ApoE ε4 carriers with dementia were observed to be 4 years younger at diagnosis than non-carriers in one study. [23] This may reflect a more aggressive disease process in these patients. 40-65% of patients with AD are thought to have this allele and there is a doubling of mortality in these patients. Approximately 19% of VaD patients and 34% of mixed dementia patients carry the allele. [13]

Study of Late onset dementia (LOAD) in genome wide association studies (GWAS) has identified a significant overrepresentation of signal pathways related to cholesterol metabolism. [25]

Two other associations from GWAS are Clusterin and PICALM (phosphatidylinositol clathrin assembly lymphoid-myeloid leukaemia). Clusterin is apolipoprotein J and has also been shown to have an association with AD in two large GWAS. Its role is unclear, but it appears to interfere with beta amyloid aggregation and neuro-inflammation. [26] The gene for PICALM has a positive association with amyloid plaque levels. Further work is needed to understand their roles in the development of AD and to target specific therapies. [27]

Other genetic causes are rarer and are strongly associated with younger onset dementia i.e., before 65 years. In particular, mutations in the genes for proteins presenilin (PSEN) 1 and

2 and for amyloid precursor protein (APP). [28] They can cause an autosomal dominant early onset AD.

C-Reactive Protein

Inflammatory neurodegenerative processes in AD have been linked to elevated C-reactive protein (CRP) in pathological brain studies of AD patients. One prospective study has also shown an association between serum CRP and an increased risk of AD. [29] It is been proposed that generalised inflammation in the brain could lead to atherogenic processes. An elevated CRP has also been linked to an increased risk of cardiovascular disease.

However, once AD has been diagnosed the association changes to one of a lower CRP, compared to non-AD patients. It is unclear if this is due to a reduction in immune system behaviour as a result of physiological aging, or that the neurodegenerative processes have reduced. Trials using salicylic acid as an anti-inflammatory drug and cholinesterase inhibitors have not shown a beneficial effect. A higher CRP in AD may still be associated with more significant cognitive impairment and reduced survival, even when compared to non-AD persons. [29]

Cognitive Reserve

Cognitive reserve is the theory that high premorbid levels of education and hence neurological functioning may be protective of AD and delay its presentation. If the brain has more neuronal networking and more efficient pathways, it may be more resilient to neuronal damage. A high level of education may also mask an early diagnosis of dementia, compared to a less educated one. This may lead to a seemingly higher mortality in better educated patients, because they are diagnosed later in the disease process. A study observed that the mortality rate was lower in dementia patients who had worked in manual jobs, as opposed to those who had not. [11]

Education

Low levels of educational attainment are also associated with poor levels of general health, and higher levels of smoking and alcohol consumption, which are adverse vascular risk factors and contributed to increased VaD. [30] Those living in deprived areas have an increased risk of dementia. [31] A study showed that poor literacy was associated with a HR of 1.72 for developing AD. However, a systematic review concluded that there was not a conclusive link between educational level and mortality in AD. [32, 33]

Traumatic brain injury e.g., as a result of boxing can result cognitive impairment. Severe traumatic brain injury is associated with a 4.5 times increased risk of AD. [30]

Ethnicity

A multi-ethnic study looking at dementia survival identified that mortality is higher in Caucasian dementia patients, followed by African Americans and lowest in Hispanics. This was thought to be as a result of lower education attainment among Hispanics and the diagnosis occurring earlier in the disease, rather than an actual difference in survival. [34]

Diet

A diet that is low in saturated fat and has recommended quantities of fruit and vegetables may be associated with a reduced incidence of dementia. This may be because of an advantageous vascular risk profile. [30] A diet with less than 2 portions of fruit and vegetables per day is associated with a HR of 1.26 for developing dementia over 7 years. Those who eat a Mediterranean type diet (a higher proportion of fruit, vegetables, cereal., fish, with less meat and a moderate alcohol) have a lower risk of AD (HR 0.6-0.91). [35]

Depression

Depression has also been shown to be a risk factor for dementia. It is associated with an adjusted HR of 1.39 for developing dementia. [33] However, it has also been observed that patients suffering both problems have a longer survival time. One possible explanation is that their diagnosis presents earlier as their symptoms may be more pronounced. A different study demonstrated a higher mortality in females with both dementia and depression RR 2.4. [11]

Education, diet and depression are interesting, as they are all potentially modifiable. This presents the opportunity to reduce the incidence of new cases of dementia via improved public health programmes. [33]

Management Strategies

The management of dementia, which is an incurable, progressive disease and causes morbidity and increased mortality, is not straight forward. It is based upon increasing public and physician awareness, early diagnosis, initiation of appropriate treatment, providing information for the patient and care-giver, supporting the patient to live in their own environment for as long as possible, and planning for the future. Charities such as the Alzheimer's Society and Alzheimer's Research Trust have important roles in raising public awareness of the condition, campaigning, and research.

People aged over 65 years are more concerned about developing dementia than cancer, heart disease, or stroke. [36] In the UK, only a third of dementia sufferers are diagnosed and often at a late stage, therefore missing out on early diagnosis. The benefits of an early diagnosis include awareness and education opportunity for the patient and family, healthcare staff, appropriate support can be offered, and early pharmacological treatment which can improve symptoms. The cost of caring for dementia patients varies from country to country, ranging from an average of €6000 in France to €19,500 in Norway. [37] Differing family support structures, rates of diagnosis and the range of care offered for dementia may account for some of this variation. Caring for patients in their own home can be up to five times cheaper than in institutions. [38] The cost of care also increases with dementia severity. One Scandinavian report estimated the cost of care for mild dementia at US$7,500, rising to US$46,350 for severe dementia. [37]

Diagnosis

The diagnosis and management of dementia ideally should involve a dementia specialist team. These specialists may include old age Psychiatrists, Geriatricians and Neurologists, as well as specialist nurses, occupational therapists, physiotherapists, psychologists, social services and carers. It can be community or secondary care based. The care should be patient centred and seek to facilitate the wishes of the patient and also include the family and carers perceptions. [39]. The UK body the National Institute for Health and Clinical Excellence (NICE) supports this strategy and has several recommendations:

In making the diagnosis, the team need access to screening bloods for reversible causes of cognitive impairment (such as hypothyroidism), an accurate collateral history, and neuroimaging. Neuroimaging should be performed to exclude structural pathology using a CT scan or preferably MRI. Single-photon emission computed tomography (SPECT) or CT PET scanning can help to differentiate AD, VaD and FTD if the diagnosis is unclear. These scans are not always universally available. [40] Electroencephalogram (EEG) and cerebrospinal fluid analysis are not routinely recommended, but may be useful in diagnosing atypical dementias, such as variant CJD dementia.

Genetic Testing

Genes predictable for AD are useful for screening and also to target therapeutic treatments. Research into LOAD i.e., over 65 years is on-going and the most commonly associated gene is ApoE ε4. Routine screening for AD is not recommended. However, referral for genetic counselling can be considered for families of persons who suffer from FTD, or early onset AD (less than 65 years). [40]

In families where clusters of AD occur, three genes have been strongly associated APP, PSEN1, PSEN2. These are all involved in beta amyloid production. Research into genome wide association studies (GWAS) aims to identify further specific genes which can help in the diagnosis and treatment of AD and the other dementias. [41]

Research

In the preclinical stages of AD, when cognition is normal., it is possible to identify biomarkers. CSF can be tested for amyloid and Tau and along with cognitive testing, it is possible to diagnose a state of preclinical AD (NIA-AA criteria). Preclinical AD biomarkers were common in sampled patients over 65 years (31%). There is evidence that the presence of these increases the risk of developing AD, compared to normal individuals. Mortality is also increased in these patients. [42]

Biomarkers which are present in the preclinical phase of MCI and AD, would be useful in screening for AD and targeting potential therapies. By targeting beta- amyloid modifying therapies in the preclinical phase, it may be possible to prevent beta amyloid related neuro-degeneration and possibly AD. [43] Further research is needed.

Table 2. Drugs commonly used in Dementia

Drug Type	Drug	Indication	Relevant Side Effect
Cholinesterase Inhibitor	Donepezil Rivastigmine Galantamine	Mild to moderate AD	Cholinergic-Nausea, vomiting, diarrhoea Heart block (rare)
NMDA receptor antagonist	Memantine	Moderate to severe AD, or as an alternative to AD	Collapse (rarely)
Anti-psychotic	Haloperidol Chlorpromazine Atypical antipsychotics e.g., Risperidone, Olanzapine	Severe BPSD	Extra-pyramidal symptoms Increase stroke risk Sedation Increased falls risk

Pharmacological Treatment

Early use of the two main relevant pharmacological medications can be helpful, though there is not always a uniform response. The aim in early treatment is to maximise cognitive and functional ability in AD. [38] Cholinesterase inhibitors (CIs) and the NMDA receptor antagonist memantine are the mainstay of treatment (see table 2). There is a loss of cholinergic synaptic conduction in AD. The use of CI has been shown to improve cognition and maximise functional ability, delay and moderate behavioural and psychological symptoms in dementia (BPSD), and delay time to institutionalisation. [44]

There are three approved CIs for AD. In the UK, NICE allows the initiation of these drugs by a specialist for mild to moderate AD. The main side effects are cholinergic gastrointestinal (nausea, vomiting, and diarrhoea) and are dose related. Topical rivastigmine patches can improve tolerability and may be of use if there are issues with tablet compliance. If one CI isn't tolerated another may be tried. There is also a rare risk of heart-block, so a baseline ECG should be performed. NICE does not recommend their use for VaD unless part of a clinical trial, however there is some evidence that they are beneficial. In cases of mixed dementias, the disease is managed according to the predominant causative aeitology. [40] Rivastigmine is beneficial in Parkinson's Dementia and DLB, where there is greater cholinergic loss than in AD. [44] Whether to stop CIs in more advanced dementia is unclear, as some patients will suffer a rebound effect in adverse symptoms.

Memantine is a NMDA receptor antagonist used for moderate to severe AD. NICE has recommended memantine in moderate to severe AD and can be used as in addition to a CI, or instead if a CI can't be used or is poorly tolerated. There is evidence of improved cognition and reduction in BPSD in some patients. There is some evidence that withdrawal of these medications can cause adverse symptoms to recur and cognition can deteriorate. [45]

Anti-psychotic medication is used for its sedative properties for agitation. BPSD cause difficulties in managing and caring for patients and are a significant cause for institutionalisation. There is an associated increased risk of cerebrovascular disease, infections and death with the long-term use of these medications. Therefore it is recommenced that they are only used if absolutely necessary for severe BPSD, at the lowest dose needed and for a limited duration. Newer atypical antipsychotics such as Risperidone are more often used, as they tend to have less adverse side effects in the elderly. In the UK Risperidone is the only antipsychotic that has a licence for use, for treating agitation in dementia. [40] Anti-psychotics should be avoided in dementia with Lewy bodies as they can exacerbate the disease symptoms.

Regular review of these patient's medications, optimisation of beneficial CI treatment and rationalising adverse cognitive medications such as commonly prescribed anti-cholinergic medication, will help improve cognition and minimise patient morbidity. [44]

Non-Pharmacological Strategies

Souvenaid is a drink reinforced with nutrients needed for synapse formation. There is increased synaptic loss in AD. There is some evidence that use of this supplement in "drug-naive" mild AD patients improves cognition. No benefit was found in later stages of dementia. [46]

Axona is a 'medical food' rich in medium triglycerides, which are metabolised into ketones after ingestion. There is some evidence that there is reduced brain neuronal glucose metabolism in patients who have ApoE ε4, or who have a maternal history of AD. The reason is unclear. This treatment provides an alternative ketonic energy supply to brain tissue, which may optimise neurone function and prevent damage from hypoglycemia. [47]

Non-Pharmacological strategies do not alter the disease course of dementias, but they can improve the BPSD. These include, agitation, poor sleep and wandering. Various studies have assessed different non-pharmacological methods of improving the BPSD, but they are often small trials, with mixed results.

A meta-analysis of studies found that most successful were multicomponent interventions, tailored to the needs of the patient and care giver and followed up. This strategy is endorsed by NICE. [5, 40]

Cognitive Stimulation

Reminiscence has been shown to reduce BPSD and may utilise long term memory storage not yet damaged. Exercise as part of behaviour management strategy has been shown to improve physical health and mood in AD. [48]

Public Health and Health and Care Services

Accurate prognostic population data for the inevitable increase in the prevalence of dementia is helpful for health authorities in planning services and even public buildings, including hospitals, which will need to be "dementia friendly". There will need to be an increase in the availability of specialists who can diagnose and manage patients with dementia.

While planning for managing dementia and costs associated with it, several things need to be considered, including medical care for hospital costs, drugs, community and institutional care, informal carer costs from family and friends, and the loss of economic output that results.

Dementia patients have three times as many hospital admissions as dementia-free persons and their stay in hospital can be up to a third longer. [5] It is estimated that in 2014 dementia will cost the US $214 Billion in healthcare and formal care costs. [49]

A lot of the management of patients with more advanced dementia involves one-on-one care. This is either provided in the person's natural environment, or in an institution. Informal care from family and friends undoubtedly makes up the majority of this care. Data from the US in 2013 estimated unpaid (informal) care for patients with AD accounting for 17.7 billion hours and at an estimated cost of $220 Billion. The proportion of female carers was estimated at 65%, with 21% themselves aged over 65yrs. [5]

Dementia is one of the main causes for care need and admission to nursing homes. A study of AD patients in nursing homes found they had survived a long time with the illness and had more functional impairment than community AD patients. There was not a significant difference in mortality however, highlighting the non-standard disease projection. [50]

Conclusion

Faced with a future global epidemic of dementia, health and social care services must meet growing demands in an already aging population. The main stay of care is increasing public education and awareness, early diagnosis with open access to dementia specialist services, treatments and support. Early diagnosis allows early treatment with cognitively beneficial medications and a better chance to allow suffers to remain in their own environment with support, which is what most patients seek and is also less costly than institutional care. Governments need to have a dementia strategy. Research into biomarkers, better diagnostic tests and genetic testing, will help improve diagnosis and may result in new treatments.

References

[1] Kipps CM et al. Cognitive assessment for Clinicians. *J. Neurol. Neurosurg. Psychiatry* 2005;76(Suppl I):i22–i30.

[2] American Psychiatric Association. Highlights of Changes from DSM-IV-TR to DSM-5. American Psychiatric Publishing 2013.

[3] McKhann G. et al. "Clinical diagnosis of Alzheimer's disease: report of the NINCDS-ADRDA Work Group under the auspices of Department of Health and Human Services Task Force on Alzheimer's Disease". *Neurology* 34 (7): 939–44.

[4] Hyman BT et al. National Institute on Aging–Alzheimer's Association guidelines for the neuropathologic assessment of Alzheimer's disease. *Alzheimer's and Dementia: The Journal of the Alzheimer's Association*, 2012;8,1:1-13.

[5] Alzheimer's Association. 2014 Alzheimer's Disease Facts and Figures. *Alzheimer's & Dementia*;10,2.

[6] Todd SA et al. Survival in Dementia and predictors or mortality: a review. *International Journal of Geriatric Psychiatry* 2013.

[7] Hebert LE et al. Alzheimer's disease in the United States (2010-2050) estimated using the 2010 Census. *Neurology* 2013;80(19):1778–83.

[8] Hebert LS et al. Alzheimer's disease in the U.S. population: Prevalence estimates using the 2000 census. *Arch. Neurol.* 2003;60:1119–22.

[9] Seshadri S. et al. The lifetime risk of stroke: Estimates from the Framingham Study. *Stroke* 2006;37(2):345–50.

[10] Rait et al. Survival of people with clinical diagnosis of dementia in primary care: cohort study. *BMJ* 2010;341c3584.

[11] Guehne U. et al. Mortality in Dementia. *Neuroepidemiology* 2005;25:153-162.

[12] Rascovsky K. et al. Rate of progression differs in frontotemporal Dementia and Alzheimer's disease. *Neurology* 65 2005: 397-403.

[13] Fitzpatrick AL et al. Survival Following Dementia onset: Alzheimer's disease and vascular dementia. *Journal of the neurological Sciences* 229-230 (2005) 43-49.

[14] Russ et al. Cognitive and behavioural predictors of survival in Alzheimer's disease: results form a sample of treated patients in a tertiary-referral memory clinic. *International Journal of Geriatric Psychiatry* 2012; 27:844-853.

[15] Heun R. et al. Alzheimer's disease and co-morbidity: Increased prevalence and possible risk factors of excess mortality in a naturalistic 7-year follow up. *European Psychiatry* 28 (2013) 40-48.

[16] Ives DG et al. Surveillance and ascertainment of cardiovascular events. the cardiovascular health study. *Ann. Epidemiology* 1995;5:278-85.

[17] Ganguli et al. Alzheimer's Disease and Mortality. *Arch. Neurology* 2005;62:779-784.

[18] Todd S. et al. Cause of death in Alzheimer's disease: a cohort study. *Q. J. Med.* May 2013:1-7.

[19] Cereda E. et al. Alzheimer's disease and mortality in traditionally long-term care facilities. *Archives of Gerontology and Geriatrics* 56 (2013):437-441.

[20] Brookmeyer R. et al. Survival Following a Diagnosis or Alzheimer's Disease. *Arch. Neruol*; 59:1764-1767.

[21] Barr S, Todd S. et al. Mortality and Alzheimer Disease: Rate and predictive factors of mortality in a community dwelling population. Unpublished data.

[22] Moschetti K. et al. Burned on Alzheimer's Disease-related mortality in the United States, 1999-2008. *JAGS* 60(2012): 1509-1514.

[23] Beydoun MA et al. Apolipoprotein E ε4 Allele Interacts with sex and cognitive status to Influence all-cause mortality and cause-specific mortality in U.S. older adults. *JAGS* 61 (2013);525-534.
[24] Honig LS et al. Association of shorter Leukocyte Telomere Repeat Length with dementia and mortality. *Arch. Neurology*;69 (2012):1332-1339.
[25] Jones L, Holmans PA, Hamshere ML, Harold D, Moskvina V, et al. (2011) Correction: Genetic Evidence Implicates the Immune System and Cholesterol Metabolism in the Aetiology of Alzheimer's Disease. *PLoS ONE* 6(2): 10.1371.
[26] YU JT et al. The role of clusterin in Alzheimer's disease: pathways, pathogenesis, and therapy. *Mol. Neurobiol.* 2012 Apr;45(2):314-26.
[27] Baig S. et al. Distribution and expression of picalm in Alzheimer disease. *J. Neuropathol. Exp. Neurol.* 2010 Oct;69(10):1071-7.
[28] Alzheimer's Society. *Genetics of Dementia.* http://www.alzheimers.org.uk/factsheet/405 July 2012.
[29] Nilsson K. et al. C-Reactive Protein level is decreased in patients with Alzheimer's disease and related to cognitive function and survival time. *J. Clinical Biochemistry* 44 (2011); 1205-1208.
[30] Reitz C, Brayne C, Mayeux R. Epidemiology of Alzheimer disease. *Nat. Rev. Neurol.* 2011;7(3):137–52.
[31] Rait G et al. Survival of people with clinical diagnosis of dementia in primary care: cohort study. *BMJ* 341(2010);337.
[32] Paradise M. et al. Systemic review of the effect of education on survival in Alzheimer's disease. *International Psychogeriatrics* (2009);21:25-32.
[33] Ritchie K. et al. Designing prevention programmes to reduce incidence of dementia: prospective cohort study of modifiable risk factors. *BMJ*;342(2010):336.
[34] Helzner EP et al. Survival in Alzheimer's disease. *Neurology* 2008;71:1489-1495.
[35] Scarmeas et al. Mediterranean diet and risk for Alzheimer's disease. *Ann. Neurol.* Jun 2006;56(6);912-921.
[36] Williamson WT. Dementia. Out of the shadows. London: Alzheimer's Society 2008.
[37] Jonsson L. et al. Determinants of costs of care for patients with Alzheimer's disease. *Int. J. Geriatric Psychiatry*, 2006;21:449-459.
[38] Todd S, Passmore P. Alzheimer's Disease- The Importance of Early Detection. *European Neurological Review* 2008;2-5.
[39] Todd SA, Passmore AP. Alzheimer's disease in the United Kingdom. *European Geriatric Medicine* 1 (2010): 182-185.
[40] National Institute for Health and Clinical Excellence. Dementia clinical guideline 42: Dementia: Supporting people with dementia and their carers in health and social care. 2006. http://www.nice.org.uk/nicemedia/pdf/cg042niceguideline.pdf
[41] Bertram L. et al. *Hum. Mol. Genet.* (2009) 18 (R2):R137-R145.
[42] Vos et al. Preclinical Alzheimer's disease and its outcome: a longitudinal cohort study. *Lancet Neurol.* 2013;12:957-965.
[43] Sperling RA et al. Toward defining the preclinical stages of Alzheimer's disease: recommendations from the National Institute on Aging-Alzheimer's Association workgroups on diagnostic guidelines for Alzheimer's disease. *Alzheimer's Dement.* 2011 May;7(3):280-92

[44] Todd S, Passmore AP. Best practice in dementia care: assessment, diagnosis and treatment. *Neurology Insights Europe* 2009:11-16.
[45] Doody RS et al. Donepezil study group. Open label, multi-centre stage3 extension study of safety and efficacy of donepezil in patients with Alzheimer's disease. *Arch. Neurol.* 2001;58:427-33.
[46] Scheltens P. et al. Efficacy of Souvenaid in mild Alzheimer's disease: results from a randomized, controlled trial. *J. Alzheimer's Dis.* 2012;31(1):225-36.
[47] Cunnane SC et al. Brain fuel metabolism, aging and Alzheimer's disease. *Nutrition.* Jan 2011;27(1):3-20.
[48] Teri L. et al. Exercise plus behaviour management in patients with Alzheimer's disease: a randomised controlled trial. *JAMA* 2003;290:2015-22.
[49] Jack CR et al. Introduction to the recommendations from the National Institute on Aging–Alzheimer's Association workgroups on diagnostic guidelines for Alzheimer's disease. *Alzheimer's Dement* 2011;7(3):257–62.
[50] Guhne U. et al. Incident Dementia cases and Mortality. *Dement. Geriatr. Cogn. Disord.* 2006;22:185-193.

About the Authors

Andrew Linton is a graduate from Queens University Belfast Medical School. Dr Linton is a Specialty trainee in Geriatric and General Internal Medicine, a member of the British Geriatric Society and an Honorary Tutor for medical students at Queens University Belfast.

Emma Cunningham is a Clinical Research Fellow investigating cognitive disorders at the Centre for Public Health, Queen's University Belfast. Dr Cunningham trained at Queens University Belfast and has worked in clinical medicine in Northern Ireland, the Republic of Ireland and Uganda. She is also a Specialty Trainee in Geriatric and General Internal Medicine and also a member of the British Geriatric Society.

Peter Passmore is a Consultant in administrative charge of the Memory Clinic at Belfast City Hospital. His main research interest is the clinical and molecular/genetic basis of Alzheimer's disease, stroke, vascular dementia and behavioural disorders in dementia. His most recent publications are in these areas, including papers in Nature Genetics, The Lancet, Stroke, Annals of Neurology, the Journal of Neurology, Neurosurgery, and Psychiatry and the International Journal of Geriatric Psychiatry. Dr Passmore is a graduate of Queen's University Belfast. He trained as a junior doctor in the Northern Ireland rotational scheme. An early interest in pharmacology resulted in the award of his MD in 1987. Dr Passmore combined his interest in pharmacology with a clinical interest in care of older people and progressed through the higher medical training programme in Northern Ireland. During this period he was a locum consultant and senior lecturer in geriatric medicine at the University of Sydney, Australia, between 1990 and 1991.

Stephen Todd is a Senior Clinical Research Fellow at Queen's University of Belfast and an Honorary Consultant Geriatrician to the Belfast City Hospital. He is a member of the

British Geriatrics Society and the Ulster Medical Society. Dr Todd was awarded a Paul B Beeson Career Development Award in 2008 from the Beeson Ireland programme to continue researching platelet β-secretase activity in Alzheimer's disease. Previous work in this area led to the award of his MD in 2008. Dr Todd trained in the Northern Ireland Deanery Higher Medical Training Programme in Geriatric Medicine and General (Internal) Medicine.

In: Dementia
Editor: Pamela Tanner
ISBN: 978-1-63321-928-1

Chapter 9

Effects of Occupational Therapy Based Rehabilitation in Alzheimer's Disease: Current Advances

Juan Rodríguez Mansilla[1]*, Patricia Martín Romo-Morcillo[2], María Jiménez Palomares[1], Antonio María Flores Nieto[1], Elisa María Garrido Ardila[1] and María Victoria González López-Arza[1]

[1]Department of Medical-Surgical Therapy, Medicine Faculty, Extremadura University, Badajoz, Spain
[2]Encinar de las Cruces Senior Center, Don Benito, Badajoz, Spain

Abstract

Alzheimer's disease is a primary degenerating brain condition. Its etiology is unknown and it is characterized by the presence of neuropathological and neurochemical features. This condition generally starts slowly and in an insidious way and it progresses gradually along a period of time, normally years.

The clinical symptoms include a progressive and total deterioration of the cognitive function which is often accompanied by personality and behavior changes. This leads to a reduction of the capacity to carry out activities of daily living (ADL) by the person affected.

Currently, Alzheimer's disease is the most common type of dementia. The consequences of this condition are devastating. The patient will have his cognitive function affected, his normal behavior altered and he will progressively need help to perform the ADL. These consequences also extend to the family who also suffer the impact of the effects of dementia. The family will be absolutely essential in order to provide the care needed by the patient during the time of the condition and its progression.

* Phone number: 0034 924289300 ext: 86150 ; e-mail: jrodman@unex.es

Nowadays, there are studies that have analyzed and compared the effectiveness of different rehabilitation approaches. These techniques have shown improvements of the ADL performance and the quality of life of the patients diagnosed with Alzheimer's disease. From the rehabilitation approach of Occupational Therapy, the objective is to maintain as long as possible the independence of the person to perform ADL. Slowing down the progression of the disability and improving the quality of life of the person and his family is of crucial importance. This can only be achieved with a holistic approach that allows the management of the complexity of Alzheimer's disease from the psychological., physical and social view, including as well the environment as all these factors have an influence on the performance of ADL.

Considering the reported benefits of rehabilitation on the quality of life of these patients, the objective of this chapter was to analyse the results obtained by different authors in relation to the effects that rehabilitation, with a special focus on Occupational Therapy, has on subjects diagnosed with Alzheimer's disease. The results obtained showed that there is scientific literature that indicates that Occupational Therapy has a positive effect on persons with this condition. The main improvements were seen in behavior and emotional aspects, in carer burden, in the quality of life, independence, cognitive function and the institutionalisation of the subjects.

1. Introduction

Alzheimer's disease is considered as one of the epidemic of the 20th century and it has become a health problem of the first order. This condition has an impact on family, society and health professionals [1].

Alzheimer's disease is characterized by different symptoms which include progressive and total deterioration of the cognitive functions (memory loss, language deficits, loss of sense of orientation and executive functions) frequently accompanied by personality and behavior changes. All this leads to a reduction of the person's capacity to perform activities of daily living [2].

The onset of this condition begins with small disorders that initially go unnoticed but gradually, they become ostensible affecting the person severely. The progression of the disease differs from patient to patient regarding the symptoms and the speed of development. However, three common stages of the progression can be established: mild, moderate and severe stage [1].

Important syndromes are associated to Alzheimer's disease such as the following: memory deficits; communication problems; perception disorders (hallucination, pathological delusions, and delirious ideas); behavior disorders (emotional lability, aggressive or violent behavior, persecution and repetitive behaviors, vagrancy, lost inhibition); sleep patterns disturbances such as wakefulness (hypersomnia, day and night rhythm disorders, agitation during the night and insomnia, including onset insomnia, maintenance insomnia, early morning insomnia and early awakening); mood disorders (depression), disturbances of consciousness and eating disorders [1].

The progression of the disease is slow and it can vary between 3 to 20 years. A patient is considered to be able to live for 8 to 10 years from the time when the diagnosis is made. The progress will be faster the younger the person is when he or she was diagnosed [3].

Three different levels of severity of Alzheimer's disease can be described [4]:

- Level I, or mild dementia: Characterized by progressive memory disturbances, normal motor assessment, incapacity to perform complex social tasks (finance or work), new jobs or tasks that are not in the normal routine although the performance of home activities is preserved. Other deficits such as complex calculations, anomia and executive functions disturbances begin to be apparent. The duration of this phase is usually between 1 to 3 years, although it varies.
- Level II, or moderate dementia: dementia causes mental confusion and extrapyramidal symptoms are frequent. The patient starts requiring assistance for basic activities of daily living and at home. The memory loss is present and even temporal disorientation is usual (confusion phase), clear cortical deficits (reading difficulties, dysphasia and dyspraxia) and behavior alterations (misplacements, irritability and apathy) start to appear. This phase usually lasts for 2 to 5 years.
- Level III, or severe dementia: The dementia is established completely and there are motor dysfunctions. This phase is characterized by the need of constant supervision and help. The patient is incontinent, mainly bladder incontinent, forgets everything, is not able to reason and does not recognize people close to him/her. Language is progressively reduced and there is a total deterioration of the personality. The duration of this phase varies from 2 to 4 years.

These stages are in many patients preceded by a pre-clinic phase characterized by cognitive deterioration without dementia, with complaints of memory loss, frequent forgetfulness, cognitive deficits and functional capacity not clearly affected [4].

The treatment of Alzheimer's disease requires a multidisciplinary intervention answering all the problems of the patients and considering the stage of the condition. Therefore, the treatments that are currently used focus on different aspects including preserving mental function, management of behavior related symptoms and delay or prevention of the condition [5].

In the absence of a curative treatment, a multidimensional approach is needed. This approach should include pharmacological therapy and non-pharmacological interventions that focus on optimizing the cognition, behavior and function of the subjects with dementia. It should also consider and address the needs of the carers [6].

The increase of incidence of this condition has led to a rise of interest on the use of non-pharmacological therapies for its management. These therapies facilitate the optimization and maintenance of the cognitive abilities of the patients with dementia [7].

Non-pharmacological therapies (NPT) or cognitive interventions are those that achieve a relevant improvement of the patients or their carers without the use of psychopharmacological substances [7].

NPT started to be used in the management of dementia by various groups of professionals (occupational therapists, psychologists, physiotherapists, etc.) with the aim to alleviate the effects of the condition. The first related study was published with the title: 'Experimental treatment of persistent senile confusion'. Nowadays, the intervention that was applied in the study to improve social and domestic activities would be called occupational therapy (Cosin et al., 1958) [8].

Afterwards, the first communications related to the benefits of reality orientation were published. Today, this approach would be engulfed within the broader concept of cognitive stimulation (Taulbee y Folsom, 1966) [9].

From the 1980's, the concept of 'caregiver's burden', which was coming from psychiatry, started to be used in the field of dementia. Also, different support programmes for family carers were developed (Zarit et al.,1987) [10].

NPT in dementia is based on a combination of structured approaches, specific techniques applied on specific problems and good intuition of the caregiver in order to respect the tolerance level of the patient. NPT include among others, occupational therapy which mainly works on improving basic and instrumental ADL [11].

Non-Pharmacological Therapies [12]

Non-pharmacological therapies focusing on subjects with dementia:

- Terapias no farmacológicas para mejorar la cognición.
- NPT to improve cognition
  - Reality orientation and reminiscence therapy
  - Cognitive stimulation, training and rehabilitation
- NPT to improve ADL

In order to acquire the abilities required for the performance of ADL, the practice and repetition of tasks are needed. The improvement is clearer if the therapy programmes include: the repeated practice of the capacities to reinforce, stimulation through multiple sensory channels and lesser cognitive demands. In this way, basic ADL are more prone to improve than instrumental ADL [12].

Among the interventions that have shown better results we can highlight programmed urination to decrease bladder incontinence, gradual assistance to improve independence and positive feedback to increase feeding autonomy [12].

- NPT focusing on behavior symptoms
  - Care programmes focused on the people
  - Musical therapy
  - Snoezelen (multisensory stimulation)
  - Multicomponent intervention on the patient
- Other NPT
  - Physical exercise
  - Enviromental modifications

NPT focusing on the caregiver

- Multicomponent intervention focused on the patient and the carer.
- Caregiver support
- Training and education

- Counseling and case management
- Respite care

Now, the current situation of occupational therapy applied as an NPT for the management of Alzheimer's disease is described.

2. Occupational Therapy

Occupational therapy is a young discipline in many aspects. However, since ancient times, there are many references in health science literature and at the beginning of neurology and psychiatry that referred to the origins and the main basis of this profession. Examples can be found that illustrate how philosophy and occupational therapy clinical practice have its origins in the humanization of medical assistance [13].

Benjamin Rush was the first physician in the U.S.A. who used the concept of occupation and moral treatment. He is frequently considered as the father of psychiatry in U.S.A. Occupation emerged at the early days of the 20th century under the term of occupational therapy [13].

Some therapists continued with the ideas of industrial and working therapy applied in the field of psychiatry rehabilitation and many studies related to occupational therapy were published [13].

In the First World War, the need to provide assistance to all the injured had to be faced and occupational therapy was introduced by Dr. Henderson in 1919 in a modern psychiatric hospital in Scotland, the Gartnavel Royal Mental Hospital. With the observation and analysis of the occupational therapy practice, the discipline was included in different centres and the American Association of Occupational Therapy was created [13,14].

There are many definitions of occupational therapy. Each professional society, each training school and even each professional have their own definition of occupational therapy. Among all of them, the definition from 1986 of the American Association of Occupational Therapy is probably the most known: Occupational therapy is the therapeutic use of the self-care, work and leisure activities in order to achieve independent function, improve development and prevent disability. It can include the adaptation of tasks and environment to accomplish maximum independence and to improve quality of life [14].

The concept of occupation has evolved over the history of the profession and it can be defined as: 'Daily activities that reflect cultural values and provide life structure and meaning to individuals; those activities are related to self-care human needs, enjoyment and participation in society' [15].

The occupational therapists support that wellbeing and health is achieved and maintained when clients are able to partake in occupations and activities that allow the participation needed at home, in school, in the working place and during community life. When occupational therapists work with their clients, they take into consideration the different types of occupation in which the person will be involved. The great variety of existing activities and occupations are classified in 'occupational areas': ADL, instrumental ADL, rest and sleep, education, work, games, leisure and social participation [16].

- Activities of daily living: bathing, showering, bladder and bowel care, dressing, eating and nutrition, functional mobility, assistive devices care, personal hygiene and grooming, sexual activity, toileting.
- Instrumental ADL: Others people's care, pet care, bringing up children, communication management, mobility in the community, finance management, health management and maintenance, home management, cooking and cleaning, religious practice, security and emergency response, shopping.
- Rest and sleep: rest, sleep, get ready for bed and sleep participation.
- Education: participation in formal education, non-formal training needs assessment, participation in non-formal education.
- Work: interests and activities for employment search, searching and finding a job, work performance, preparation and adaptation for retirement, volunteering assessment and analysis, participation as a volunteer.
- Game: game analysis, game participation, leisure and time off, leisure assessment and analysis, leisure participation.
- Social participation: participation in the community, participation in the family, participation with peer and friends [16].

In occupational therapy, the intervention and rehabilitation is carried out through activity itself. Activities are applied as intervention techniques to improve any ability required for leisure, work or ADL.

The occupational therapist designs activities to encourage abilities that the person is losing or to train other capacities that have the same function. The main objective is functionality in order to help the person to be as independent as possible. In this way, the professional reinforces the abilities that are still present and provides the person other tools to develop daily functions [17].

The intervention is based on the facilitation of the participation in occupation related to health through the actions taken by the professionals in collaboration with the client. This process is divided into three steps: intervention planning, implementation and evaluation [10].

The types of interventions that are acknowledged in the occupational therapy framework are the following [16]:

- Therapeutic use of oneself
- Therapeutic use of occupations and activities
- Counselling process
- Education and training process
- Self-management

The professional body of knowledge consists of a group of theories selected from different areas of knowledge, including those developed from the occupational therapy's clinical practice. When theories are brought together, they are the Theoretical Reference Frameworks [18].

Each reference framework guides and directs the occupational therapists actions allowing the professional activity to be effective and coherent. It always needs to be in accordance to the needs and reality of the clients and considering the environment [19].

The occupational therapy reference frameworks are classified, according to Hagedorn (1997) referred to by Romero, in the following [18]:

- Primary physiological reference framework: Supports that the cause of the disease is the alteration of the internal and external balance of the person leading to dysfunction. These alterations can affect perception, feelings, cognition, movement and functional activities performance. These specific problems can be treated thought the principles of the reference frameworks: Bio-mechanic, neurodevelopment or motor control, perceptive-cognitive.
- Psychological reference framework: It is based on different theories: psychoanalytic, phenomenological., behavioral and humanistic. These theories guide the analysis of the behavior and the psyche of the human being having a strong influence in the field of mental health. This area is approached by occupational therapists through the principles of the reference frameworks: psychodynamic, humanist and behavioral-cognitive.

Objectives of Occupational Therapy in Dementia

The contribution of occupational therapy caring for the person with senile dementia is focused on the use and encouragement of those abilities that are intact. The assessment is performed to confirm the strengths and difficulties that the person has. The activities are analyzed in order to adjust them to the capacities of the person within their daily routine, their interests and their social interactions [20].

The main objectives of occupational therapy, when applied to persons with dementia, are [21]:

a) To maintain, restore or improve functional capacity
b) To promote the participation in activities that optimize mental and physical health.
c) To facilitate care activities

The specific type of intervention depends on the stage of the disease and the clinical manifestations of the cognitive deterioration in relation to ADL [21].

In particular, the occupational therapist working with Alzheimer's disease patients is responsible for the holistic assessment and the posterior observation of the relation between the cognitive and physical losses and the environmental factors that can influence in the progression [21,22].

In this way and through different types of activities, the aim is to maintain the independence as much as possible and to help the person have a better quality of life at home or at the residential home.

The development of these activities is essential as well as their need to be significant for the person because, if that is the case, the wellbeing level and the accomplishment of the set goals will be more successful [22].

As the disease progresses, the person will be dependent for the performance of ADL and for most of the instrumental ADL. In some cases, the person may only need supervision or minimal assistance to perform a task appropriately while in some others, the person may need maximum help from another person [22].

The assessment of the functional capacities of the individual is necessary in order to identify the deficits and abilities and use it as the base to formulate the objectives and plan the treatment.

The occupational therapists can use a combination of methods to analyse the functional profile of the person. The main methods are questionning, tests and observation.

When working with persons diagnosed with dementia such as Alzheimer's disease, we do not refer to the terms rehabilitation, unless it is an exceptional cases. Instead, the terms maintaining, preserving, keeping, stimulating, encouraging, facilitating, etc., are used [22].

In Alzheimer's disease, apathy and mood swings are very frequent and therefore, the intervention should focus on the improvement of these symptoms as it will have an impact on the performance of activities [22].

The occupational therapist will carry out a therapeutic intervention based on different types of activities in order to achieve the previously set objectives. These activities will be selected and adapted according to the level of deterioration of the person [22].

3. Effectiveness of Occupational Therapy in Alzheimer's Disease

Considering the need to analyse the evidence of effectiveness of occupational therapy, the clinical effects reported in different studies regarding the improvement of the quality of life of the person with Alzheimer's disease are now described.

a. Effects of Occupational Therapy on Independence

Regarding the benefits of the occupational therapy intervention on Independence and autonomy of persons with Alzheimer's disease performing ADL, five studies analyse this outcome measure.

Rogers JC et al. [23], carried out a clinical trial with 86 patients with Alzheimer's disease. The results showed that occupational therapy intervention based on behavior rehabilitation improved ADL. In particular, the patients significantly improved the time spent dressing without help, the global participation in ADL and the inadequate behavior patterns decreased. It was also observed that the improvements were maintained if the behavior rehabilitation intervention continued.

The conclusion of the study was that individualized behavior rehabilitation, when it is designed to identify ADL deficits and to maintain the abilities trained, decreases the physical assistance that these patients need for their personal care.

Dooley NR, Hinojosa J [24] conducted a study with 40 subjects diagnosed with Alzheimer's disease and their caregivers. Although the main objective of the study was to observe the improvement accomplished in relation to the quality of life of the person and the caregiver's burden, the secondary outcome measure was the impact on ADL.

The authors found that the training of the carers on environmental modifications, accessibility and helping their siblings in daily activities was more beneficial than just the information provided without training.

The training of theses caregivers increase the independence of their family member with Alzheimer's disease in the performance of ADL.

However, Voigt – Radloff S et al. [25] affirmed that 10 sessions of community occupational therapy were not more beneficial in relation to the daily functionality of patients with Alzheimer's disease than periodic consultations in the short and long term.

In this randomized controlled trial, the participants were allocated to an intervention group that received 10 sessions of domiciliary occupational therapy with a duration of 1 hour each session for a period of 5 weeks. The sessions were divided into a diagnostic phase, to identify de ADL deficits or problems; a decision making phase, when the therapeutic goals and objectives for the patients and the caregiver were established; and a last phase of treatment when the required compensations and environmental modifications were done as a management approach of the functional problems. The control group received information sessions focusing on the same ADL problems. The authors concluded that there were no significant differences between the intervention and the control group. During the follow up period, the need of help increased in both groups and therefore, the hours of assistance provided by the carers for ADL performance also increased.

Callahan CM et al. [26] also included the main caregivers in their study and the total of participants was 180 including them and the patients. They carried out an intervention programme where the experimental group received occupational therapy and primary health care and the control group only received primary health care. The objective of this trial was to delay the functional deterioration, help the patients and their caregivers in the performance of ADL and encourage self-care abilities. There are no results available in the literature as the study has not been completed yet.

Regarding the comparison of the benefits of occupational therapy in Alzheimer's disease with other types of dementia, the study of Baldelli MV et al. [27] must be highlighted. They compared the effects of a therapeutic ADL programme during 40 days on 20 patients with Alzheimer's disease and 14 patients with vascular dementia. The results of the study showed significant improvements on the 'The Ronchi Brief Evaluation Battery'[54] (occupational therapy scale that assesses ADL including washing, dressing, eating and toileting) after the intervention. However, they observed that the improvements were superior in the case of the patients with vascular dementia.

b. Effectiveness of Occupational Therapy on the Caregiver's Burden and Quality of Life

In relation to the benefits of occupational therapy on the caregiver's burden and the quality of life of the patient and the caregiver, 3 studies refer to this outcome measure.

Glitin LN et al. [28] did a randomized controlled trial with 127 main caregivers of patients with Alzheimer's disease. The objective was to assess if the occupational therapy intervention helped to decrease the caregiver's burden and allow them to have the capacities to perform the appropriate environmental modifications to assist the independent function of the patients. They compared an experimental group that received 6 sessions of occupational therapy with a control group that had the routine health care services.

The conclusion of the study were that after 6 weeks of intervention, the participants required less assistance (p = 0,043) from the carer and had less behavior incidents (p = 0,019) as compared to the control group. In addition, after 12 months follow up check, the improvements were maintained (p = 0,033).

Dooley NR, Hinojosa J [24] conducted a study with 40 persons diagnosed with Alzheimer's disease and their caregivers. They found that the participant's training on care, environmental modifications, accessibility and the intervention made in relation to the items of the Assessment of Instrumental Function improved the quality of life of persons with Alzheimer's disease and decreased the workload of the caregivers in comparison to the intervention that was based on counselling and information to the carers without training.

This study shows that the assessment and training of functional capacities have better outcomes than when therapy is applied with no previous evaluation of the affected functions.

Other authors who focused their research on the benefits of occupational therapy on the quality of life are Viola LF et al. [29]. The main objective of their study was to find out if an intervention combining cognitive stimulation, occupational therapy, physiotherapy and fun activities improved the cognitive functions of patients with dementia. However, the results of the secondary outcome measures showed that intervention combined with psychoeducation group sessions and psychological therapy was beneficial for the quality of life of the patients.

c. Effectiveness of Occupational Therapy on Cognitive Function

Two studies analyzed this outcome measure. Regarding the comparison of the benefits of cognitive rehabilitation with other types of therapy and/or no other treatment, we can highlight the research done by Clare L et al. [30]. They conducted a randomized controlled trial with 69 subjects with Alzheimer type dementia or mixed Alzheimer and vascular dementia and their 44 family carers.

The experimental group received 8 individual weekly sessions of cognitive rehabilitation, control group 1 followed a relaxation therapy programme and control group 2 was not given any treatment.

The assessment was done through the Canadian Occupational Performance Measure, mood and quality of life questionnaires and a brief range of neuropsychological tests. The results showed that cognitive rehabilitation caused a significant improvement of the objective performance indexes of the cognitive tests and the satisfaction of the patients. This improvement was also observed in behavior.

On the other hand, Viola LF et al. [29] proved in their double blind study conducted with patients diagnosed with Alzheimer's disease that the cognitive rehabilitation programme that they applied did not improve the cognitive functions when compared to those who did not follow the programme but instead the functions were maintained. The control group did not maintain the cognitive functions and they even became worse.

The intervention consisted on computer assisted cognitive rehabilitation, cognitive training, speech therapy, occupational therapy, art therapy, physical education, physiotherapy and cognitive stimulation through reading and logical games. The group sessions for the caregivers included psychological therapy and psychoeducation focusing on the clinical aspects of the disease, the progression and the expected loss of independence of the patient.

d. Effectiveness of Occupational Therapy on Behavior and Emotional Changes

No studies that analyzed the effects of occupational therapy on behavior changes in Alzheimer's disease have been found published in the literature. Only 3 studies assessed this outcome measure as a secondary objective of the research.

The intervention on the ADL conducted by Rogers JC et al. [23] showed that an occupational therapy programme based on behavioral rehabilitation not only achieved improvements of the independence but also significantly decreased the inadequate behavior of the patients.

Glitin LN et al. [28] obtained a reduction of the incidences related to behavior with 6 sessions of occupational therapy.

Lastly, Clare L et al. [30] concluded that 8 sessions of cognitive rehabilitation improved global cognitive function and the behavior of subjects diagnosed with Alzheimer's type dementia, mixed dementia and vascular dementia.

e. Effects of Occupational Therapy on Intitutionalisation

One study analyses if occupational therapy can delay the admission to residential homes or not. Brodaty H et al. [31] carried out a randomized controlled trial during 8 years to assess the long term effectiveness of an intensive training programme for the caregivers of patients with dementia. All the participants followed a 10 day programme based on memory training, occupational therapy and relaxation techniques. The caregivers were allocated into three groups: two experimental groups (10 days of immediate training or delayed training after 6 months) and a control group. The 10 day sessions for the carers were informal sessions led by health professionals.

The authors found out that the intense 10 day training programme and follow up for the caregivers delayed the admission into residential homes of the patients with Alzheimer's disease.

References

[1] Álvarez C. El Alzheimer: La enfermedad y su entorno. Madrid (Spain): Ediciones Eneida; 2002.

[2] Gutiérrez Pérez A. 2011 año de la investigación en el Alzheimer. 2011; 4(135): 47-49.

[3] Peña J. Enfermedad de Alzheimer. Del diagnóstico a la terapia: conceptos y hechos. Barcelona (Spain) : Fundación "la caixa"; 1999.

[4] Ouedraogo A, Ouango, JG. Clinical aspects of adult schizophrenia in the psychiatric service al the Salgado Ouedraogo Nacional Hospital Center de Ouagadougou (Burkina Faso). *Dakar Medical.* 1998; 43: 194-197.

[5] Alzheimer's Disease Fact Sheet. [Internet]. [Consultado el 9 de Junio de 2013]. Disponible en: www.nih.gov/Alzheimers/Publications/adfact.htm

[6] Woods,RT. Non-pharmacologial techiniques. En:Qizilbash N, Schneider LS, Cui E, Tarior P, Brodaty H, Kaye J, Erkinjuyi T. Evidence-based Dementia Practice. Ed: Blackwell Science Ltd. Oxford 2003: 428-446.

[7] Arroyo-Anlló E M, Poveda Díaz-Marta J, Chamorro Sánchez J. Técnicas de rehabilitación neuropsicológica en demencias: hacia la ciber-rehabilitación neuropsicológica. *Pensamiento psicológico.* 2012; 10(1): 107-127.

[8] Cosin LZ, Mort M, Post F, Westropp C, Williams M. Experimental treatment of persistent senile confusion. Int J Soc Psychiatry 1958; 4: 24-42.

[9] Taulbee LR, Folsom JC. Reality orientation for geriatric patients. *Hosp Community Psychiatry* 1966; 17: 133-5.

[10] Zarit SH, Anthony CR, Boutselis M. Interventions with care givers of dementia patients: comparison of two approaches. *Psychol. Aging* 1987; 2: 225-32.

[11] Guía de Recomendaciones Clínicas. Demencia. Dirección General de Organización de las Prestaciones Sanitarias Consejería de Salud y Servicios Sanitarios del Principado de Asturias; 2008.

[12] Manual de Actuación en la enfermedad de Alzheimer y otras demencias. Consejería de Sanidad Servicio Canario de la Salud. Dirección General de Programas Asistenciales. Gobierno de Canarias; 2011.

[13] Pérez de Heredia M, Brea M, Martínez R M. Origen de la terapia ocupacional en España. *Revista de neurología.* 2007: 45(11): 695-698.

[14] Durante Molina P. Conceptos básicos de terapia ocupacional. En: Polonio López B, directora. Conceptos fundamentales de terapia ocupacional.1ºed. Madrid: Médica Panamericana; 2001. 13-24.

[15] Crepeau, E., Cohn, E., & Schell, B. (Eds.) Willard and Spackman's occupational therapy. Philadelphia: Lippincott Williams & Wilkins; 2003

[16] Ávila Álvarez A, Martínez Piédrola R, Matilla Mora R, Máximo Bocanegra M, Méndez Méndez B, Talavera Valverde MA et al., Marco de Trabajo para la práctica de la Terapia Ocupacional: Dominio y proceso. 2da Edición [Traducción]. www.terapia-ocupacional.com [portal en internet]. 2010 [10/05/2014]; [85p.]. Disponible en: http://.terapia –ocupacional.com/aota2010esp.pdf Traducido de: American Occupational Therapy Asociation (2008). Occupational therapy practice framework: Domain and process (2nd Ed.).

[17] Redondo Garcés A. Terapia Ocupacional en Alzheimer y otras demencias. Nuevos puntos de vista para un cuidador. AFAL. Mayo 2005.

[18] Romero A, Moruno M. Terapia Ocupacional. Teoría y técnicas. Barcelona (Spain): Masson, S.A; 2003.

[19] Santana Jorge Z. Marcos de referencias aplicación en terapia ocupacional. [Internet]. [Acceso 30 Mayo 2013]. Disponible en: http://www.espaciotovenezuela.com/pdf_to/ marcos_de_refencias.pdf

[20] Durante Molina P, Altimir Losada S. Demencia senil. En: Durante Molina P, Pedro Tarrés P editores del libro. Terapia ocupacional en geriatría: principios y práctica. 1ª ed. Barcelona (Spain): Masson; 1998.117-132.

[21] Statement: Occupational Therapy Services for persons with Alzheimer´s disease and other dementias. *Am. J. Occup. Ther.* 1994; 48(11): 1029-1031.

[22] Pérez Muñano C, Pérez Muñoz A, Rodríguez Pérez I. Intervención desde el área de terapia ocupacional. Guía práctica para profesionales que trabajan con enfermos de Alzheimer. Centro Alzheimer Fundación Reina Sofía. Madrid. 32-51.

[23] Rogers JC, Holm MB, Burgio LD, Granieri E, Hsu C, Hardin JM, et al., Improving morning care routines of nursing home residents with dementia. *J. Am. Geriatr. Soc.* 1999 ;47(9):1049-1057.

[24] Dooley NR, Hinojosa J. Improving quality of life for persons with Alzheimer's disease and their family caregivers: brief occupational therapy intervention. *Am. J. Occup. Ther.* 2004 ; 58(5):561-569.

[25] Voigt-Radloff S, Graff M, Leonhart R, Schornstein K, Jessen F, Bohlken J, et al., A multicentre RCT on community occupational therapy in Alzheimer's disease: 10 sessions are not better than one consultation. *BMJ Open* 2011 Aug 9;1(1):e000096-2011-000096.

[26] Callahan CM, Boustani MA, Schmid AA, Austrom MG, Miller DK, Gao S, et al., Alzheimer's disease multiple intervention trial (ADMIT): study protocol for a randomized controlled clinical trial. *Trials* 2012; 27;13:92-6215-13-92.

[27] Baldelli MV, Boiardi R, Ferrari P, Bianchi S, Bianchi MH. Dementia and occupational therapy. *Arch. Gerontol. Geriatr* 2007;44 Suppl 1:45-48.

[28] Gitlin LN, Hauck WW, Dennis MP, Winter L. Maintenance of effects of the home environmental skill-building program for family caregivers and individuals with Alzheimer's disease and related disorders. *J. Gerontol. A. Biol. Sci. Med. Sci.* 2005 ;60(3):368-374.

[29] Viola LF, Nunes PV, Yassuda MS, Aprahamian I, Santos FS, Santos GD et al., Effects of a multidisciplinary cognitive rehabilitation program for patients with mild Alzheimer's disease. *Clinics* (Sao Paulo). 2011; 66(8):1395-400.

[30] Clare L, Linden DE, Woods RT, Whitaker R, Evans SJ, Parkinson CH, et al., Goal-oriented cognitive rehabilitation for people with early-stage Alzheimer disease: a single-blind randomized controlled trial of clinical efficacy. *Am. J. Geriatr. Psychiatry* 2010 ;18(10):928-939.

[31] Brodaty H, Gresham M, Luscombe G. The Prince Henry Hospital dementia caregivers training programme. *Int. J. Geriatr. Psychiatry.* 1997 ; 12 (2):183-92.

In: Dementia
Editor: Pamela Tanner

ISBN: 978-1-63321-928-1

Chapter 10

Normal Pressure Hydrocephalus

F. C. G. Pinto[1], M. F. Oliveira[2,*] and R. M. Pereira[3]
[1]Division of Functional Neurosurgery of the Institute of Psychiatry, Hospital das Clínicas, Universidade de São Paulo, São Paulo, Brazil
[2]Department of Neurosurgery.Hospital do Servidor Público Estadual de São Paulo, São Paulo-Brazil
[3]Medical student at Universidade Anhembi Morumbi, São Paulo, Brazil

Abstract

Idiopathic normal pressure hydrocephalus (INPH) is characterized by progressive gait apraxia, cognitive dysfunction and urinary incontinence (Hakim-Adams syndrome). INPH is associated with communicating hydrocephalus (as demonstrated by brain CT or MRI) and cerebrospinal fluid (CSF) pressure within the normal range (7-24 cm H2O). The clinical triad of Hakim-Adams syndrome is present in approximately 50% of cases; however, only one or a combination of two symptoms should be considered for diagnostic investigation. It is a differential diagnosis for most of the dementia syndromes and occurs mainly in elderly populations and it is one of the causes of potentially reversible dementia. Treatment of INPH is based in three pillars: conservative, ventriculoperitoneal shunt (VPS) and endoscopic third ventriculostomy (ETV). **Conclusion:** Appropriate and well designed high-level evidence studies are still lacking, but the current gold standard treatment of INPH is performed with VPS.

Keywords: Endoscopic third ventriculostomy, cerebrospinal fluid shunts, idiopathic normal pressure hydrocephalus

* Corresponding author: Matheus Fernandes de Oliveira, Av. Pedro de Toledo, 1800 – Vila Clementino, São Paulo – São Paulo – Brazil. Email: mafernoliv@yahoo.com.br.

1. Introduction

Normal pressure hydrocephalus (NPH) is a neurological syndrome which manifests typically between 60 and 80 years of age, characterized by a triad of symptoms consisting of gait apraxia, dementia and urinary incontinence, associated with ventriculomegaly (detected radiologically) and normal pressure of the cerebrospinal fluid (CSF) [1-3]. The neurosurgeon Salomón Hakim was the first to report such syndrome in Hospital San Juan de Dios, Bogota, Colombia, in 1964.

NPH can be divided into two categories: idiopathic and secondary. The secondary NPH occurs in the context of neurological events such as subarachnoid hemorrhage (SAH), intraventricular hemorrhage caused by trauma or aneurysm rupture and meningitis. In contrast, idiopathic NPH usually occurs between the sixth and eighth decades of life and does not have its pathophysiological mechanisms completely understood [4-6].

Once NPH is a rare case of reversible dementia, it is essential to have an adequate clinical assessment, early diagnosis and proper treatment in such cases [4-7]. Standard treatment is accomplished through the implantation of a ventricular shunt, offering the possibility of significant neurological improvement [7].

2. Epidemiology

The incidence and prevalence of NPH are still not accurate and many studies have reported different values. This fact is due to the absence of a universal consensus on the steps for diagnosis of the disease, which results in underdiagnosis and misdiagnosis, since NPH can be "confused" with other etiologies of similar presentation, especially when the characteristics of the triad do not manifest at the same time [8-12].

The known incidence is approximately 6 per 100,000 and it has a prevalence of 22 per 100,000 for suspected iNPH. There are associations with hypertension, cerebrovascular disease and Alzheimer disease [13, 14].

3. Physiopathology

Although NPH was described 50 years ago, its pathophysiology is still not fully defined. Great efforts were made to elucidate the mechanisms of installation and various some hypotheses have been the basis for current comprehension. These assumptions vary widely and include impaired CSF absorption, ischemia of the deep white matter, redistribution of vascular pulsations and decreased compliance of the brain parenchyma, blood vessels and the subarachnoid space [15, 16, 17, 18].

4. Clinical Features

NPH manifests itself in general through clinical triad of gait apraxia, dementia and urinary incontinence combined with radiographic findings of ventriculomegaly and CSF normal pressure. Signs and symptoms typically develop insidiously, bilaterally, but may appear lateralized when superimposed by coexisting conditions such as cerebrovascular accident (CVA), peripheral neuropathy and radiculopathy and usually occur between the sixth and eighth decades of life [8-14]

Because NPH is a disease primarily of the elderly population , age group in which the difficulty of gait, dementia and urinary incontinence are relatively common , a variety of diagnoses of individual symptoms should be considered , including neurodegenerative diseases , vascular etiologies and urological disorders. A list of differential diagnosis of NPH is shown in Table 1 , and before such diagnoses , it is clear the importance of a proper clinical evaluation , both by general practitioners , as by geriatricians and neurologists who are finally assisting patients who have characteristics of NPH , since early diagnosis and, above all , correct, closely related to the therapeutic success [8-14].

4.1. Gait Disturbing

Generally, the disturbance of gait and some other symptoms are required for diagnosis, and tends to be the most recognizable feature of NPH. Although no pathognomonic feature is present, it is usually a broad-based, short steps with your feet drag on the ground (like a "magnetic gait"), difficulty turning gait [17, 18]. No motor weakness is present but patients often have a history of falls. Imbalance and decreased gait speed (due to the short steps and gait apraxia) are also common. However, the arm swing when walking is preserved, which may help in distinguishing with Parkinsonian gait [17, 18]. Patients may complain of difficulty rising from a chair, weakness of the lower extremities and fatigue when walking. Moreover, often show an inability to climb on the exam table or in their own beds [17, 18].

The origin of changes in gait is not fully understood, but several hypotheses have been suggested. One of the hypotheses suggests that the increase of the ventricles in NPH causes a compression and / or deformation of the fibers of the upper motor neurons that pass through the medial portion of the corona radiata [15, 16].

Table 1. Differential diagnosis of NPH [(28)]

Degenerative	Vascular dementia	Other causes
Alzheimer Disease	Multiple infarcts	Obstructive hydrocephalus
Parkinson Disease	Small vessel disease	Congenital hydrocephalus
Lewy Body Disease	Binswanger disease	Spinal tumors
Huntington Disease	Vertebro-basilar insufficiency	Deficiency of vitamin B12
Frontotemporal dementia		Spinal stenosis
Multiple systems atrophy		Traumatic brain injury
Spongiform encephalopathy		
Corticobasal degeneration		

Other conditions that cause abnormalities of gait should be considered when making the diagnosis of NPH as lumbar canal stenosis, peripheral neuropathy, cerebrovascular disease, Alzheimer's disease (AD), tumors, trauma, Parkinson's disease, Lewy bodies dementia, depression, chronic alcoholism, vitamin B12 and folic acid deficiency. Furthermore, the abnormality of gait is the most responsive to treatment with signal implementation of a CSF shunt system [15, 16].

4.2. Cognitive Impairment

Cognitive changes are generally the second manifestation of NPH after progressive gait disturbance. It is characterized by a progressive impairment of the functions of subcortical and frontal areas, manifested as psychomotor retardation, decreased attention and concentration, executive dysfunction and spatial vision and memory impairment, and impaired executive function in the early disease course [8-18].

Deficits of cortical area as apraxia, agnosia and aphasia are rare. Severity of such deficits seen in NPH may vary from minimally detectable to severe deep and significant improvement of symptoms can be obtained after the shunt, thus being one of the few reversible causes of dementia [19, 20, 21].

Mini mental state examination (MMSE) may show deficits for performing calculations, concentration, writing sentences, copy the intersecting pentagons, and follow a three-stage command. Slowed mental processing may be apparent due to increased test time. The test performance of the clock can also be changed, showing a poor space planning and organization. Behavioral disorders have also been reported associated with NPH as depression, mania, aggression, obsessive compulsive disorder, psychosis including paranoia, hallucinations and disorders of impulse control [19, 20, 21].

Nevertheless, MMSE may be normal in some cases with early behavioral and executive symptoms. It is suggested that other tests should be applied, such as Montreal Cognitive Assessment Test (MOCA) and Cambridge Cognitive Test (CAMCOG). These tests present higher sensitivity in detecting early global deficits [19, 20, 21].

Depressive symptoms in patients with NPH may be a consequence of neurochemical brain disorder. However, it may appear in response to physical and mental disability. The site of dysfunction responsible for dementia in NPH remains uncertain, although the frontostriatal system has been implicated by some investigators. Others emphasize the importance of other subcortical structures, including projection fibers passing near the lateral ventricles [19, 20, 21].

The differential diagnosis can be particularly difficult due to the similarity of cognitive changes such as Alzheimer disease (AD). Generally, the latter is most associated with memory impairment, learning and guidance, while NPH is more often associated with decreased psychomotor and fine motor speed. Both diseases can lead to a loss of executive function, attention and concentration, but NPH hardly cause early changes of language. The existence of AD and concomitant NPH is not uncommon, and the probability of each increases with the presence of advanced age and hypertension. Subtle clinical details associated with neuroimage tools and predictive tests may help to differentiate diagnoses [19, 20, 21].

4.3. Urinary Incontinence

Urinary incontinence is usually observed in advanced stages of the disease and appears to occur by a disruption of periventricular neuronal pathways that are directed to the sacral center of the bladder leading to overactivity of the detrusor muscle, which can result primarily in urinary urgency and urinary frequency. It may also occur due to gait, apraxia and bradykinesia that prevent the patient from reaching the toilet in time and in extremely advanced cases, disorder can result from a lack of concern for micturition, suggesting that incontinence is associated with a frontal executive dysfunction [15, 16, 17, 18].

A study revealed that 95% of patients had evidence of detrusor overactivity, 93% had symptoms of lower urinary tract. Such symptoms included storage symptoms in 93 % of patients and voiding symptoms in 71% of patients. This study demonstrated that in the early stages urinary urgency may precede incontinence in patients with NPH [15, 16, 17, 18].

Incontinence is not a fixed component of the disease and may intermittently occur rarely or only in some cases. Pollakiuria and nocturia may also be present. Incontinence can also be caused by diseases that affect the autonomic control of the bladder, such as diabetic neuropathy. Other frequent causes are the use of diuretics and drugs with anticholinergic effect and multifactorial loss of bladder control as enlarged prostate and pelvic organ prolapsed [15, 16, 17, 18].

5. Diagnosis

Diagnosis of NPH requires converging evidence from clinical history, physical examination and neuroimaging studies, including computed tomography (CT) and MRI. MRI is superior to CT.

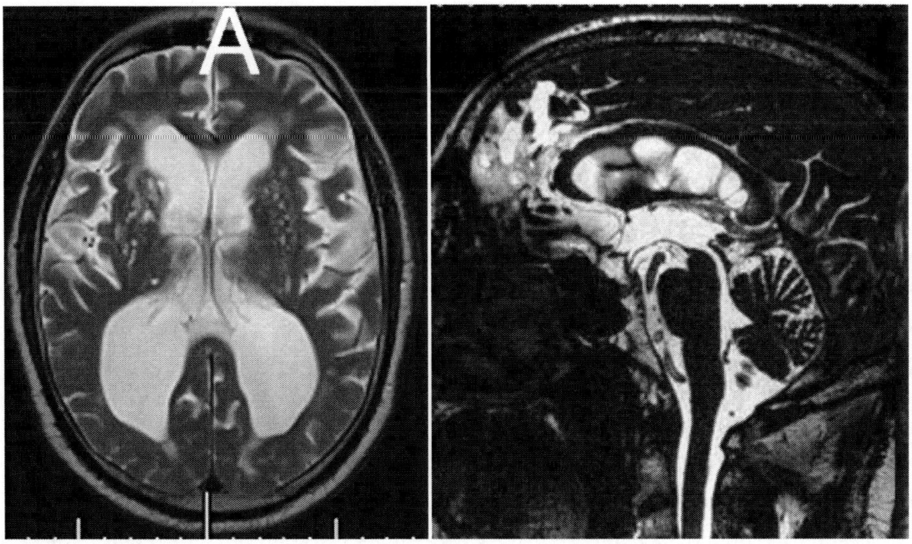

Figure 1. Typical neuroimage evaluation of NPH patient. Ventriculomegaly associated with cortical atrophy.

A CT scan can exclude the hypothesis of NPH and is useful for initial screening, while MRI provides more accurate information, allows the identification of structural abnormalities and cause of NPH. In addition, MRI can be used to obtain additional physiological information, such as CSF flow estimate using T2-weighted images [15, 16, 17, 18].

Ventricular enlargement (Evans index ≥ 0.3) in neuroimaging is needed, however, is not sufficient to establish the diagnosis of NPH. Results of neuroimaging (Figure 1) require interpretation associated with the clinical history and physical findings for the diagnosis [15, 16, 17, 18].

As for the physiological assessment, the opening pressure of the CSF, determined by lumbar puncture or a comparable procedure should be in a range 105-190 mm H2O, and appropriate measures of higher pressure or lower than this range are not consistent with the diagnosis of NPH [15, 16, 17,18].

Despite the importance of clinical evaluation for the diagnosis of NPH, the degree of certainty provided only by clinical diagnosis, related to improved patient after implantation of a CSF shunt system ranges from less than 50 % to 60 %. Therefore, because such surgery is an invasive procedure that can lead to complications, especially in elderly patients, it becomes necessary to use additional tests for two purposes: (1) confirm the diagnosis and (2) identify patients most likely to improve after surgery and predict with greater accuracy the likelihood of this improvement. The additional tests most commonly used are Tap test, cerebrospinal fluid infusion test, External lumbar drainage, continuous monitoring of intracranial pressure, assessment of the volume of cerebrospinal fluid ejection in the midbrain aqueduct (Aqueduct stroke volume) [8-14].

Treatment

Surgery, Rehabilitation Therapy or Conservative

Treatment of NPH based in current evidence lies in three pillars: conservative, endoscopic third ventriculostomy (ETV) and ventriculoperitoneal shunt (VPS). The conservative option has fallen after several studies which revealed good outcomes after surgical intervention. Thus, it is widely accepted that surgical treatment of patients with INPH is mandatory because surgery has been associated with a positive impact on the course of the disease, implicating in the life quality of patients and caregivers [22-25].

Rehabilitation strategies must always be included in the treatment of INPH. However it is considered a complementary treatment option.

Endoscopy or Shunt Surgery

Surgical interventions can be done by endoscopic or shunt approach. VPS is by far the most common method used to treat INPH worldwide. Once INPH is comprehended as a classic communicant hydrocephalus, ETV has been somehow not encouraged in its management. Different types of CSF shunt may be used, but the most common is the VPS [22-25].

However, VPS presents both the inconvenience of a prosthesis implant and medium- to long-term risk of complications requiring reoperation, such as infection, mechanical malfunction and overdrainage. If INPH patients could be treated by ETV with the same long-term effects as the VPS, the risk of long term complications would be reduced. The reduction of long term complications would be an advantage for elderly patients, who often have comorbidities [22-25].

The Italian multicenter retrospective study published in 2008 by Gangemi caused great debate in the neurosurgical community. This study showed a success rate of 69.1% for ETV treatment in 110 patients with INPH after a follow-up period of at least 2 years. Much of the criticism of this work originated from the following reasons: there was a lack of a clear distinction between the cases of idiopathic NPH and possible cases of secondary NPH, and the predictive functional test used was the monitoring of intracranial pressure, rather than the tests that are more widely used in the literature, such as the Tap Test (TT), the lumbar infusion test and external lumbar drainage monitoring for 72 hours [22-25].

Additionally, a study compared VPS with ETV and found higher perioperative mortality and complication rates in ETV group. This consideration is important to weight against the potential benefit of ETV: avoiding long-term shunt dependence. Prospective, randomized studies are needed to clarify some contradictory results [22-25].

In 2013, Pinto et al. conducted a randomized clinical trial to solve these conflicting facts comparing radiological and clinical patterns of evolution according to the treatment modality adopted (VPS x ETV). Both treatment modalities of INPH could reach benefits, and VPS revealed to be superior (76% versus 50%). In VPS group, however, there was 19% of complications (subdural hematomas) compared to no complications in ETV group. In this study, the valve applied was a fixed pressure valve [22-25].

Fixed Pressure, Programmable Pressure or Flow Regulated Valves

Programmable valves are increasingly recommended for the treatment of iNPH, since the drainage pressure can be adjusted according to clinical setting of the patient, in order to achieve maximum improvement and minimum complications such as overdrainage due to siphoning effect. So far, no randomised clinical trials comparing flow-regulated versus programmable valves were published and programmable valves are considered gold standard treatment to NPH, but an important point is that no cost-effectiveness study concerning NPH and its treatment modalities have been designed and conducted to the best of our knowledge [22-25].

Conclusion

NPH may be a cause for dementia in up to 10% of patients. Once it is a reversible etiology, effort is increasing in comprehending its physiopatholy and improve its diagnosis. Currently, there are still no uniform treatment protocol uniformely applied. However, there is strong evidence for response with shunt surgery.

References

[1] Adams RD, Fisher CM, Hakim S, Ojemann RG, Swett WH: Symptomatic occult hydrocephalus with "normal" cerebrospinal-fluid pressure: a treatable syndrome. *N. Engl. J. Med.* 273:117-126, 1965.

[2] Hakim CA, Hakim R, Hakim S: Normal-pressure hydrocephalus. *Neurosurg. Clin. N. Am.* 12:761-773, ix, 2001.

[3] Hakim S, Adams RD: The special clinical problem of symptomatic hydrocephalus with normal cerebrospinal fluid pressure. Observations on cerebrospinal fluid hydrodynamics. *J. Neurol. Sci.* 2:307-327, 1965.

[4] Toma AK, Stapleton S, Papadopoulos MC, Kitchen ND, Watkins LD: Natural history of idiopathic normal-pressure hydrocephalus. *Neurosurg. Rev.* 34:433-439, 2011.

[5] Boon AJ, Tans JT, Delwel EJ et al: Dutch Normal-Pressure Hydrocephalus Study: randomized comparison of low- and medium-pressure shunts. *J. Neurosurg.* 88:490-495, 1998.

[6] McGirt MJ, Woodworth G, Coon AL., Thomas G, Williams MA, Rigamonti D: Diagnosis, treatment, and analysis of long-term outcomes in idiopathic normal-pressure hydrocephalus. *Neurosurgery* 62 Suppl 2:670-677, 2008.

[7] Petersen RC, Mokri B, Laws ER: Surgical treatment of idiopathic hydrocephalus in elderly patients. *Neurology* 35:307-311, 1985.

[8] Vanneste J, Augustijn P, Dirven C, Tan WF, Goedhart ZD: Shunting normal-pressure hydrocephalus: do the benefits outweigh the risks? A multicenter study and literature review. *Neurology* 42:54-59, 1992.

[9] Weiner HL, Constantini S, Cohen H, Wisoff JH: Current treatment of normal-pressure hydrocephalus: comparison of flow-regulated and differential-pressure shunt valves. *Neurosurgery* 37:877-884, 1995.

[10] Marmarou A, Bergsneider M, Klinge P, Relkin N, Black PM: The value of supplemental prognostic tests for the preoperative assessment of idiopathic normal-pressure hydrocephalus. *Neurosurgery* 57:S17-28; discussion ii-v, 2005.

[11] Relkin N, Marmarou A, Klinge P, Bergsneider M, Black PM: Diagnosing idiopathic normal-pressure hydrocephalus. *Neurosurgery* 57:S4-16; discussion ii-v, 2005.

[12] Brean A, Eide PK: Prevalence of probable idiopathic normal pressure hydrocephalus in a Norwegian population. *Acta Neurol. Scand.* 118:48-53, 2008.

[13] O'Kane MC, Richards H, Winfield P, Pickard JD: The United Kingdom Shunt Registry. *Eur. J. Pediatr. Surg.* 7 Suppl 1:56, 1997.

[14] Kestle J, Drake J, Milner R, Sainte-Rose C, Cinalli G, Boop F, Piatt J, Haines S, Schiff S, Cochrane D, Steinbok P, MacNeil N: Long-term follow-up data from the Shunt Design Trial. *Pediatr. Neurosurg.* 33:230-236, 2000.

[15] Ishikawa M, Hashimoto M, Kuwana N, Mori E, Miyake H, Wachi A, Takeuchi T, Kazui H, Koyama H: Guidelines for management of idiopathic normal pressure hydrocephalus. *Neurol. Med. Chir* (Tokyo). 2008;48 Suppl:S1-23.

[16] Mori K: Management of idiopathic normal-pressure hydrocephalus: a multiinstitutional study conducted in Japan. *J. Neurosurg.* 95:970–973, 2001.

[17] Shprecher D, Schwalb J, Kurlan R: Normal Pressure Hydrocephalus: Diagnosis and Treatment. *Curr. Neurol. Neurosci. Rep.* 2008 September ; 8(5): 371–376.

[18] Kazui H, Mori E, Hashimoto M, Ishikawa M, Hirono N, Takeda M: Dement Geriatr Cogn Disord. 2011 May 27;31(5):363-370. Effect of Shunt Operation on Idiopathic Normal Pressure Hydrocephalus Patients in Reducing Caregiver Burden: Evidence from SINPHONI.

[19] Eide PK, Sorteberg W: Changes in intracranial pulse pressure amplitudes after shunt implantation and adjustment of shunt valve opening pressure in normal pressure hydrocephalus. *Acta Neurochir* (Wien). 2008 Nov;150(11):1141-7; discussion 1147. Epub 2008 Oct.

[20] Bakker SL, Boon AJ, Wijnhoud AD, Dippel DW, Delwel EJ, Koudstaal PJ: Cerebral hemodynamics before and after shunting in normal pressure hydrocephalus. *Acta Neurol. Scand.* 2002 Sep;106(3):123-7.

[21] Freimann FB, Streitberger KJ, Klatt D, Lin K, McLaughlin J, Braun J, Sprung C, Sack I: Alteration of brain viscoelasticity after shunt treatment in normal pressure hydrocephalus. *Neuroradiology*. 2011 May 3.

[22] Gangemi M, Maiuri F, Naddeo M et al: Endoscopic third ventriculostomy in idiopathic normal pressure hydrocephalus: an Italian multicenter study. *Neurosurgery* 63:62-67; discussion 67-69, 2008.

[23] Oliveira MF, Saad F, Reis RC, Rotta JM, Pinto FC. Programmable valve represents an efficient and safe tool in the treatment of idiopathic normal-pressure hydrocephalus patients. *Arq. Neuropsiquiatr*. 2013 Apr;71(4):229-36.

[24] Zemack G, Romner B. Adjustable valves in normal-pressure hydrocephalus: a retrospective study of 218 patients. *Neurosurgery*. Dec 2002;51(6):1392-1400; discussion 1400-1392.

[25] Pinto FC, Saad F, de Oliveira MF, Pereira RM, de Miranda FL, Tornai JB, Lopes MI, Ribas ES, Valinetti EA, Teixeira MJ. Role of Endoscopic Third Ventriculostomy and Ventriculoperitoneal Shunt in Idiopathic Normal Pressure Hydrocephalus: Preliminary Results of a Randomized Clinical Trial. *Neurosurgery*. 2013 May;72(5):845-54.

In: Dementia
Editor: Pamela Tanner

ISBN: 978-1-63321-928-1

Chapter 11

Basal Ganglia Calcifications and Cognitive Decline

J. R. M. Oliveira[1] *and M. F. Oliveira*[2,*]
[1]Neuropsychiatric Department,
Federal University of Pernambuco (UFPE),
Recife, Pernambuco, Brazil
[2]Neurosurgery Residency Program,
Hospital do Servidor Público Estadual de São Paulo,
São Paulo, SP, Brazil

Abstract

Basal ganglia calcifications (BGC) may be present in various medical conditions, such as infections, metabolic, psychiatric and neurological diseases, associated with different etiologies and clinical outcomes, including parkinsonism, psychosis, mood swings and dementia. A literature review was performed highlighting main neuropsychological findings of BGC, with particular attention to clinical reports of cognitive decline. Neuroimaging studies combined with neuropsychological analysis show that some patients present progressive disturbances of selective attention, declarative memory and verbal perseveration. Therefore, the calcification process might represent a putative cause for demential syndromes, suggesting a probable link between calcinosis, the aging process and eventually with neuronal death. The increasing number of reports available will foster a necessary discussion about cerebral calcinosis and its role in determining symptomatology in demential patients.

Keywords: basal ganglia, dementia, calcinosis

* Corresponding author: Matheus Fernandes de Oliveira, MD., Department of Neurosurgery, Hospital do Servidor Público Estadual de São Paulo. Rua Pedro de Toledo, 1800 - São Paulo, Zip Code: 04029-000. Phone: 55-11-985467815 Fax: 55-11-50888379. e-mail: mafernoliv@yahoo.com.br.

Introduction

Basal ganglia calcifications (BGC) may be present in various medical conditions, such as infections, metabolic, psychiatric and neurological diseases, associated with different etiologies and clinical outcomes, including parkinsonism, psychosis, mood swings and dementia [1, 2] (Table 1). They may be present in up to 12% of patients screened with a routine Skull tomography (CT) [3]. Nosologic distinction is made between idiopathic form (also called Fahr´s disease), when there is no clear cause for the symptoms; and secondary form when a known disorder such as endocrinopathy or infection is identified [1, 2].

BCG is usually diagnosed between 30 and 60 years old. Some authors reported different clinical forms of BGC according to the age of onset for symptoms: A childhood form, with precocious manifestation in the first years of life, an early adult onset type with presentation between 20 and 40 years of age, manifesting as a schizophrenia-like psychosis and finally a late-onset variety, presenting between the ages of 40 and 60, with dementia and parkinsonism [4, 5]. However, the study of familial BGC shows that clinical heterogeneity is very common even among relatives, developing symptoms, sometimes, in those three different moments of life [6, 7, 8, 9, 13, 14, 15].

Neuropathological analysis suggests that basal ganglia calcinosis implicate in neuronal loss, hypometabolism, hypoperfusionand impairment of neurochemmical activity. A connectivity impairment of basal ganglia with frontal lobe, corticobasal structures and interhemispheric relations, generates psychiatric, cognitive, and behavioral changes [1, 10, 11, 12]. Depletions in variable grades in dopamine, glutamate and acetylcholine synapses are the main chemical findings. Limbic structures and temporal lobe may also be enrolled, leading to mood swings and memory disturbances [1, 10, 11, 12].

Neuropsychological and Cognitive Assessment

Some examples come from specific clinical cases and neuropsychological tests show severe deficits in mental flexibility, executive, as well as in verbal memory in a 50-year-old patient, suggesting participation of the dorsolateral prefrontal loop. He showed no deficits in motivation or drive, withsocially appropriate behavior, intact language abilities and upper average verbal intelligence [16].

Palilalia and dysarthria might be found as a language impairment [11]. Idiopathic BGC (IBCG) has been associated with personality changes due to frontal-subcortical dysfunction [2]. Lopez-Villegas et al. (1996) described relevant impairments in executive functions, visuospatial skills, and selected memory functions [17] (Table 2).

Konupcíková et al. (2008) reported a case of a 62-year-old manpresenting extensive brain calcifications, including BGC but with mild movement disorders , mild calcium metabolism abnormalities and severe dementia [18]. Weisman et al. (2007) also described the case of a 66-year-old man, without any metabolic alterations but with diffuse brain calcification and progressive dementia for 5 years, showing early signs of frontal impairment [19].

Table 1. Events associated with BGC

Endocrine / metabolic	Congenital / development	Inflammatory / infectious	Toxic / anoxic	Miscellaneous
Hypoparathyroidism	Cockayne Syndrome	AIDS	Radiation therapy	Aging. Over 50 years
Pseudohypoparathyroidism	Syndrome of microcephaly, demyelination, and striopallidodentate calcification	Epstein–Barr virus infection	Carbon monoxide poisoning	Syphilis
Pseudo-pseudohypoparathyroidism		Meningoencephalitis	Lead intoxication	Hematoma
Hyperparathyroidism		Mumps encephalitis	Methotrexate therapy	
Addison's disease	Developmental Angiomatous malformation with vein of Galen aneurysm	Cytomegalic inclusion	Methanol intoxication	Wilson's disease
Kallman's syndrome		Toxoplasmosi	Mercury poisoning	
Dihydropteridine reductase deficiency		Cysticercosis		Huntington's chorea
		Tuberculosis		
	Down's Syndrome	Congenital rubella		Systemic lúpus
MELAS syndrome				
Post-hypoxic/ischemic	Oculocraniosomatic disease (Kearns–Sayre Syndrome)			Scleroderma
				Folate deficiency
	Aicardi–Goutieres syndrome			Celiac disease
	Coat's disease			
	Diffuse cerebral microangiopathy			
	Tuberous sclerosis			

Table 2. Main neuropsychological findings in basal ganglia calcifications patients

Author	Neuropsychological and cognitive profile
Delazer	Deficits in mental flexibility, problem solving and planning, verbal memory
Lopez-Villegas	Impairments in executive functions, visuospatial skills, and selected memory functions
Konupcíková	Severe demential state
Weisman	Progressive dementia
Paschali	progressive gait disturbances, memory impairment, speech difficulty, and reduced psychomotor speed
Hempel	disturbances of selective attention, verbal perseveration and declarative memory
Geschwind	impaired cognitive flexibility, figural., and working memory
Cartier	Impaired verbal and visual-spatial memory, planning, attention and concentration capacities and visual constructive skills

Several patients will present a combined motor and cognitive impairment, such as the patient reported by Paschali et al. (2009), a 56-year-old woman with IBGC, progressive gait disturbances, reduced psychomotor speed, speech difficulty and memory impairment. Reduced glucose uptake in PET in basal ganglia, frontal., temporal and parietal cortex was also detected. The Dopamine transporter (DAT) SPECT/TC combined with a low-dose x-ray computerized tomography transmission (hybrid SPECT/CT) and 99^{m}Tc-D,L hexamethylpropylene amine oxime (99^{m}Tc-HMPAO) revealed a reduction in DAT binding in both striation regions coinciding with bilateral calcifications in the basal ganglia, correlating well with the clinical condition of the patient.

The comorbidity with unusual situations should also be considered and there is a particular report of a case of a patient with previous poliomyelitis coexisting with IBGC [18]. Severe and diffuse cognitive impairment at age 67 was consistent with the diagnosis of dementia in patient. He had severe executive dysfunction with an attention deficit, intrusions, perseverations, reduced verbal fluency and loss of cognitive flexibility. Working memory was impaired, as well as visual and verbal episodic memory, judgment and performance on visuo-spatial tasks [18].

Neuroimage Studies

Computerized tomography is the best exam to detect brain calcifications but neuroimaging studies combined with neuropsychological analysis show that some patients present progressive disturbances of selective attention, declarative memory and verbal perseveration [20].

A reduced uptake in striatum bilaterally, the frontal., temporal and parietal cortices was detected through PET in a patient presenting with BGC, hyperkinetic-hypotone syndrome, impaired cognitive flexibility, figural memory and constructive praxis [21]. On the contrary, reduced glucose uptake in PET was not only restricted to the left basal ganglia, but also involved the right temporoparietal and the right cerebellar cortices corresponding to the impaired cognitive flexibility, figural., and working memory [22].

In other familial study, eight patients were analyzed over 3 generations with IBGC detected on brain CT scan, showing an autosomal dominant mode of inheritance and predominant psychiatric and cognitive impairment, 3 of them also going under a FDG brain metabolic analysis. Cortical dysfunction might be detected early in patients with idiopathic BGC, suggesting that retrosplenial hypometabolism might be involved in the episodic memory deficit [23].

FDG PET brain scan in a 50 year old man presenting with a 6 month history of personality change and an impairment of planning and memory functions showed that significant reductions of glucose metabolism in basal ganglia and frontal lobes, particularly the dorsolateral., orbitofrontal., and ventromedial cortex. No significant hypometabolism was seen in the temporal or parietal cortex [23, 24, 25].

Future

Due to a ramping use of neuroimaging techniques, particularly CTs, brain calcifications are detected more often than previously. Before such availability, the only resource to detect brain calcification *in vivo* was regular radiography, suitable only for the most massive calcifications that would be seen through the skull as cloudy patches [1-14]. Indeed, even the standardized protocol applied in most reference centers as well as in this essay might underestimate the prevalence of calcifications. Multiple detectors scanners are able to perform 0.5 mm thickness slices and thus smaller calcifications may not be detected (Figure 1).

An intriguing consequence is the incidental finding of BGC during the investigation of milder symptoms, some of them with transient symptomatology, in asymptomatic subjects with massive calcifications and positive family history, in emergency rooms or even randomly during the investigation of other pathologies affecting the patient´s face [1-14].

This suggests that this phenotype is more common than previously assumed and a growing number of cases have been systematically reported in several countries, especially those where neuroimaging equipment and imaging facilities are recently more available due to lower price per exam.

Basal ganglia calcification (BGC) in its idiopathic or secondary form is more classically labeled as a subcortical cause of dementia. Cognitive and behavioral findings might also include mood disorders, psychosis, mood swings, with significant impairment on tests of frontal-executive functions, resembling other degenerative diseases with basal ganglia dysfunction [1, 2]. A marked presence of motor symptoms, especially a rigid hypokinetic syndrome, helps to differentiate this condition from other subcortical syndromes [10].

Therefore, the calcification process might represent a putative cause for demential syndromes, suggesting a probable link between calcinosis, the aging process and eventually with neuronal death [6, 7, 8, 9].

The increasing number of reports available will foster a necessary discussion about cerebral calcinosis and its role in determining symptomatology in demential patients.

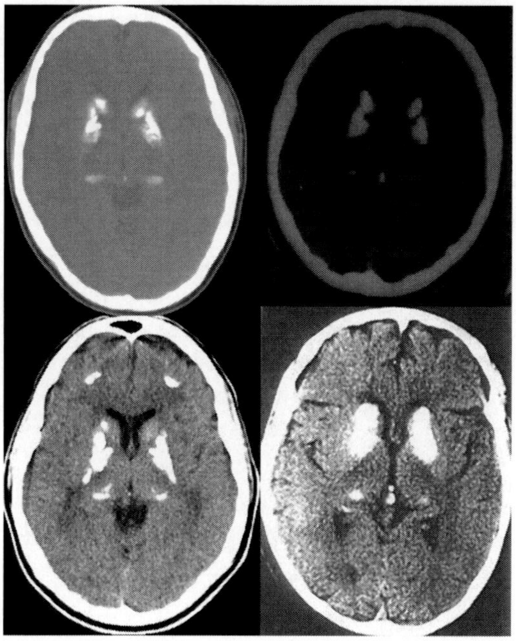

Figure 1. Skull computed tomography of subjects with BGC. The two above are of a 45 year-old man and a 68 year-old woman, both with parkinsonism features. The two below are of a 26 year-old man and a 48 year-old woman, both asymptomatic.

References

[1] Manyam BV. What is and what is not 'Fahr's disease'. *Parkinsonism Relat. Disord.* 2005; 11(2):73-80.

[2] Geschwind DH, Loginov M, Stern JM. Identification of a locus on chromosome 14q for idiopathic basal ganglia calcification (Fahr disease). *Am. J. Hum. Genet.* 1999; 65:764–72.

[3] Gomille T, Meyer RA, Falkai P, Gaebel W, Königshausen T, Christ F. Prevalence and clinical significance of computerized tomography verified idiopathic calcinosis of the basal ganglia. *Radiologe*. 2001 Feb;41(2):205-10.

[4] Brodaty H, Mitchell P, Luscombe G, Kwok JJ, Badenhop RF et al. Familial idiopathic basal ganglia calcification (Fahr's disease) without neurological., cognitive and psychiatric symptoms is not linked to the IBGC1 locus on chromosome 14q. *Hum. Genet.* 2002; 110:8-14.

[5] Cummings JL, Gosenfeld LF, Houlihan JP, McCaffrey T. Neuropsychiatric disturbances associated with idiopathic calcification of the basal ganglia. *Biol. Psychiatry.* 1983; 18: 591–601.

[6] Oliveira JRM, Spiteri E, Sobrido MJ, Hopfer S, Klepper J et al. Genetic heterogeneity in Familial Idiopathic basal Ganglia Calcification ("Fahr's disease"). *Neurology*. 2004; 63: 2165-2167.

[7] Lemos RR, Oliveira MF, Oliveira JRM. Reporting a new mutation at the SLC20A2 gene in familial idiopatic basal ganglia calcification. *Eur. J. Neurol.* 2013 Mar;20(3):e43-4.

[8] Hsu SC, Sears RL, Lemos RR, Quintáns B, Huang A, Spiteri E, Nevarez L, Mamah C, Zatz M, Pierce KD, Fullerton JM, Adair JC, Berner JE, Bower M, Brodaty H, Carmona O, Dobricić V, Fogel BL, García-Estevez D, Goldman J, Goudreau JL, Hopfer S, Janković M, Jaumà S, Jen JC, Kirdlarp S, Klepper J, Kostić V, Lang AE, Linglart A, Maisenbacher MK, Manyam BV, Mazzoni P, Miedzybrodzka Z, Mitarnun W, Mitchell PB, Mueller J, Novaković I, Paucar M, Paulson H, Simpson SA, Svenningsson P, Tuite P, Vitek J, Wetchaphanphesat S, Williams C, Yang M, Schofield PR, de Oliveira JR, Sobrido MJ, Geschwind DH, Coppola G. Mutations in SLC20A2 are a major cause of familial idiopathic basal ganglia calcification. *Neurogenetics*. 2013 Feb;14(1):11-22.

[9] Oliveira JRM, Lemos RR, Oliveira MF. Updating Genetic studies in familial idiopathic basal ganglia calcification. *Southern Medical Journal*. 2009 Sep;102(9):989.

[10] de Oliveira MF, Steinberg SS, de Oliveira JR. The challenging interpretation of genetic and neuroimaging features in basal ganglia calcification. *Gen. Hosp. Psychiatry*. 2013 Mar-Apr;35(2):210-1.

[11] Keller A, Westenberger A, Sobrido MJ, García-Murias M, Domingo A, Sears RL, Lemos RR, Ordoñez-Ugalde A, Nicolas G, da Cunha JE, Rushing EJ, Hugelshofer M, Wurnig MC, Kaech A, Reimann R, Lohmann K, Dobričić V, Carracedo A, Petrović I, Miyasaki JM, Abakumova I, Mäe MA, Raschperger E, Zatz M, Zschiedrich K, Klepper J, Spiteri E, Prieto JM, Navas I, Preuss M, Dering C, Janković M, Paucar M, Svenningsson P, Saliminejad K, Khorshid HR, Novaković I, Aguzzi A, Boss A, Le Ber I, Defer G, Hannequin D, Kostić VS, Campion D, Geschwind DH, Coppola G, Betsholtz C, Klein C,Oliveira JR. Mutations in the gene encoding PDGF-B cause brain calcifications in humans and mice. *Nat. Genet.* 2013 Sep;45(9):1077-82.

[12] de Oliveira JR, de Oliveira MF. Brain resilience and obsessive-compulsive disorder: defining the neuroanatomical pathways of vulnerability. *J. Neuropsychiatry Clin. Neurosci.* 2013 Fall;25(4):E19-21.

[13] Cartier L, Passig C, Gormaz A, López J. Neuropsychological and neurophysiological features of Fahr's disease. *Rev. Med. Chil.* 2002 Dec;130(12):1383-90.

[14] Sobrido MJ, Hopfer S, Geschwind DH. 2007. Idiopathic basal ganglia calcification. GeneReviews: Genetic Disease Online Reviews. www.geneclinics.org.

[15] Saiki M, Saiki S, Sakai K, Matsunari I, Higashi K, Murata KY, et al. Neurological deficits are associated with increased brain calcinosis, hypoperfusion, and hypometabolism in idiopathic basal ganglia calcification. *Mov. Disord.* 2007; 22(7): 1027-30.

[16] Delazer M, Domahs F, Lochy A, Karner E, Benke T, Poewe W. Number processing and basal ganglia dysfunction: a single case study. *Neuropsychologia*. 2004; 42(8):1050-62.

[17] Lopez-Villegas D, Kulisevsky J, Deus J, Junque C, Pujol J, Guardia E, et al. Neuropsychological alterations in patients with computed tomography-detected basal ganglia calcification. *Archs. Neurol.* 1996; 53: 251–256.

[18] Konupcíková K, Masopust J, Valis M, Horácek J. Dementia in a patient with Fahr's syndrome. *Neuro Endocrinol. Lett.* 2008 Aug;29(4):431-4.

[19] Weisman DC, Yaari R, Hansen LA, Thal LJ. Density of the brain, decline of the mind: an atypical case of Fahr disease. *Arch. Neurol.* 2007 May;64(5):756-7.

[20] Paschali A, Lakiotis V, Messinis L, Markaki E, Constantoyannis C, Ellul J, et al. Dopamine transporter SPECT/CT and perfusion brain SPECT imaging in idiopathic basal ganglia calcinosis. *Clin. Nucl. Med.* 2009; 34(7):421-3.

[21] Oliveira MF, Oliveira JRM. A Comorbid Case of Familial Idiopathic Basal Ganglia Calcification (``Fahr´s Disease``) Associated with Post-Polio Syndrome. *J. Neuropsychiatry Clin. Neurosci.* 2012 Mar 1;24(2):E14-5.

[22] Hempel A, Henze M, Berghoff C, Garcia N, Ody R et al. PET findings and neuropsychological deficits in a case of Fahr's disease. *Psychiatry Res.* 2001; 108(2): 133-40.

[23] Yulug B. A Case of Idiopathic Basal Ganglia Calcification Presenting With only Acting-Out Attacks and Mild Cognitive Impairment: PET Findings. *J. Neuropsychiatry Clin. Neurosci.* 2007, 19 (3): 348-349.

[24] Le Ber I, Marié RM, Chabot B, Lalevée C, Defer GL. Neuropsychological and 18FDG-PET studies in a family with idiopathic basal ganglia calcifications. *J. Neurol. Sci.* 2007; 258(1-2):115-22.

[25] Benke T, Karner E, Seppi K, Delazer M, Marksteiner J, Donnemiller E. Subacute dementia and imaging correlates in a case of Fahr's disease. *J. Neurol. Neurosurg. Psychiatry.* 2004; 75(8):1163-5.

In: Dementia
Editor: Pamela Tanner

ISBN: 978-1-63321-928-1

Chapter 12

Virtual Reality Training Improves Spatial Navigation Disorientation in Dementia Patients

Daniel Serrani*

Facuty of Psychology, National University of Rosario,
Rosario, Argentina

Abstract

Background: Spatial disorientation (SD) is a severe and persistent impairment of spatial navigation in familiar as well as new environments and a trait marker of dementia (DA). Virtual reality (VR) provides a tool for the assessment and improvement of SD. In VR training program different degrees of motor control over navigation may be implemented (i.e., more passive spatial navigation vs. more active). Increasing demands of active motor control may overload those failing visuo-spatial resources necessary for learning spatial orientation and navigation. In the present study we used a VR-based verbally-guided passive navigation training program to improve general spatial abilities in DA patients with spatial disorientation.

Methods: Forty DA patients which showed deficits in spatial orientation, as well as 20 healthy controls performed a route finding training in a virtual environment. Participants learned and recalled different routes for navigation in a virtual city over nine training sessions. Before and after VR training, general spatial abilities were assessed with standardized neuropsychological tests.

Results: Route finding ability in the VR task increased over the ten training sessions. Moreover, both groups improved different aspects of spatial abilities after VR training in comparison to the spatial performance before VR training.

Conclusions: Verbally-guided passive navigation training in VR enhances general spatial cognition in DA patients with spatial disorientation as well as in healthy controls and can therefore be useful in the rehabilitation of spatial deficits associated with SD.

* Contact: danielserrani@argentina.com. Address: Estanislao Zeballos 1625 (2000) Rosario.

Keywords: Spatial disorientation, dementia, route-finding training, rehabilitation, virtual reality, visuo-spatial memory, visual navigation

Background

Subjective memory deficits have long been established as a hallmark of patients with dementia (DA). However, spatial memory deficits and disorientation have received less attention until recently (Lithfous et al., 2013; Vlček & Laczó, 2014). Unfortunately, despite multiple reported memory deficits, those related to spatial memory have yielded mixed results (Chan et al., 2012; Kessels et al., 2011). Confusion is due, in part, to various methodological flaws, including ascertainment limitations, patients and controls matching methods, patients being assessed during illness´ different phases, medication confounds, and multifaceted nature of spatial ability measurement. Usually spatial memory abilities are assessed asking the person to remember items position in an array. These tasks, however, focus solely on one aspect of spatial cognition and do not provide an ecological frame resembling real life challenging situations. Navigation tasks based on virtual reality (VR), instead, may provide a more accurate and sensitive measure of deranged spatial ability in complex and dynamic situations. Beside the use of VR as an assessment tool for spatial deficits, there are also scarce studies using VR for training spatial abilities in patients with orientation problems. Virtual training environments offer the possibility to train specific spatial deficits associated with MCI, such as egocentric or allocentric (e.g., landmark agnosia) disorientation problems [2,7-9]. This method has been applied in cases of amnesia for route finding in a hospital unit (Cherrier et al., 2001), in other real world scenarios (Kalová et al., 2009), physically disabled children (Foreman et al., 2003; Stanton et al., 1996), in brain damaged patients (Kessels et al., 2005). Superiority of VR training over real world learning has been attributed to several reasons: more intensive and frequent virtual trails performance compared to real world, overcoming physical disabilities in a VR environment, which can be attuned to different degrees of motor or sensory coordination, depending on individual disabilities; self pacing of the task using different devices such as joystick (Antonova et al., 2011), Keyboard (Morganti et al., 2013), verbal instructions (Maguire et al., 1998) or passive guidance (Pine et al., 2002), when participants are unable to control navigation tasks. In line with those assumptions, we tested the hypothesis that specific cognitive deficits including spatial navigation disorientation, associated with MCI could be amenable to training using a virtual reality device. We administered a novel virtual reality navigation task to patients with spatial disorientation and healthy controls, in order to improve spatial navigation performance.

Method

Participants

Participants were recruited from three outpatient public community mental health services. The subjects included 40 patients; aged between 61 to 75 years with a diagnosis of dementia, defined as a Mini-Mental State Examination (MMSE) score between $\leq$ 17. There was no attempt made to diagnose the cause of the cognitive impairment except to exclude delirium or psychotic features, as assessed by the Structured Clinical Interview for DSM-V (SCID). Healthy controls (N=20) were age and gender matched and were selected between caregivers of the dementia patients. All participants had no acute medical illnesses. Participants with dementia that render them incapable of understanding virtual reality training rules were also excluded. Subjects from the comparison group were excluded on the basis of the presence of current or past psychiatric or neurological illness, any medical condition that could affect cognitive performance, and a family history of psychiatric illness; none had a history of substance abuse. Given a likely relationship between familiarity with video games and the outcome measure, individuals reporting high expertise in video games were excluded (Richardson et al., 2011). The local ethical committee review board accepted the test protocol, which followed the declaration of Helsinki for ethical issues. After a complete description of the study to the subjects, written informed consent was obtained. Consent of the treating physicians was also obtained.

Statistical Method

Independent-sample t tests were used to evaluate differences between the patients and comparison subjects on the outcome measures (i.e., number of locations found on the navigation task and performance on the Spatial Working Memory task) and demographic characteristics. Pearson r correlations were used to examine the relationships between independent variables and the outcome measures. All statistics were evaluated at $p \leq 0.05$, two-tailed.

Procedure

The present study employed a virtual reality town (Figure 1).

On day 1, the subjects were oriented to the town for 20 minutes. After that they were given 20 minutes to navigate the town through a computer-generated sequence of destinations. At the end of this period, the subjects had to find at least three predetermined destinations within the town during five 3-minute practice rows. If the subjects succeeded to do so, training period *was* terminated. If not, they were given an additional 20 minutes to explore the town again to ensure adequate familiarity with the various locations. Three days later, participants explored the town for 20 minutes in order to familiarize themselves again with the task. Four hours later, they were tested on their memory of the town (as assessed by the number of locations found) in a manner identical to that used in the practice sessions but during nine 3-minute rows and beginning at different locations. The software recorded the locations visited. Preliminary data from a group of healthy participants revealed high test-retest reliability on this task ($r=0.81$, $N=15$, $p<0.001$). Additionally, patients and comparison group also completed the Spatial Working Memory task, a component of the Cambridge Automated Neuropsychological Testing Battery (Cambridge Cognition, Cambridge, U.K.). This tests taps both frontal and hippocampal functions, which have been proposed as neural substrates of spatial navigation (Burgess et al., 2002; Rankin et al., 2007).

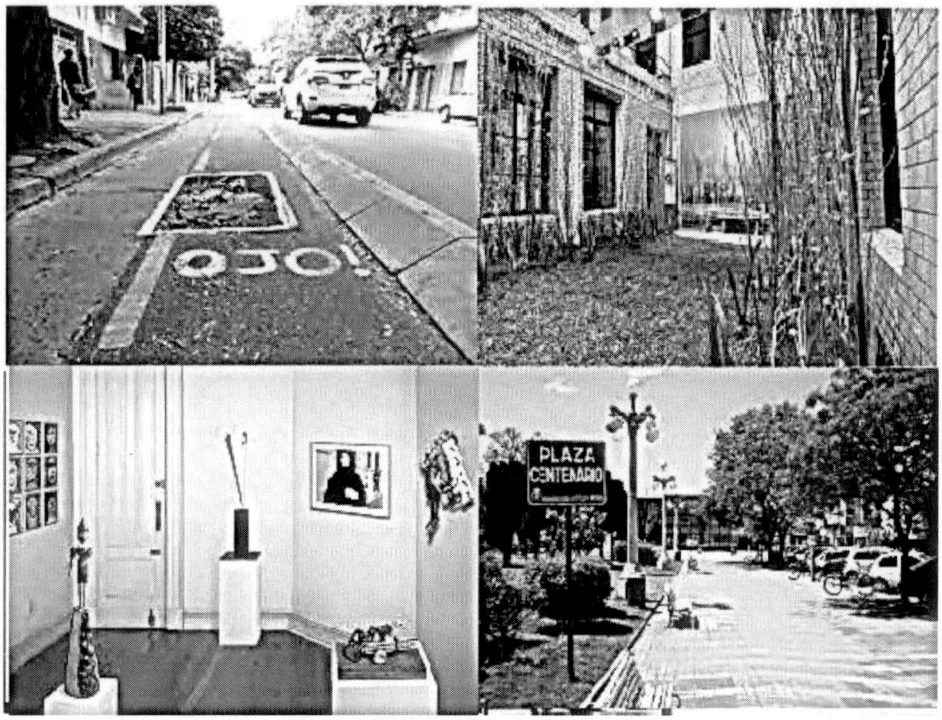

Figure 1. Sample views of the virtual environment used for the VR-based spatial navigation training, which was a real district of Buenos Aires, Argentina.

Results

There were no significant differences in age or gender between patients with dementia and comparison subjects (Table 1).

Table 1. Demographic and clinical characteristics DA and HC

group	Gender		Age (years)		Instruction (years)		MMSE		Illness length	
	M	F	Mean	SD	Mean	SD	Mean	SD	Mean	SD
Patients (N=40)	19	22	68.3	8.2	6.3	2.4	18.3	2.3	6.8	3.2
HC (N=20)	12	8	63.1	5.2	6.9	2.6	27.3	2.6		

MMSE (mini mental state examination)= normal values range from 23 to 30, ≤17 suggest cognitive impairment.

Patients found significantly fewer locations (mean=2.4, SD=1.7) than healthy controls (mean=3.8, SD=2.0) on the spatial navigation task (t=–2.70, *df*=47, p=0.01). There was no significant difference between men and women (t=–0.01, *df*=47, p=0.99). Among patients only, the number of locations found was correlated with the score on the MMSE (r=–0.33,

N=30, p=0.02) such that the more severely impaired patients performed worse. On the Spatial Working Memory task, the number of locations found was correlated with overall task performance (r=–0.45, p=0.007). It was interesting, however, that there was no difference in scores on the Spatial Working Memory task between the patients (mean= 33.3, SD=4.8) and comparison subjects (mean=33.4, SD=6.4) (t=–0.06, df=33, p=0.95), while there remained a performance difference on the virtual reality spatial navigation task when comparing means of route findings across the 9 sessions (t=–2.36, df=33, p=0.03) (figure 2)

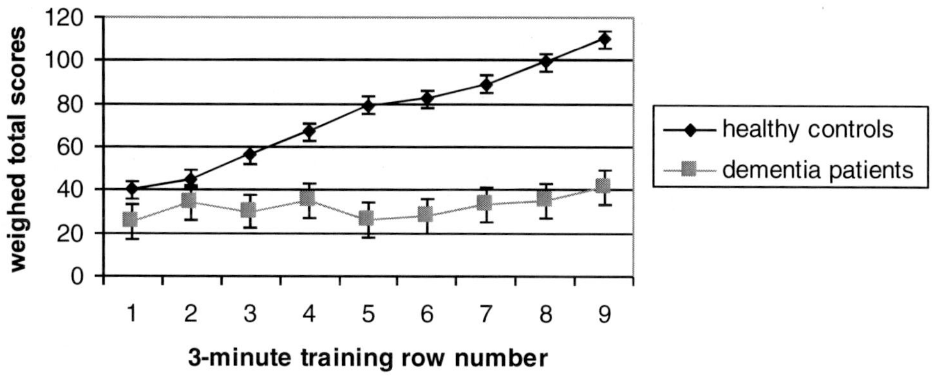

Figure 2. Comparison of means of route findings between HC and DA.

Discussion

The patients with DA performed significantly worse than the healthy comparison subjects on a novel virtual reality measure of spatial memory, which uses a navigation format based on virtual reality. This difference was manifested through a lower number of locations found in the task. An important finding was that, while performance on the navigation task was correlated with performance on the Spatial Working Memory task, the patients and comparison subjects did not differ in performance on the Spatial Working Memory test. Differences detected on the virtual reality task suggest that it may be a sensitive measure of hippocampal-related spatial memory deficits and may more clearly elucidate the relationship between that and other cognitive domain. Thus, despite the fact that the present task is more involved than existing measures, such as the Spatial Working Memory task, it has the advantage of detecting performance deficits in DA subjects. Prior research has demonstrated a robust correlation between recruitment of the hippocampus and the dependent measure used in this study. Because of the role of the hippocampus in this task and studies suggesting hippocampal volume reduction in DA, it is reasonable to speculate that the patient deficit being measured is dependent on altered hippocampal function, which was not detected on the Spatial Working Memory test. (Nedelska et al., 2012; Lövdén et al., 2012). However, while this task has previously been shown to involve the hippocampus and require normal function of the hippocampus, we cannot be certain that the differences on this task that we observed in DA patients are due to altered function of the hippocampus (as opposed to other brain areas that could be involved). The addition of supplementary control measures that target various structures within the medial temporal lobe would be necessary to more clearly delineate the neuroanatomical structures involved in the task performance (Lithfous et al., 2013; Vlček & Laczó, 2014; Konishi et al., 2013). Nevertheless, our results suggest that spatial memory performance on a virtual reality navigation task may represent a quantifiable measure to assess possible hippocampal deficits in patients with DA. This hypothesis can be further confirmed by applying spatial memory tests with a virtual reality navigation format to patients with cognitive impairment due to different causes, such as depressed patients, in order to correlate performance with structural and functional neuroimaging measures of relevant structures, such as the hippocampus.

The author reports no conflict of interest.

References

Antonova, E., Parslow, D., Brammer, M., Simmons, A., Williams, S., Dawson, G. R., & Morris, R. (2011). Scopolamine disrupts hippocampal activity during allocentric spatial memory in humans: an fMRI study using a virtual reality analogue of the Morris Water Maze. *Journal of Psychopharmacology*, *25*(9), 1256-1265.

Burgess, N., Maguire, E. A., & O'Keefe, J. (2002). The human hippocampus and spatial and episodic memory. *Neuron*, *35*(4), 625-641.

Chan, E., Baumann, O., Bellgrove, M. A., & Mattingley, J. B. (2012). From objects to landmarks: the function of visual location information in spatial navigation. *Frontiers in psychology*, *3*.10. doi: 10.3389/fpsyg.2012.00304

Cherrier, M. M., Mendez, M., & Perryman, K. (2001). Route learning performance in Alzheimer disease patients. *Cognitive and Behavioral Neurology*, *14*(3), 159-168.

Foreman, N., Stanton, D., Wilson, P., & Duffy, H. (2003). Spatial knowledge of a real school environment acquired from virtual or physical models by able-bodied children and children with physical disabilities. *Journal of Experimental Psychology: Applied*, *9*(2), 67.

Kalová, E., Vlček, K., Jarolímová, E., Bureš, J. (2009). Allothetic orientation and sequential ordering of places is impaired in early stages of Alzheimer's disease: corresponding results in real space tests and computer tests. *Behavioural brain research* 159 (2), 175-186.

Kessels RP, Feijen J, Postma, A (2005). Implicit and explicit memory for spatial information in Alzheimer's disease. *Dement Geriatr Cogn Disord.*;20 (2-3), 184-91

Kessels, R. P., Van Doormaal., A., & Janzen, G. (2011). Landmark recognition i.n Alzheimer's dementia: spared implicit memory for objects relevant for navigation. *PloS one*, *6*(4), e18611.

Lithfous, S., Dufour, A., & Després, O. (2013). Spatial navigation in normal aging and the prodromal stage of Alzheimer's disease: insights from imaging and behavioral studies. *Ageing research reviews*, *12*(1), 201-213.

Lövdén, M., Schaefer, S., Noack, H., Bodammer, N. C., Kühn, S., Heinze, H. J & Lindenberger, U. (2012). Spatial navigation training protects the hippocampus against age-related changes during early and late adulthood. *Neurobiology of aging*, *33*(3), 620-e9

Maguire EA, Burgess N, Donnett JG, Frackowiak RS, Frith CD, O'Keefe J: Knowing where and getting there: a human navigation network. Science 1998; 280:921–924.

Morganti, F., Stefanini, S., & Riva, G. (2013). From allo-to egocentric spatial ability in early Alzheimer's disease: a study with virtual reality spatial tasks. *Cognitive neuroscience*, *4*(3-4), 171-180.

Nedelska et al., Z., Andel, R., Laczó, J., Vlcek, K., Horinek, D., Lisy, J., ... & Hort, J. (2012). Spatial navigation impairment is proportional to right hippocampal volume. *Proceedings of the National Academy of Sciences*, *109*(7), 2590-2594.

Pine DS, Grun J, Maguire EA, Burgess N, Zarahn E, Koda V, Fyer A, Szeszko PR, Bilder RM: (2002). Neurodevelopmental aspects of spatial navigation: a virtual reality fMRI study. Neuroimage; 15:396–406.

Rankin, K. P., Mucke, L., Miller, B. L., & Gorno-Tempini, M. L. (2007). Spatial cognition and the human navigation network in AD and MCI. *Neurology*, *69*(10), 986-997.

Richardson, A. E., Powers, M. E., & Bousquet, L. G. (2011). Video game experience predicts virtual., but not real navigation performance. *Computers in Human Behavior*, *27*(1), 552-560.

Stanton, D., Wilson, P., & Foreman, N. (1996). Using virtual reality environments to aid spatial awareness in disabled children. In *Proceedings of the 1st European conference on disability, virtual reality and associated technologies* (pp. 93-101).

Vlček, K., & Laczó, J. (2014). Neural correlates of spatial navigation changes in mild cognitive impairment and Alzheimer's disease. *Frontiers in behavioral neuroscience*, *8*.89. doi:10.3389/fnbeh.2014.00089.

In: Dementia
Editor: Pamela Tanner

ISBN: 978-1-63321-928-1

Chapter 13

Sleep and Sleep Disorders in Dementia: An Updated Overview

Nicholas-Tiberio Economou[1], Barbara Wolgamuth[2] and Luigi Ferini-Strambi[3]
[1]Sleep Study Unit - Dept. of Psychiatry, Sleep Disorders Center, Dept. of Respiratory Medicine, University of Athens, Greece
[2]Cleveland Clinic Epilepsy Center, Neurological Institute, Cleveland, Ohio, US
[3]Sleep Disorders Center, Dept. of Neuroscience, Università Vita-Salute San Raffaele, Milan, Italy

Abstract

Changes in sleep organization are a hallmark of the normal aging process. Sleep macro- and micro-structure changes are more evident in the context of dementia. The "Sleep and neurodegeneration and/or dementia" issue contains a causality dilemma; in the context of neurodegeneration, sleep-wake promoting neurons may be affected, while in many of the neurodegenerative disorders, central respiratory drive and autonomic neurons are also degenerated and may cause primary sleep disorders. Conversely, several recent studies suggest that common sleep disorders (i.e., insomnia, daytime sleepiness and generally decreased amplitude and robustness of sleep-wake cycle), which are mostly prevalent among the cognitively impaired people, may precede clinical symptoms of dementia and may be risk factors for cognitive decline and dementia.

Here, sleep, its alteration and sleep disorders in the context not only of dementia but also in pre-dementia stages (i.e., the mild cognitive impairment - MCI) are reviewed. Moreover, the complex interactions between sleep and dementia and the previously-mentioned causality dilemma are addressed by also reviewing the existing management strategies and evidence of the impact of therapeutic approaches on sleep disorders in dementia.

Keywords: Sleep, sleep disorders, dementia

1. Introduction

Sleep is a cardinal physiologic process in which crucial restorative functions occur. With the advance of age, several sleep alterations regarding the quality and the quantity of sleep appear. These regard not only the physiology of sleep *per se'*, but also the higher occurrence of sleep disorders. Patients with neurodegenerative disorders and/or dementia present further deterioration of their sleep physiology (sleep macro-and microstructures) and a higher prevalence as far as the sleep disturbances are concerned. Over the last years, it was believed that sleep disturbances in the context of neurodegeneration were the consequence of neuropathological lesions, whereas recent data suggests that sleep and its disturbances may precede the cognitive deterioration process and impact on that. Given that sleep alterations regardless of whether they concern the healthy elderly or people suffering from neurodegenerative diseases/dementia though being very common, receive limited attention; therefore, a brief overview of sleep changes related to normal aging will be presented first.

2. Sleep in Normal Aging

Both subjective and objective sleep measures suggest that with advancing age there are sleep alterations. Basically, the main impact of age on sleep affects the sleep architecture (sleep macro-and microstructures) more than the total amount of sleep (Gillin, Ancoli-Israel 2008, Rajput). Generally, sleep tends to be lighter and more fragmented with increased arousals and awakenings with variability in duration in middle-aged and elderly adults compared to young adults.

A normal sleep polysomnographic profile reveals four cyclically distributed sleep stages (former classification comprised five stages). These are Stages: 1, 2, 3 (also called Slow Wave Sleep -SWS-, previously divided into two different stages: 3 and 4) and Rapid Eye Movement sleep -REM-). Normal sleep is characterized by the cyclic alternation of NREM sleep (Stages 1, 2, 3) and REM sleep. Stage 1, which occupies approximately 5% of total sleep time, is defined as the transition from wakefulness to sleep. In Stage 1, the alpha rhythm (8-12 Hz), which is the dominant rhythm in wakefulness with eyes closed, is replaced with a slower theta rhythm (4–7 Hz – theta rhythm). Stage 2, which represents approximately 50% of the normal sleep, is characterized by the appearance of two typical phasic features, sleep spindles and K-complexes on a background of theta waves. Stage 2 is considered an intermediate state between stage 1 and SWS, as far as the "deepness" of the sleep is concerned. Stage 3, which occupies approximately 20% of total sleep time, is the real deep sleep and is defined by delta waves of high amplitude and low-frequency (0.25–2 Hz). Finally, REM sleep, which represents the remaining 25% of the total sleep time, is characterized by a fast ''desynchronized'' low-voltage EEG of mixed frequencies (alpha, beta and theta frequencies), rapid eye movements and an absence of muscle tone (Rechtschaffen, Iber).

The common finding, as shown with objective sleep measures (polysomnography – PSG), is that healthy elderly have less deep sleep (SWS) and less REM sleep. However, a recent meta-analysis of 65 overnight sleep studies, comprising 3,577 subjects across the adult lifespan (5 to 102 years old), concluded that the percentage of lighter sleep increased with age, while REM and SWS decreased as a function of age. SWS decreases linearly at a rate of approximately 2% per decade of age, up to age 60 years (Ohayon). Interestingly, SWS seems to remain relatively constant from age 60 to the mid-90s, although sleep efficiency (which is the amount of sleep relative to the amount of the time spent in bed) showed a continuous decrease. The reduction of SWS is a cardinal age-related PSG feature (Feinberg, Bliwise 1993, Reynolds), demonstrated also with studies focusing on the spectral power of the delta band (Cajochen, Carrier). This reduction of SWS is mostly prominent in the frontal lobe (Munch) and concerns both the amplitude and the number of delta waves (Petit, Feinberg, I., & Campbell). However, the decrease of SWS reflects mostly a decrease of delta amplitude (Crowley 2011), given that the scoring criteria for SWS require not only the presence of at least 20% slow delta activity (0.25–2 Hz) per epoch, but that the delta activity have an amplitude of at least 75 μV. Finally, regarding SWS, it seems that with aging, SWS shows a broader distribution across the whole night, rather than being mostly concentrated at the beginning of the night (in the first one or two NREM– REM cycles of the night) as usually occurs in young adults (Lombardo). Another important finding regarding SWS, is that with aging males seem to lose more SWS than females (Fukuda).

As stated before, across the lifespan, reduction of SWS and possibly of REM sleep implies that sleep gets lighter, that there is more time spent in NREM stage 1 and possibly in stage 2. Nevertheless, the cardinal features of stage 2, namely, sleep spindles and K complexes present notable alterations; sleep spindles are transient 12–15 Hz oscillations that are seen in NREM stages 2 and 3 sleep. They originate in the thalamus, thanks to membrane hyperpolarization of thalamocortical neurons (Steriade), while K complexes are considered to be an incomplete form of delta waves. With normal aging, sleep spindles are reduced in number, frequency, amplitude and generally are less well-formed (Wauquier, Crowley 2002b, Petit), while K complexes are of reduced number and amplitude (Crowley 2002a, b). Finally, regarding other sleep microstructure features, although REM percentage reduces slightly across the lifespan (Floyd, Ohayon), REM density, which is defined as the number of rapid eye movements per unit time, seems to be considerably decreased (Darchia).

Age-related chronobiological changes are the result of the altered function in the interaction of the two main sleep-wake regulatory mechanisms, which are the circadian pacemaker and the homeostatic process. Briefly, the circadian pacemaker is located in the suprachiasmatic nucleus (SCN) of the hypothalamus. SCN provides a wake-promoting signal., which is strong during the day and reaches its peak at approximately 21.00–22.00, while it decreases drastically with the nocturnal melatonin secretion (Dijk). The homeostatic process represents the need for sleep; thus, it increases during wakefulness and it decreases with sleep. SWS is considered to be a marker of this process (Daan). With normal aging, these two mechanisms go across several alterations therefore, the normal sleep-wake cycle gets compromised with poorer night sleep consolidation or fragments of sleep during wakefulness. Nevertheless, it is not completely clear if the disturbed circadian rhythms of the elderly are to be attributed to the reduced sleep consolidation to the altered sleep-wake timing, or to the reduced SWS (Crowley 2011). However, the most typical chronobiological phenomenon in the healthy elderly is the phase advance of the normal circadian cycle. Therefore, elderly people tend to have an anticipated sleep onset and consequently an earlier morning wake signal (Wolkove, Carrier). As far as the primary sleep disorders are concerned, there seems to be an elevated prevalence of these compared to that of young adults (i.e., 49%

of adults aged 53–97 years had at least one insomnia trait (either difficulty getting to sleep, frequent awakenings or waking up too early)) (Schubert).

2. Sleep in Dementia

2.1. Sleep Structure Alterations

Generally, sleep changes in dementia are quite similar, but definitely more pronounced (especially in the advanced phases of dementia), to those appearing in the healthy elderly.

Sleep disturbances are usually linearly correlated with the severity of dementia (Petit, Bombois); nevertheless, there are few published data, suggesting that sleep disturbances in dementia show an inverted U-shape pattern, with moderately demented persons showing more impaired sleep than patients in early and late disease stages (McCurry). As dementia progresses, there is an increased number and duration of awakenings, an increased arousal index, an increased sleep latency and wakefulness after sleep onset (WASO), a decreased sleep efficiency and total sleep time, an increased light sleep (mostly Stage 1) and a decreased SWS (in advanced dementias and in tauopathies a marked decrease also of REM sleep). SWS in demented patients did not show the normal decline that is observed in normal sleep. NREM stage 2 spindles and K complexes diminish in number, frequency, amplitude, and morphological integrity. As the disease further progresses, the number of REMs further reduces, while the background rhythm in REM gets slower due to the increase of delta and theta power at the expense of alpha and beta (Petit, Bliwise 1993, Bombois, Bonanni, Chockroverty, Rauchs, Gagnon, Raggi, Ancoli-Israel 2008).

2.2. Common Sleep Disorders in Dementia

In demented people several sleep disorders may be observed, including insomnia, excessive daytime sleepiness/hypersomnia (EDS), circadian rhythm disruption, sleep-related breathing disorders, sleep-related movement disorders and other abnormal nocturnal motor behaviors. Sleep disorders in dementia may be multifactorial; neuropathological changes related to different types of dementia, high medical co-morbidity (affective disorders, medication adverse effects, chronic pain), primary sleep disorders and circadian dysregulation are the main causes (Guarnieri). The majority of the above-mentioned disorders are not specific for any given type of dementia, thus they may occur in all forms of dementia. Nevertheless, the association of a specific sleep disorder with a certain neurodegenerative disease and/or process (i.e., REM Behavior Disorder – RBD and synucleinopathies) may be of extreme importance in order to raise awareness of specific sleep-related issues more common in particular dementia syndromes (Table 1). The severity of sleep disorders in dementia is rather correlated to the severity of dementia itself (Moe, Happe, Wolkove).

Insomnia

Insomnia is defined as difficulty falling or staying asleep for at least one month, which results in impairment of daytime functioning and is more frequent in elderly people (Rajput).

It is well known that insomnia may be primary or secondary to medical co-morbidities (i.e., anxiety, depression, chronic pain, bladder dysfunction, heart and lung diseases), moreover, several drugs may cause and/or worsen insomnia (Table 2). The latter type of insomnia is more common in demented patients (Bombois), who experience difficulty falling asleep or difficulty in sleep maintenance with repeated nighttime awakenings. This sleep pattern is particularly pronounced among Alzheimer's disease (AD) patients (Tractenberg), while awakenings during the night is the most common sleep burden in Parkinson's disease (PD) patients (Porter); moreover, PD patients also experience delayed sleep onset, with these insomnia-related disturbances attributed to severe nocturia, stiffness and drug side-effects (Mehta). Finally, though sleep in Progressive Suprauclear Palsy (PSP) has not been investigated to the same degree as that of AD and/or PD, there is evidence that insomnia in PSP is very prevalent and that insomnia associated with PSP appears to be worse than insomnia in Parkinson's disease or AD patients; the latter may be due to several factors including difficulties with rigidity, nocturia and swallowing, with underlying changes in brain-related sleep mechanisms that are more affected in that disease process (i.e., prominent brainstem pathology) (De Bruin).

EDS

Excessive daytime sleepiness, at times together with fatigue, is a common complaint among patients suffering from dementia and its nature is multifactorial: reduced sleep at night and/or poor sleep quality, drug-induced somnolence, irregular sleep wake rhythms, primary sleep disorders. Hypersomnia can also be due to an intrinsic disorder affecting the sleep-wake cycle that is particularly evident in certain types of dementia (mostly in synucleinopathies – PD and Dementia Lewy Body (DLB), and Multiple System Atrophy (MSA)-) (Braga-Neto, Friedman, Comella, Arnulf 2005, Ghorayeb 2002, Boddy). Comparative studies assessing hypersomnia in dementia have shown that EDS is much more prominent in synucleinopathies compared to tauopathies (AD, PSP, etc.). A study that has used the principal objective sleep tool to assess EDS, that is Multiple Sleep Latency Test (MSLT), found that the mean sleep latency in patients suffering from DLB was half the time of AD patients (5 versus 10 minutes) (Ferman). Other studies performed with standardized sleep inventories, suggested that daytime sleepiness was more prominent among DLB patients compared to AD patients (Grace, Boddy). Finally, in PSP patients with EDS, the use of the Epworth Sleepiness Scale (the most common questionnaire used to assess sleepiness) has not verified any difference compared to healthy elderly (Arnulf I & Merino-Andreu M 2005). EDS prevalence in PD ranges from 29% to 40% and even more in advanced stages, while male patients with advanced disease, cognitive impairment, drug-induced psychosis and orthostatic hypotension are most at risk for developing EDS (Gagnon, Raggi). PD patients suffer not only from fatigue and reduced alertness, but there may be also "sleep attacks", which are defined as sudden episodes of sleep that appear without warning in a background of normal alertness. The latter symptom is similar to the sudden-onset sleep, which is the cardinal feature of narcolepsy/cataplexy. In the latter disease, with the sudden sleep-onset episodes there are also visual hallucinations. These two symptoms may occur also in PD and in DLB, suggesting that the loss of alertness and arousal in these neurodegenerative diseases may have a common neuropathological pathway with narcolepsy/cataplexy, namely a dysfunction of the lateral hypothalamus. This brain area contains orexin/hypocretin neurons, which are crucial for maintaining alertness during the day. As a matter of fact, recent investigations showed that hypocretin levels, in accordance with the findings in narcolepsy/cataplexy, are reduced also in PD and in DLB (Fronczek, Thannickal). Daytime sleepiness and its severity in PD seem to occur regardless of possible sleep deprivation and nighttime sleep quality, which implies that EDS is rather driven by a central mechanism. Moreover, though primary sleep disorders (i.e., Periodic Leg Movement Disorder -PLMD-, Restless Legs Syndrome -RLS-, Sleep-Disturbed Breathing –SDB-) may disrupt nighttime sleep in patients with synucleinpathies, the degree of EDS in these patients does not necessarily correlate with these primary sleep disorders (Arnulf 2002, Rye).

Finally, another common feature between narcolepsy and PD and DLB is RBD; narcoleptic patients are at a higher risk to develop RBD, which is the cardinal sleep disorder in synucleinopathies.

Table 1. Drugs involved in sleep disruption

CNS stimulants (modafinil, methylphenidate, dextroamphetamine)
Antidepressants with stimulating action (SNRI, buproprion, protriptyline, MAO inhibitors)
Antihypertensives (Beta-Blockers, Alpha-Blockers, Reseprine, Ca^{++}channel blockers – verapamil, amlodipine, diltiazem)
Bronchodialators (theophylline)
Corticosteroids (Dexamethasone, Prednisone)
Other (Thyroxine)

Table 2. Sleep disturbances according to different neurodegenerative diseases

	Insomnia	EDS	SDB	RBD	RLS/PLM	CRD	Sundowning
AD	+	+	++	-	+	++	+++
PSP	++	++		-			
FTD				-		+++	
PD	++	+++		++	+		
DLB		++		++	++	++	
MSA				+++			
VaD			+++				
MCI	+		+		n.a.	+/-	

EDS: Excessive Daytime Sleepiness, SDB: Sleep Disturbed Brteathing, RBD: REM Behavior Disorder, RLS/PLM: Restless Legs Syndrome/Periodic Leg Movement CRD: Circadian Rhythm Disruption

AD: Alzheimer's Disease, PSP: Progressive Sopranuclear Palsy, FTD: Frontotemporal dementia, PD: Parkinson's Disease, DLB: Lewy-Body dementia, MSA: Multiple System Atrophy, VaD: vascular Dementia, MCI: mild Cognitive Impairment

- (absent), +/- (debatable presence), + (present), ++ (prominent), +++ (very prominent).

SDB

Sleep-related breathing disorders are comprised of snoring, respiratory related arousals (RERAs) and Sleep Apnea (SA), which can be of three types: obstructive (OSA), central and mixed. With aging, the weakening and loss of tone of upper airway muscles during sleep predisposes individuals to airway obstruction that leads to snoring, or even worse to OSA. In the elderly and/or in the demented patients, OSA is the most common SDB burden; OSA is characterized by complete cessation (apnea) and/or partial decreases (hypopnea) in respiration during sleep as a result of pharyngeal collapse. Generally, untreated OSA is accompanied by EDS, reduced sleep quality, mood disorders, and overall reduced quality of life.

SDB may be more common in AD than in the general population (Bliwise), and it seems that dementia may be a risk factor for OSA; a study performed in institutionalized patients with dementia showed a very high prevalence (over 70%) of sleep apnea defined as apnea hypopnea index (AHI) of greater than 5 events per hour (Ancoli-Israel 1991). Similarly, it has been suggested that OSA is more prevalent among institutionalized elderly adults, especially those with dementia, with a prevalence ranging from 33 to 70% compared with elderly people living independently (Gehrman). It has been suggested that the lipoprotein allele APO E4, which is associated with a higher risk for AD, is related also with a higher risk for OSA; the latter suggestion is still under debate (Kadotani, Gottlieb, Saarelainen, Foley). SDB and OSA are quite frequent in synucleinopathies as well. It is debatable whether OSA in PD is more prevalent compared to healthy elderly (Maria, De Cock), while it seems that daily impairment, nocturia and cognitive impairment in PD are rather to be attributed to other mechanisms than the apneic ones. Conversely, sleep-related breathing disorders have also been extensively reported in MSA (Vetrugno, Ghorayeb 2001), and nocturnal stridor and central apnoeas are the most common clinical features. Noctural stridor, which rarely gets confounded with snoring, is a harsh and strained high-pitched sound. Though OSA in MSA is quite prevalent (15-37%) (Vertugno, Plazzi), nevertheless, central apnoeas contribute more severely than OSA to the dysfunction in respiratory regulation; the latter may be due to the fact that the cholinergic and serotoninergic systems, which are crucial for the normal respiratory drive, are associated with damages in the MSA process (Ghorayeb 2005). Finally, in MSA patients Cheyne– Stokes respirations occur frequently, which is a factor further aggravating the scenario and why these patients may die of respiratory insufficiency despite tracheostomy (Silber).

RBD

REM behavior disorder (RBD) is another sleep disorder quite common among the elderly and definitely more common in the context of the neurodegenerative process. RBD is a parasomnia defined as a dream-enacting motor behavior due to the loss of the normal skeletal muscle atonia which characterizes REM sleep. In this context, RBD sufferers may experience vigorous and sophisticated motor behaviors (i.e., talking, yelling, crying, laughing, singing, punching, kicking, sitting on the bed, jumping out of bed) as a consequence of the "acting-out" of the (usually unpleasant) dream. RBD can be suspected during the sleep interview, but diagnosis is done with the use of the Video-PSG, which reveals the presence of phasic and/or tonic electromyographic activity during REM sleep in accordance of dream-enacting activity (AASM ICSD 2). RBD affects mostly men and occurs primarily in the second half of the night, where REM sleep is more pronounced. RBD may be elicited and/or get worse with several substances; Antidepressants (Tricyclic, selective serotonin reuptake inhibitors (SSRIs), venlafaxine, mirtazapine, biperiden) excessive caffeine or chocolate intake and benzodiazepines or alcohol withdrawal can produce an acute RBD syndrome (Trotti). RBD may be found in the context of various neurological diseases of the elderly: subarachnoic hemorrhage, ischemic cerebrovascular disease and of course neurodegenerative diseases (Ancoli-Israel 2008). Regarding the latter category, RBD regards strictly synucleinopathies (PD, DLB and MSA) and is also considered a marker for these three diseases (Postuma).

RBD may precede the appearance of any other clinical manifestation of synucleinopathies by more than 10 years (Boeve 2003). RBD is very prevalent in PD; RBD in idiopathic PD ranges from 15-45% and from 46-58% if diagnosed from the sleep interview or polysomnographically, respectively (Raggi). The prevalence of RBD is even more increased among DLB patients (50-83%) (Boeve); hence in the diagncotic criteria for DLB, RBD pathology has been added as a suggestive disease for DLB (McKeith). Finally, RBD in MSA seems to be even more prevalent with respect to the other two synucleinopathies, ranging from 90.5% to 100%. RBD in MSA is associated with more severe motor symptoms, longer disease duration, depression and longer duration of levodopa treatment with respect to PD (Raggi). The association between RBD and synucleinopathies is closely associated especially when that disorder affects the pontine region. The pericoeruleus region sends glutaminergic projections to the medullary magnocellular reticular nucleus, and this in turn activates glycinergic neuron projections that inhibit anterior horn cell spinal neurons. When pericoeruleus regions are affected by synuclein disease, the spinal neurons could become less inhibited, and allow patients to act out their dreams (Boeve, Raggi, Gagnon).

RLS – PLM

Restless Legs Syndrome (RLS), as occurs in the adult population is similarly a commonly underdiagnosed cause of disrupted sleep in the elderly (Ancoli-Israel 2008), thus its detection may be even more challenging in the demented people. RLS is characterized by a great variety of dysesthesia/paresthesia symptoms mostly in the lower limbs (at times also in the upper limbs), occurring with a circadian pattern (late in the afternoon/evening) in a restful, relaxed state and is associated with an urge to move (Walters). RLS increases with age and is more common in women (Berger). RLS prevalence in the general population is between 10% and 15%, while the prevalence increases linearly with aging (prevalence is estimated as 16% in the age 60-69 and 19% in the age > 80years) (Berger, Phillips). Approximately 80% of RLS patients have co-morbid periodic leg movements (PLMs) during sleep. PLM is characterized by periodic episodes of repetitive and stereotyped limb movements (dorsiflexion of the foot) that occur during sleep, usually about every 20 to 40 seconds. An index of movements/hour above 5 is considered pathological. Prevalence of PLMs increases drastically with age (5%–6% in young adults, 45% in the elderly) (Phillips). Though robust data on the prevalence of RLS and PLM disorder in dementia are lacking, it seems that the latter disease is more common in the synucleinopathies (Raggi). On the other hand, a recent epidemiological study, reported no differences in the prevalence of RLS among the various types of dementia (Guarnieri). In a study assessing RLS in PD, prevalence of RLS was found between 7.9 and 20.8% (Ondo). As far as PLMs in cognitively impaired elderly people (mean age 81.8 years, mean MMSE 17.3), PLM index was found to be 17.3 and one third of the participants scored over 15 (Richards).

Circadian Rhythm Disturbances

Circadian rhythms are 24-hour biological rhythms that control many physiological functions, such as sleep/wake cycle, core body temperature and the secretion of several hormones. Circadian rhythms are controlled by an internal mechanism (the suprachiasmatic nucleus in the anterior hypothalamus), which gets synchronized to the 24 hour day, following various mostly external stimuli, the so-called "*zeitgebers*" (i.e., light, diurnal activities). Across the life span, either due to neurodegeneration processes (e.g., the suprachiasmatic nucleus degenerates, with tangles and neuronal cell loss with reactive gliosis (Stopa, Swaab)), or due to less light exposure and/or due to neurosensory dysfunctions (especially the visual ones – retinopathies, cataracts), the above-mentioned sleep/wake circadian rhythm get disrupted and less synchronized (Stopa, Zhou). Moreover, evidence of impairment in the endogenous pacemaker has been implied by studies on melatonin in patients with AD; these studies have shown alteration in the melatonin secretion and/or a reduction of its levels in the cerebrospinal fluid in the presence of an intact pineal gland, potentially implying an alteration of the suprachiasmatic nucleus output (Wu, Cardinali). As a result of these alterations, sleep/wake cycles in the elderly and even more in the demented patients usually shifts, or advances; patients go to sleep in the early evening and wake up in the early morning hours, leading to complaints of waking up in the middle of the night and being unable to return to sleep. In frontotemporal dementia (FTD) the sleep-wake cycle seems to undergo important alterations. Harper et al. have suggested that the sleep-wake rhythm is highly fragmented and is phase-advanced despite normal timing of core body temperature rhythm, suggesting a dysfunction of the SCN (Harper). Another study on FTD performed with the use of actigraphs (Anderson) suggested a different pattern of sleep disturbance compared to that of AD. Concerning the distribution of activity across the day and evening, the patients with AD of an earlier study of the same group (Hatfield) consistently showed less activity in the morning compared with the FTD group, but persisted with greater activity during the evening and into the night. In a study of ours, comparing the sleep of equally cognitively impaired FTD and AD by means of PSG, we concluded that FTD patients had several sleep parameters similarly or more affected by neurodegeneration, but in a shorter time span (Bonakis). Given that these findings were not related to primary sleep disorders, a centrally originating sleep deregulation was hypothesized. Thus, a study of sleep spindles, which are hallmarks of sleep microstructure was consequently conducted, which evidenced that similarly to the macrostructure findings, sleep microstructure in FTD may be equally or even more disturbed compared to that in Alzheimer's disease (Economou, Ktonas, submitted).

Sundowning

Sundowning phenomenon is the result of sleep-wake cycle disruptions. Sundowning syndrome is characterized by the origin or aggravation of neuropsychiatric behaviors comprising agitation, anxiety, confusion, and aggressiveness in the late afternoon, evening, or at night. The severity of sundowning is related to the severity of cognitive impairment that may be one of the important predisposing factors in the development of the syndrome (Khachiyants). The prevalence of sundowning in institutionalized patients with AD ranges from 10% to 25% (Evans, Martin) but, in community-dwelling patients, it may reach 66% (Gallgher-Thompson). Sundowning may be aggravated by reduced lighting, increased shadows, fatigue/exhaustion, changes in environments and caregivers.

3. Sleep in Mild Cognitive Impairment – MCI

Mild Cognitive Impairment – MCI is a transitional stage between normal aging and dementia, which consists in a clinical situation of subjective memory complaints and objective evidence of MCI without signs of dementia (Petersen). MCI could be of two types, amnestic – aMCI and non amnestic – naMCI; possible cognitive progression of aMCI is towards AD and that of naMCI is towards Lewy-Body, vascular or frontotemporal dementia (Bombois).

Sleep, its patterns and its disturbances in MCI have not been systematically assessed (Beaulieu-Bonneau). The existing data in the literature regards primarily studies performed with inventories/questionnaires that have assessed the neuropsychiatric features of MCI e.g., sleep disturbances (Beaulieu-Bonneau), but very few studies exist, which have been conducted with the use of objective tools e.g., PSG. Data on sleep, sleep patterns and sleep disorders in MCI compared either to demented people or to healthy elderly are inconclusive. Some authors suggest that sleep in MCI is equally (Peters) or more (Geda, Tatsch) disturbed with respect to that of healthy elderly. Lyketsos et al. (Lyketsos) suggest that the prevalence of sleep disorders in MCI is in between that of healthy elderly and demented patients. Other authors suggest that sleep disorders in MCI may be equally compared to those of patients with vascular dementia and early-AD (Chiu, Lopez). Finally, only four PSG studies exist that have assessed sleep patterns in MCI, with results similar to those previously described, thus rather inconclusive. Three of those have comparable sleep patterns of MCI to those of healthy elderly (Jae Kim, Westerberg 2012, Hita-Yañez 2012), while one is comparable to the sleep of healthy elderly, MCI and AD (Yu).

Kim et al. (Kim) by comparing 30 MCI patients vs 30 HE did not find any significant difference among the sleep parameters, but they referred a positive correlation of SWS amount with neuropsychological performances. Similarly, Yu et al. (Yu) who compared 10 mild AD, vs 12 MCI vs 13 HE, did not report major differences regarding the sleep parameters in these three groups; only sleep efficiency was found to be slightly different only if the comparison was done between HE and a unique group called “cognitively impaired group” (formed by both MCI and AD patients). However, this study has some methodological issues (e.g., AD patients were under cholinesterase inhibitors therapy, no adaptation night was performed), which may have had an impact on the results. Hita-Yañez et al. (Hita-Yañez), compared sleep parameters of 25 MCI vs 25 HE; they concluded that there was significant REM% reduction in the MCI group, especially when referring to MCI ApoE+ carriers. Furthermore, they also referred to significant SWS fragmentation (as expressed by the SWS arousal index). The authors used these findings, which showed impaired sleep years before the AD diagnosis, which attributed a predictive value. Westenberg et al. (Westenberg 2012) by studying both sleep macro- and microstructure (spectral analysis of theta, delta and sleep spindle ‘s’ bands) in 10 MCI patients vs. 18 HE, reported that SWS in MCI was markedly decreased, while borderline changes in REM, REM latency, WASO and sleep efficiency were reported as well. Furthermore, given that the EEG bands under investigation are implicated in the declarative memory mechanisms, the authors concluded that the considerable reduction of power shown in MCI patients has an impact also in memory consolidation. Finally, unpublished data of ours (Economou, Papageorgiou, submitted) on a PSG study on sleep and cognition of 30 aMCI vs 18 mild-moderate AD vs 24 HE, concluded that along with cognitive decline (from HE through MCI to mild-moderate AD) sleep appears to be linearly impaired. In other words, as cognitive status declines, sleep performances are impaired as well.

4. Disturbed Sleep and Sleep Disorders As Aggravating or Risk Factors for Cognitive Decline and Dementia

As shown previously, there is robust evidence that overall sleep and sleep/wake cycle in dementia (all types) are disturbed. The latter seems to occur also in predementia forms (MCI). In well-established dementia the detection of sleep abnormalities is useless in order to evaluate if sleep abnormalities play a role in the origin or in the aggravation of the cognitive decline, or conversely, if the progression of dementia contributes to sleep disruption. Thus, it is of extreme importance to investigate sleep in predementia states; the goal is twofold: firstly, to explore the possibility of sleep to act as a marker of early detection of dementia and secondly, to prevent and/or arrest dementia by performing intervention in disrupted sleep.

The link between sleep and cognitive impairment has been demonstrated on molecular and clinical levels. Naidoo et al. (Naidoo) suggested that cellular neuropathologies (e.g., amyloid plaques and neurofibrillary tangles in AD, Lewy bodies in PD and DLB, inclusion bodies in Huntington's disease) accumulate over wakefulness and, conversely, that sleep may inhibit their aggregation. Thus, sleep deprivation in the context of sleep disorders, may enhance the onset of neurodegeneration; in experimental models, it has been proven that the amyloid-ß plaques, which is a cardinal finding in AD pathology, are increased following experimentally induced sleep deprivation (Kang). In a recent study in 26 healthy adults who underwent 1-night total sleep deprivation, it was shown that sleep deprivation (or prolonged wakefulness) counteracted the normal decrease of Aβ42, which occurs during unrestricted sleep (Ooms). Greater beta-amyloid load was associated with shorter sleep and poorer sleep quality in HE as shown in positron emission study (Spira). Sleep deprivation could lead to abnormal accumulation of endogenous substances as in AD, due to the reduced interstitial fluid and associated metabolite clearance rate which normally occurs during sleep (Xie).

Disrupted sleep predicts poor cognitive performances and/or dementia in healthy elderly and for deterioration in mild cognitively impaired people.

In a large epidemiological study with 3000 elderly, it was shown that advanced sleep phase was predictive of low cognitive performances as measured with the MMSE (Auyenberg), while in the elderly aged 65-95 years, poor sleep quality as measured by the Pittsburgh Sleep Quality Index and by the mean sleep duration predicted MMSE scores compatible with cognitive impairment at 12-month follow-up (Potvin). Other parameters of sleep disruption i.e., reduced mean sleep duration, EDS and sleep fragmentation, increased the risks of cognitive decline and/or AD in elderly who have been followed for several years (Keage, Lim). In preclinical forms of dementia, specific sleep disturbances and disorders may act as early predictors of progression (Hita-Yanez 2012, Hita-Yanez 2013, Mander). In an actigraphic study performed in 30 MCI patients and 28 age-matched controls, it was seen that melatonin secretion was burdened, thus MCI patients presented similarly to AD patients circadian misalignment of advanced-phase sleep type (Naismith). In a large prospective actigraphic study, which was performed in 300 MCI patients, it was shown that sleep-disordered breathing itself was an independent risk factor for incident MCI or dementia (Yaffe). In more studies sleep disordered breathing (SDB) has been correlated with cognitive decline and/or dementia (Dealberto, Cohen-Zion). In a large community study, in healthy elderly over 65 years self-reported insomnia predicted cognitive deterioration after 3 years of follow-up (Cricco). Finally, it is widely known that idiopathic RBD itself is a strong predictor for the development of neurodegenerative diseases of synclein type (Iranzo 2006, Postuma 2009), but there is additional evidence that specific peculiarities in idiopathic RBD (iRBD) patients i.e., a marked EEG slowing, may be a marker for the development of cognitive impairment among patients with iRBD (Iranzo 2010).

5. Management of Disturbed Sleep and Sleep Disorders in Dementia

The management of sleep disorders in the context of dementia is similar to that recommended for the elderly. Firstly, management should be addressed toward treatment of any co-morbid condition (medical/psychiatric, drugs etc.) and/or towards the primary neurologic disease, as these conditions may be responsible for the appearance or aggravation of the sleep disorders. Lifestyle intervention i.e., elimination of substances that disrupt sleep like alcohol, or caffeine, avoidance of excess evening fluid intake and particular attention to the sleep environment, exposure in the day-time light etc., are of extreme importance (Wolkove, Chokroverty, Vitiello, Gitlin).

In case of insomnia, medical/psychiatric/neurologic and/or drugs adverse effects should be firstly addressed. Lifestyle interventions and non-pharmacologic treatments are preferred, while pharmacological treatment should be appropriately selected; benzodiazepines, mostly those with long action, should be avoided especially in case of severe cognitive impairment or in case of sleep apnea. Melatonin trials (3-5 mg) are suggested, but results are inconsistent, while antidepressants, especially those with sedative effects (i.e., trazodone 50-100 mg, mirtazapine 15 mg, mianserin 15-60 mg) are safe and possibly recommended. EDS should be cause-addressed.

If EDS is due to primary sleep disorders (RLS/PLMD, SDB, insomnia), or due to drug-related side effects, these should be managed first. Lifestyle interventions i.e., light-exposure, physical activity are generally recommended. In case of EDS of other origin (i.e., central origin) stimulants (low-dose modafinil, methylphenidate or selegiline) may be considered, but they should be used with caution due to side effects.

SDB (all types of sleep apnea, Cheyne Stokes breathing) should be assessed as for the adult or the healthy elderly. CPAP is the first line treatment and it seems that the CPAP compliance in the demented population is about the same as that of the healthy elderly (Ayalon). In cases of low-tolerance, auto-adjust CPAP or Bi-PAP trials should be given. SDB should be particularly treated with cases of vascular dementia, as SDB is an aggravating vascular factor. Interestingly, in AD and co-morbid OSA, the combination of CPAP and donepezil improved both cognitive impairment and SDB (Moraes).

RBD treatment should be started with lifestyle interventions focusing on minimizing injuries. Pharmacologic approach is as for the elderly; clonazepam is the treatment of choice, though dosage preferably should not exceed 1 mg. Melatonin (3-12 mg) can be used as an alternative treatment either as sole therapy or in conjunction with clonazepam. There is scarce evidence for other drugs that have been used in small trials (i.e., cholinesterase inhibitors, pramipexole, levodopa, triazolam, etc.) and should be used with caution and closely monitored.

RLS/PLM treatment should be started with removing possible aggravating factors (drugs, alcohol, primary disorders that induce RLS/PLM i.e., iron deficiency with levels of ferritin < 50 μg/L). Then, as for the adult population, dopamine-agonists in a first place and L-Dopa or gabapentin/pregabalin may be used at the same dosages.

The main approach for the circadian rhythm disturbances is light therapy (evening bright therapy for phase-advance condition and EDS) and melatonin (taken at 1-2 p.m.).

References

American Academy of Sleep Medicine. The international classification of sleep disorders. 2nd ed. Westchester, IL: American Academy of Sleep Medicine (2005).

Ancoli-Israel, S; Ayalon, L; Salzman, C. Sleep in the Elderly: Normal Variations and Common Sleep Disorders. *Harv Rev Psychiatry*, 2008, 16(5), 279-86.

Ancoli-Israel, S; Klauber, MR; Butters, N; et al. Dementia in institutionalized elderly: relation to sleep apnea. *J Am Geriatr Soc*, 1991, 39, 258–263.

Anderson, KN; Hatfield, C; Kipps, C; Hastings, M; Hodges, JR. Disrupted sleep and circadian patterns in frontotemporal dementia. *Eur J Neurol*, 2009, 16, 317–323.

Arnulf, I. Excessive daytime sleepiness in parkinsonism. *Sleep Med Rev*, 2005, 9, 185-200.

Arnulf, I; Konofal., E; Merino-Andreu, M; et al. Parkinson's disease and sleepiness" an integral part of PD. *Neurology*, 2002, 58, 1019–1024.

Arnulf, I; Merino-Andreu, M; Bloch, F; Konofal., E; Vidailhet, M; Cochen, V; et al. REM sleep behavior disorder and REM sleep without atonia in patients with progressive supranuclear palsy. *Sleep*, 2005, 28, 349-354.

Auyeung, TW; Lee, JS; Leung, J; Kwok, T; Leung, PC; et al. Cognitive deficit is associated with phase advance of sleep-wake rhythm, daily napping, and prolonged sleep duration-a cross-sectional study in 2,947 community-dwelling older adults. *Age* (Dordr), 2013, 35(2), 479-486.

Ayalon, L; Ancoli-Israel, S; Stepnowsky, C; et al. Adherence to continuous positive airway pressure treatment in patients with Alzheimer disease and obstructive sleep apnea. *Am J Geriatr Psychiatry*, 2006, 14(2), 176–180.

Beaulieu-Bonneau, S; Hudon, C. Sleep disturbances in older adults with mild cognitive impairment. *Int Psychogeriatr*, 2009, 21(4), 654-666.

Berger, K; Luedemann, J; Trenkwalder, C; Ulrich, J; Kessler, C. Sex and the risk of restless legs syndrome in the general population. *Arch Intern Med*, 2004, 164, 196–202.

Bliwise, D. L. Sleep in normal aging and dementia. *Sleep*, 1993, 16, 40–81.

Bliwise, DL. Sleep apnea, ApoE4, and Alzheimer's disease: 20 years and counting? *J Psychosom Res*, 2002, 53, 539–546.

Boddy, F; Rowan, EN; Lett, D; O'Brien, JT; McKeith, IG; Burn, DJ. Subjectively reported sleep quality and excessive daytime somnolence in Parkinson's disease with and without dementia, dementia with Lewy bodies and Alzheimer's disease. *Int J Geriatr Psychiatry*, 2007, 22, 529-535.

Boeve, BF; Silber, M; Parisi, JE; et al. Synucleinopathy pathology and REM sleep behaviour disorder plus dementia or parkinsonism. *Neurology*, 2003, 61, 40–45.

Bombois, S; Derampure, P; Pasquier, F; Monaca, C. Sleep disorders in aging and dementia. *J Nutr Health Aging*, 2010, 14(3), 212-217.

Bonakis, A; Economou, NT; Paparrigopoulos, T; Bonanni, E; Maestri, M; Carnicelli, L; Di Coscio, E; Ktonas, P; Vagiakis, E; Theodoropoulos, P; Papageorgiou, SG. Sleep in frontotemporal dementia is equally or possibly more disrupted, and at an earlier stage, when compared to sleep in Alzheimer's disease. *J Alzheimers Dis*, 2014, 38(1), 85-91.

Bonanni E; Di Coscio, E; Maestri, M; Carnicelli, L; Tsekou, H; Economou, NT; et al. Differences in EEG delta frequency characteristics and patterns in slow-wave sleep between dementia patients and controls: a pilot study. *J Clin Neurophysiol*, 2012, 29, 50–54.

Braga-Neto, P; da Silva-Junior, FP; Sueli Monte, F; de Bruin, PF; de Bruin, VM. Snoring and excessive daytime sleepiness in Parkinson's disease. *J Neurol Sci*, 2004, 217(1), 41–45.

Cajochen, C; Munch, M; Knoblauch, V; Blatter, K; Wirz-Justice, A. Age-related changes in the circadian and homeostatic regulation of human sleep. *Chronobiol Int*, 2006, 23, 461–474.

Cardinali, DP; Brusco, LI; Liberczuk, C; Furio, AM. The use of melatonin in Alzheimer's disease. *Neuro Endocrinol Lett*, 2002, 23, 20-23.

Carrier, J; Land, S; Buysse, DJ; Kupfer, DJ; Monk, TH. The effects of age and gender on sleep EEG power spectral density in the middle years of life (ages 20–60 years old). *Psychophysiology*, 2001, 38, 232–242.

Carrier, J; Monk, TH; Buysse, DJ; Kupfer, DJ. Sleep and morningness- eveningness in the 'middle' years of life (20-59 y). *J Sleep Res*, 1997, 6, 230-237.

Chiu, PY; Liu, CH; Tsai, CH. Neuropsychiatric manifestations in vascular cognitive impairment patients with and without dementia. *Acta Neurol Taiwan,* 2007, 16, 86-91.

Chocroverty S. (2009). Sleep and Neurodegenerative Diseases. *Semin Neurol*, 2009, 29(4), 446-467.

Cochen De Cock, V; Abouda, M; Leu, S; Oudiette, D; Roze, E; Vidailhet, M; Similowski, T; Arnulf, I. Is obstructive sleep apnea a problem in Parkinson's disease? *Sleep Med*, 2010, 11(3), 247-252.

Cohen-Zion, M; Stepnowsky, C; Marler Shochat, T; et al. Changes in cognitive function associated with sleep disordered breathing in older people. *J Am Geriatr Soc*, 2001, 49, 1622–1627.

Comella, CL. Sleep disorders in Parkinson's disease: an overview. *Mov Disord*, 2007, 22(Suppl 17), S367-373.

Cricco, M; Simonsick, EM; Foley, DJ. The impact of insomnia on cognitive functioning in older adults. *J Am Geriatr Soc*, 2001, 49, 1185–1189.

Crowley, K. Sleep and Sleep Disorders in Older Adults. *Neuropsychol Rev*, 2011, 21(1), 41-53.

Crowley, K; Trinder J; Kim, Y; Carrington, M; Colrain, IM. The effects of normal aging on sleep spindle and K-complex production. *Clin Neurophysiol*, 2002b, 113, 1615–1622.

Crowley, K; Trinder, J; Colrain, IM. An examination of evoked K-complex amplitude and frequency of occurrence in the elderly. *J Sleep Res*, 2002a, 11, 129–140.

Daan, S; Beersma, D. Circadian gating of human sleepwake cycles. In MC; Moore-Ede, CA; Czeisler (Eds.), Mathematical models of the circadian sleep-wake cycle, 1984, 129–158. New York: Raven

Darchia, N; Campbell, IG; Feinberg I. Rapid eye movement density is reduced in the normal elderly. *Sleep*, 2003, 26, 973–977.

De Bruin, VS; Machado, C; Howard, RS; Hirsch, NP; Lees, AJ. Nocturnal and respiratory disturbances in Steele-Richardson-Olszewski syndrome (progressive supranuclear palsy). *Postgrad Med J*, 1996, 72(847), 293–296.

Dealberto, MJ; Pajot, N; Courbon, D; et al. Breathing disorders during sleep and cognitive performance in an older community sample: the EVA study. *J Am Geriatr Soc*, 1996, 44, 1287–1294.

Dijk, DJ; Cajochen, C. Melatonin and the circadian regulation of sleep initiation, consolidation, structure, and the sleep EEG. *Journal of Biological Rhythms*, 1997, 12, 627–635.

Economou, NT; Ktonas, P; Konsta, A; et al. Sleep microstructure in frontotemporal dementia may be equally or even more disturbed compared to that in Alzheimer's disease: A sleep spindle study. (submitted).

Economou, NT; Papageorgiou, SG; Maestri, M; Di Coscio, E; et al. From normal elderly, through MCI to Alzheimer's Disease: A progression based on polysomnographic findings. (submitted)

Evans, LK. Sundown syndrome in institutionalized elderly. *J Am Geriatr Soc*, 1987, 35(2), 101–108.

Feinberg, I. Functional implications of changes in sleep physiology with age. *Neurobiol Aging*, 1976, 23–41.

Feinberg, I; Campbell, IG. Kinetics of non-rapid eye movement delta production across sleep and waking in young and elderly normal subjects: theoretical implications. *Sleep*, 2003, 26, 192–200.

Ferman, T; et al. Presented at the American Academy of Neurology 62nd Annual Meeting. Toronto (Canada), April, 10–16, 2010.

Floyd, JA; Janisse, JJ; Jenuwine, ES; Ager, JW. Changes in REM-sleep percentage over the adult lifespan. *Sleep*, 2007, 30, 829–836.

Foley, DJ; Masaki, K; White, L; et al. Relationship between apolipoprotein E epsilon4 and sleep-disordered breathing at different ages. *JAMA*, 2001, 286(12), 1447–1448.

Friedman, JH; Millman, RP. Sleep disturbances and Parkinson's disease. *CNS Spectr*, 2008, 13(Suppl 4), 12-17.

Fronczek, R; Overeem, S; Lee, SY; et al. Hypocretin (orexin) loss in Parkinson's disease. *Brain*, 2007, 130(6), 1577–1585.

Fukuda, N; Honma, H; Kohsaka, M; Kobayashi, R; Sakakibara, S; et al. Gender difference of slow wave sleep in middle aged and elderly subjects. *Psychiatry Clin Neurosci*, 1999, 53, 151–153.

Gagnon, JF; Petit, D; Latreille, V; Montplaisir, J. Neurobiology of sleep disturbances in neurodegenerative disorders. *Curr Pharm Des*, 2008, 14(32), 3430-3445.

Gallgher-Thompson, D; Brooks, JO 3rd, Bliwise, D; et al. The relations among caregiver stress, "sundowning" symptoms, and cognitive decline in Alzheimer's disease. *J Am Geriatr Soc*, 1992, 40, 807–810.

Geda, YE; Smith, GE; Knopman, DS; et al. De novo genesis of neuropsychiatric symptoms in mild cognitive impairment (MCI). *Int Psychogeriatr*, 2004, 16, 51-60.

Gehrman, PR; Martin, JL; Shochat, T; Nolan, S; Corey-Bloom, J; Ancoli-Israel, S. Sleep-disordered breathing and agitation in institutionalized adults with Alzheimer disease. The *American Journal of Geriatric Psychiatry*, 2003, 11, 426–433.

Ghorayeb, I, Yekhlef, F; Chrysostome, V; Balestre, E; Bioulac, B; Tison, F. Sleep disorders and their determinants in multiple system atrophy. *J Neurol Neurosurg Psychiatry*, 2002, 72, 798-800.

Ghorayeb, I; Bioulac, B; Tison, F. Sleep disorders in multiple system atrophy. *J Neural Transm*, 2005, 112, 1669–1675.

Gillin, JC; Ancoli-Israel, S. The impact of age on sleep and sleep disorders. In: Salzman C, ed. Clinical geriatric psychopharmacology. 4th ed. Philadelphia: Lippincott Williams & Wilkins, 2005, 483–512.

Gitlin, LN; Winter, L; Dennis, MP; Hodgson, N; Hauck, WW. Targeting and managing behavioral symptoms in indi- viduals with dementia: a randomized trial of a nonpharmacological intervention. *J Am Geriatr Soc*, 2010, 58, 1465–1474.

Gottlieb, D; DeStefano, A; Foley, D; et al. APOE epsilon4 is associated with obstructive sleep apnea/hypopnea: the Sleep Heart Health Study. *Neurology*, 2004, 63, 664–668.

Grace, JB; Walker, MP; McKeith, IG. A comparison of sleep profiles in patients with dementia with Lewy bodies and Alzheimer's disease. *Int J Geriatr Psychiatry*, 2000, 15, 1028-1033.

Guarnieri, B; Adorni, F; Musicco, M; et al. Prevalence of sleep disturbances in mild cognitive impairment and dementing disorders: a multicenter Italian clinical cross-sectional study on 431 patients. *Dement Geriatr Cogn Disord*, 2012, 33(1), 50-58.

Happe, S; Lüdemann, P; Berger, K. on behalf of the FAQT Study Investigators. The association between disease severity and sleeprelated problems in patients with Parkinson's disease. *Neuropsychobiology*, 2002, 46, 90-96.

Harper, DG; Stopa, EG; McKee, AC; Satlin, A; Harlan, PC; Goldstein, R; et al. Differential circadian rhythm disturbances in men with Alzheimer disease and frontotemporal degeneration. *Arch Gen Psychiatry*, 2001, 58, 353-360.

Hatfield, CF; Herbert, J; van Someren, EJ; Hodges, JR; Hastings, MH. Disrupted daily activity/rest cycles in relation to daily cortisol rhythms of home-dwelling patients with early Alzheimer's dementia. *Brain*, 2004, 127, 1061–1074.

Hita-Yañez, E; Atienza, M; Cantero, JL. Polysomnographic and subjective sleep markers of mild cognitive impairment. *Sleep*, 2013, 36(9), 1327-1334.

Hita-Yañez, E; Atienza, M; Gil-Neciga, E; Cantero, JL. Disturbed sleep patterns in elders with mild cognitive impairment: The role of memory decline and ApoE ε4 genotype. *Curr Alzheimer Res*, 2012, 9(3), 290-297.

Iber, C; Ancoli-Israel, S; Chesson, AL. Quan. *The AASM Manual for the Scoring of Sleep and Associated Events: Rules, Terminology, and Technical Specifications*. Westchester, IL: American Academy of Sleep Medicine, SF, 2007.

Iranzo, A; Isetta, V; Molinuevo, JL; Serradell, M; Navajas, D; Farre, R; Santamaria Electroencephalographic slowing heralds mild cognitive impairment in idiopathic REM sleep behavior disorder. *J Sleep Med*, 2010, 11(6), 534-539.

Iranzo, A; Molinuevo, JL; Santamaria, J; et al. Rapid-eye-movement sleep behaviour disorder as an early marker for a neurodegenerative disease: a descriptive study. *Lancet Neurol*, 2006, 5, 572–577.

Jae Kim, S; Hie Lee, J; Young Lee, D; Hyoung Jhoo, J; Inn Woo, J. Neurocognitive Dysfunction Associated With Sleep Quality and Sleep Apnea in Patients With Mild Cognitive Impairment. *Am J Geriatr Psychiatry*, 2011, 19(4), 374-381.

Kadotani, H; Kadotani, T; Young, T; et al. Association between apolipoprotein Epsilon4 and sleep-disordered breathing in adults. *JAMA*, 2001, 285, 2888–2890.

Kang, JE; Lim, MM; Bateman, RJ; Lee, JJ; Smyth, LP; et al. Amyloid-beta dynamics are regulated by orexin and the sleep-wake cycle. *Science*, 2009, 326, 1005–1007.

Keage, HA; Banks, S; Yang, KL; Morgan, K; Brayne, C; Matthews, FE. What sleep characteristics predict cognitive decline in the elderly? *Sleep Med*, 2012, 13(7), 886–892.

Khachiyants, N; Trinkle, D; Son, SJ; Kim, KY. Sundown syndrome in persons with dementia: an update. *Psychiatry Investig*, 2011, 8, 275-287.

Lim, AS; Kowgier, M; Yu, L; Buchman, AS; Bennett, DA. Sleep fragmentation and the risk of incident Alzheimer's disease and cognitive decline in older persons. *Sleep*, 2013, 36, 1027–1032.

Lombardo, P; Formicola, G; Gori, S; Gneri, C; Massetani, R; et al. Slow wave sleep (SWS) distribution across night sleep episode in the elderly. *Aging* (Milano), 1998, 10, 445–448.

Lopez OL; Becker JT; Sweet RA. Non-cognitive symptoms in mild cognitive impairment subjects. *Neurocase*, 2005, 11, 65-71.

Lyketsos, CG; Lopez, O; Jones, B; et al. Prevalence of neuropsychiatric symptoms in dementia and mild cognitive impairment: results from the cardiovascular health study. *JAMA*, 2002, 288, 1475-1483.

Mander, BA. Disturbed sleep in preclinical cognitive impairment: cause and effect? *Sleep*, 2013, 36(9), 1275 1276.

Maria, B; Sophia, S; Michalis, M; et al. Sleep breathing disorders in patients with idiopathic Parkinson's disease. *Respir Med*, 2003, 97, 1151–1157.

Martin, J; Marler, M; Shochat, T; et al. Circadian rhythms of agitation in institutionalized patients with Alzheimer's disease. *Chronobiol Int*, 2000, 17, 405–418.

McCurry, SM; Reynolds, CF; Ancoli-Israel, S; Teri, L; Vitiello, MV. Treatment of sleep disturbance in Alzheimer's disease. *Sleep Med Rev*, 2000, 4, 603 628.

McKeith, IG; Dickson, DW; Lowe, J; Emre, M; O'Brien, JT; Feldman, H; Cummings, J; Duda, JE; Lippa, C; et al. Diagnosis and management of dementia with Lewy bodies: third report of the LBD Consortium. *Neurology*, 2005, 65, 1863-1872.

Mehta, SH; Morgan, JC; Sethi, KD. Sleep disorders associated with Parkinson's disease: role of dopamine, epidemiology, and clinical scales of assessment. *CNS Spectr*, 2008, 3(Suppl. 4), 6–11.

Moe, KE; Vitiello, MV; Larsen, LH; Prinz, PN. Symposium: cognitive processes and sleep disturbances: sleep/wake patterns in Alzheimer's disease: relationships with cognition and function. *J Sleep Res*, 1995, 4(1), 15–20.

Moraes, W; Poyares, D; Sukys-Claudino, L; Guilleminault, C; Tufik, S. Donepezil improves obstructive sleep apnea in Alzheimer disease: a double-blind, placebo-controlled study. *Chest*, 2008, 133, 677–683.

Munch, M; Knoblauch, V; Blatter, K; Schroder, C; Schnitzler, C; et al. The frontal predominance in human EEG delta activity after sleep loss decreases with age. *Eur J Neurosci*, 2004, 20, 1402–1410.

Naidoo, N. Cellular stress/the unfolded protein response: relevance to and sleep disorders. *Sleep Med Rev*, 2009, 13, 195–204.

Naismith, SL; Hickie, IB; Terpening, Z; Rajaratnam, SM; Hodges, JR; Bolitho, S; Rogers, NL; Lewis, SJ. Circadian misalignment and sleep disruption in mild cognitive impairment. *J Alzheimers Dis*, 2014, 38(4), 857-866.

Ohayon, MM; Carskadon, MA; Guilleminault, C; Vitiello, MV. Meta-analysis of quantitative sleep parameters from childhood to old age in healthy individuals: developing normative sleep values across the human lifespan. *Sleep*, 2004, 27, 1255-1273.

Ondo, WG; Vuong, KD; Jankovic, J. Exploring the relationship between Parkinson disease and restless legs syndrome. *Arch Neurol*, 2002, 59, 421–424.

Ooms, S; Overeem, S; Besse, K; Rikkert, MO; Verbeek, M; Claassen, JA. Effect of 1 Night of Total Sleep Deprivation on Cerebrospinal Fluid β-Amyloid 42 in Healthy Middle-Aged Men. *JAMA Neurol*, 2014, Jun 2. (Epub ahead of print)

Petersen, RC. Mild cognitive impairment as a diagnostic entity. *J Intern Med*, 2004, 256, 183-194.

Petit, D; Gagnon, JF; Fantini, ML; Ferini-Strambi, L; Montplaisir, J. Sleep and quantitative EEG in neurodegenerative disorders. *J Psychosom Res*, 2004, 56(5), 487-496.

Phillips, B; Young, T; Finn, L; Asher, K; Hening, WA; Purvis, C. Epidemiology of restless legs symptoms in adults. *Arch Intern Med*, 2000, 160, 2137-2141.

Plazzi, G; Corsini, R; Provini, F; et al. REM sleep behavior disorders in multiple system atrophy. *Neurology*, 1997, 48, 1094–1097.

Porter, B; Macfarlane, R; Walker, R. The frequency and nature of sleep disorders in a community-based population of patients with Parkinson's disease. *Eur J Neurol*, 2008, 15, 50–54.

Postuma, RB; Gagnon, JF; Vendette, M; Fantini, ML; Massicotte-Marquez, J; Montplaisir, J. Quantifying the risk of neurodegenerative disease in REM sleep behavior disorder. *Neurology*, 2009, 72, 1296–1300.

Potvin, O; Lorrain, D; Forget, H; Dube, M; Grenier, S; et al. Sleep quality and 1-year incident cognitive impairment in community-dwelling older adults. *Sleep*, 2012, 35, 491–499.

Raggi, A; Ferri, R. Sleep disorders in neurodegenerative diseases. *Eur J Neurol*, 2010, 17(11), 1326-1338.

Rajput, V; Bromley, SM. Chronic insomnia: a practical review. *Am Fam Physician*, 1999, 60, 1431-1438. Discussion: 1441-1442.

Rauchs, G; Schabus, M; Parapatics, S; Bertran, F; Clochon, P; et al. Is there a link between sleep changes and memory in Alzheimer's disease? *Neuro Report*, 2008, 19, 1159–1162.

Rechtschaffen, A; Kales, A; editors. A manual of standardized terminology, techniques, and scoring system for sleep states of human subjects. Washington, DC: US Government Printing Office, 1968. (US Public Health Service Publication No. 204).

Reynolds, CF; III, Monk, TH; Hoch, CC; Jennings, JR; Buysse, DJ; Houck, PR; et al. Electroencephalographic sleep in the healthy "Old Old"; a comparison with the "Young Old" in visually scored and automated measures. *Journal of Gerontology*, 1991b, 46, M39–M46.

Richards, KC; Roberson, PK; Simpson, K; Lambert, CW; Bliwise, DL; Cole, CS; Enderlin, C; Shue, VM; Siddiqui, N. & Williams, JS. Periodic leg movements predict total sleep time in persons with cognitive impairment and sleep disturbance. *Sleep*, 2008, 31, 224-230.

Rye, DB; Bliwise, DL; Dihenia, B; et al. FAST TRACK: daytime sleepiness in Par- kinson's disease. *J Sleep Res*, 2000, 9, 63–69.

Saarelainen, S; Lehtimaki, T; Kallonen, E; et al. No relation between apolipoprotein E alleles and obstructive sleep apnea. *Clin Genet*, 1998, 53(2), 147–148.

Schubert, C; Cruickshanks, KJ; Dalton, DS; Klein, BEK; Klein, R; Nondahl, D. Prevalence of sleep problems and quality of life in an older population. *Sleep*, 2002, 25, 889–893.

Silber, MH; Levine, S. Stridor and death in multiple system atrophy. *Mov Disord*, 2000, 15, 699–704.

Spira, AP; Gamaldo, AA; An, Y; Wu, MN; Simonsick, EM; et al. Self-reported sleep and betaamyloid deposition in community-dwelling older adults. *JAMA Neurol*, 2013, 70, 1537–1543.

Steriade, M; McCormick, DA; Sejnowski, TJ. Thalamocortical oscillations in the sleeping and aroused brain. *Science*, 1993b, 262, 679–685.

Stopa, EG; Volicer, L; Kuo-Leblanc, V; Harper, D; Lathi, D; Tate, B; et al. Pathologic evaluation of the human suprachiasmatic nucleus in severe dementia. *J Neuropathol Exp Neurol*, 1999, 58, 29-39.

Swaab, DF; Fliers, E; Pariman, TS. The suprachiasmatic nucleus of the human brain in relation to sex, age and senile dementia. *Brain Res*, 1985, 342, 37–44.

Tatsch, MF; Bottino, CM; Azevedo, D; et al. Neuropsychiatric symptoms in Alzheimer disease and cognitively impaired, non demented elderly from a community-based sample in Brazil: prevalence and relationship with dementia severity. *Am J Geriatr Psychiatry*, 2006, (14), 438 445.

Thannickal., TC; Lai, YY; Siegel, JM. Hypocretin (orexin) cell loss in Parkinson's disease. *Brain*, 2007, 130(6), 1586–1595.

Tractenberg, RE; Singer, CM; Kaye, JA. Symptoms of sleep disturbance in persons with Alzheimer's disease and the normal elderly. *J Sleep Res*, 2005, 14, 177-185.

Trotti, LM. REM Sleep Behavior Disorder in older individuals. Epidemiology, pathophysiology and management. *Drugs Aging*, 2010, 27(6), 457 470.

Vetrugno, R; Provini, F; Cortelli, P; et al. Sleep disorders in multiple system atrophy: a correlative video-polysomnographic study. *Sleep Med*, 2004, 5, 21–30.

Vitiello, MV; Borson, S. Sleep disturbances in patients with Alzheimer's disease: epidemiology, pathophysiology and treatment. *CNS Drugs*, 2001, 15, 777–796.

Walters AS; Aldrich MS; Allen R; et al. Toward a better definition of the restless legs syndrome. The International Restless Legs Syndrome Study Group. *Mov Disord*, 1995, 10, 634–642.

Wauquier, A. Aging and changes in phasic events during sleep. *Physiol Behav*, 1993, 54, 803– 806.

Westerberg, CE; Mander, BA; Florczak, SM; et al. Concurrent impairments in sleep and memory in amnestic mild cognitive impairment. *J Int Neuropsychol Soc*, 2012, 18, 1-11.

Wolkove, N; Elkholy, O; Baltzan, M; Palayew, M. Sleep and aging: 1. Sleep disorders commonly found in older people. *CMAJ*, 2007, 176 (9), 1299-1304.

Wu, YH; Swaab, DF. The human pineal gland and melatonin in aging and Alzheimer's disease. *J Pineal Res*, 2005, 38, 145-152.

Xie, L; Kang, H; Xu, Q; Chen, MJ; Liao Y et al. Sleep drives metabolite clearance from the adult brain. *Science*, 2013, 342, 373–377.

Yaffe, K; Laffan, AM; Harrison, SL; Redline, S; Spira, AP; et al. Sleep-disordered breathing, hypoxia, and risk of mild cognitive impairment and dementia in older women. *JAMA*, 2011, 306, 613–619.

Yu, JM; Tseng, IJ; Yuan, RY; Sheu, JJ; Liu, HC; Hu, CJ. Low sleep efficiency in patients with cognitive impairment. *Acta Neurol Taiwan*, 2009, 18(2), 91-97.

Zhou, JN; Hofman, MA; Swaab, DF. VIP neurons in the human SCN in relation to sex, age, and Alzheimer's disease. *Neurobiol Aging*, 1995, 16, 571-576.

Index

B

C

D

E

F

G

H

I

J

K

L

N

O

P

Q

R

S

T

U

V

W

Y